Homeland Security

Principles and Practice of Terrorism Response

Paul M. Maniscalco, PhD(c), MPA, MS, EMT/P

Senior Research Scientist and Principal Investigator
The George Washington University–Office of Homeland Security
President, International Association of EMS Chiefs
Deputy Chief/Paramedic (ret.), Fire Department of New York (FDNY)

Dr. Hank T. Christen, EdD, MPA

Education and Human Performance Technology Emergency Response
Lead Developer, FullyInvolvedFire.com
Battalion Chief (ret.), Atlanta Fire Department

JONES AND BARTLETT PUBLISHERS

Sudbury, Massachusetts

BOSTON   TORONTO   LONDON   SINGAPORE

World Headquarters

Jones and Bartlett Publishers
40 Tall Pine Drive
Sudbury, MA 01776
978-443-5000
info@jbpub.com
www.jbpub.com

Jones and Bartlett Publishers
Canada
6339 Ormindale Way
Mississauga, Ontario L5V 1J2
Canada

Jones and Bartlett Publishers
International
Barb House, Barb Mews
London W6 7PA
United Kingdom

Jones and Bartlett's books and products are available through most bookstores and online booksellers. To contact Jones and Bartlett Publishers directly, call 800-832-0034, fax 978-443-8000, or visit our website, www.jbpub.com.

Substantial discounts on bulk quantities of Jones and Bartlett's publications are available to corporations, professional associations, and other qualified organizations. For details and specific discount information, contact the special sales department at Jones and Bartlett via the above contact information or send an email to specialsales@jbpub.com.

Production Credits

Chief Executive Officer: Clayton Jones
Chief Operating Officer: Don W. Jones, Jr.
President, Higher Education and Professional
    Publishing: Robert W. Holland, Jr.
V.P., Sales: William J. Kane
V.P., Design and Production: Anne Spencer
V.P., Manufacturing and Inventory Control: Therese Connell
Publisher: Kimberly Brophy
Acquisitions Editor, EMS: Christine Emerton
Associate Editor: Amanda Brandt

Associate Editor: Karen Margrethe Greene
Associate Production Editor: Sarah Bayle
Director, Public Safety Group: Matthew Maniscalco
Director of Marketing: Alisha Weisman
Composition: Cape Cod Compositors, Inc.
Cover Design: Kristin E. Parker
Photo Research Manager: Kimberly Potvin
Associate Photo Researcher: Jessica Elias
Cover Image: Courtesy of FEMA
Printing and Binding: Courier Corporation
Cover Printing: Courier Corporation

The procedures and protocols in this book are based on the most current recommendations of responsible sources. The publisher and authors, however, make no guarantee as to, and assumes no responsibility for, the correctness, sufficiency, or completeness of such information or recommendations. Other or additional safety measures may be required under particular circumstances.

Additional photographic and illustration credits appear on page 227, which constitutes a continuation of the copyright page.

Library of Congress Cataloging-in-Publication Data

Maniscalco, Paul M.
Homeland security : principles and practice of terrorism response / Paul M. Maniscalco, Hank T. Christen.—1st ed.
    p. cm.
 Includes bibliographical references and index.
 ISBN-13: 978-0-7637-5785-4
 ISBN-10: 0-7637-5785-3
 1. Terrorism—United States—Prevention. 2. National security—United States. 3. Emergency management—United States. I. Christen, Hank T. II. Title.
 HV6432.M356 2011
 363.325'16—dc22

                                                                                              2009040337

6048
Printed in the United States of America
14 13 12   10 9 8 7 6 5 4 3 2

Brief Contents

Contents

Resource Preview

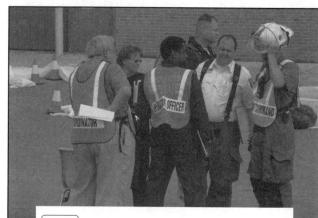

2 **National Incident Management System**

Hank T. Christen
Paul M. Maniscalco

Objectives

- Describe the evolution of the 1970s incident command system (ICS) to the modern national incident management system (NIMS).
- Diagram and define the key positions in the command staff.
- Compare and contrast incident command (IC) with unified command (UC).
- Define the key principles of ICS.
- Define the five key functions in ICS.
- Diagram the general staff and command staff in ICS.
- List and define the components in the NIMS structure that complement ICS.

19

CHAPTER OBJECTIVES are listed at the beginning of each chapter and provide readers with a clear map of information pertaining to each topic.

Other means of disseminating the agent are more likely. Insecticides are sprayed from airplanes and helicopters in both crop dusting (**FIGURE 8-1**) and mosquito eradication. This is an obvious and expensive way to disseminate an agent, but it is effective for spreading it over a large area providing the weather and winds are favorable. Vehicle-mounted spray tanks can be driven through the streets of a target area to disseminate an agent. For example, in Matsumoto, the agent was spread from the back of a vehicle in which a container of agent was heated (to help it to evaporate), and the vapor was blown through the street by a fan. Indoor areas might be attacked by putting an agent in the air system, and rooms could be thoroughly and quickly contaminated by the use of a common aerosol spray can. There are other methods of disseminating liquids.

Nerve Agents

Nerve agents are toxic materials that produce injury and death within seconds to minutes. The signs and symptoms caused by nerve agent vapor are characteristic of the agents and are not difficult to recognize with a high index of suspicion. Very good antidotes that will save lives and reduce injury if administered in time are available.

Nerve agents are a group of chemicals similar to, but more toxic than, commonly used organophosphate insecticides such as Malathion. Nerve agents were developed in Germany during the 1930s for wartime use, but they were not used in World War II. They were used in the Iran–Iraq war. They were also used by the religious cult Aum Shinrikyo in Japan on two occasions; the first use injured about 300 people and killed seven in Matsumoto in June 1994; the second killed

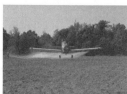

FIGURE 8-1 Crop dusting is an obvious and expensive way to disseminate an agent, but it is effective for spreading it over a large area providing the weather and winds are favorable.

CRITICAL FACTOR

Remember that it does not take an explosive device to disseminate chemical agents. There are multiple methods of disseminating chemical agents over a wide area.

12 and injured over 1,000 in the Tokyo subways in March 1995.

The common nerve agents are tabun (GA), sarin (GB), soman (GD), GF, and VX (GF and VX have no common names) (**CP FIGURE 8-2**).

The nerve agents are liquids (not nerve gases) that freeze at temperatures below 0°F and boil at temperatures above 200°F (**CP FIGURE 8-3**). Sarin (GB), the most volatile, evaporates at about the rate of water, and VX, the least volatile, is similar to light motor oil in its rate of evaporation. The rates of evaporation of the others lie in between. In the Tokyo subway attack, sarin leaked out of plastic bags and evaporated. Serious injury was minimized because the rate of evaporation of sarin is not rapid, so the amount of vapor formed was not large. If the sarin had evaporated more rapidly (e.g., like gasoline or ether), much more vapor would have been present, and more serious injury in more people would have occurred.

Nerve agents produce physiological effects by interfering with the transmission between a nerve and the organ it innervates or stimulates, with the end result being excess stimulation of the organ. Nerve agents do not actually act on nerves. Instead, they act on the chemical connection of the nerve to the muscle or organ. Normally, an electrical impulse travels down a nerve, but the impulse does not cross the small synaptic gap between the nerve and the organ. At the end of the nerve, the electrical impulse causes the release of a chemical messenger, a neurotransmitter, which travels across the gap to stimulate the organ. The organ may be an exocrine gland, a smooth muscle, a skeletal muscle, or another nerve. The organ responds to the stimulus by secreting, by contracting, or by transmitting another message down a nerve. After the neurotransmitter stimulates the organ, it is immediately destroyed by an enzyme so that it cannot stimulate the organ again. Nerve agents inhibit or block the activity of this enzyme so that it cannot destroy the neurotransmitter or chemical messenger. As a result, the neurotransmitter accumulates and continues to stimulate the organ. If the organ is a gland, it continues to secrete; if it is a muscle, it continues to contract; or if it is a nerve, it continues to transmit impulses. There is hyperactivity throughout the body.

CRITICAL FACTOR boxes reinforce the strongest messages of the text and highlight vital safety information.

WRAP UP End-of-chapter activities reinforce important concepts and improve students' comprehension.

CHAPTER QUESTIONS Open-ended questions succinctly summarize the knowledge contained within the chapter.

CHAPTER PROJECTS Broad assignments call on students to apply information from the chapter to address complex problems as well as interact with their own local community and state governments

VITAL VOCABULARY The terms that are bolded and underlined throughout the text are defined in the Wrap Up for students' reference. Vocabulary terms and definitions also appear in the glossary at the end of the textbook.

Wrap Up

Chapter Questions

1. List the four goals in the NRF strategy.
2. Describe the relationship of the NRF and NIMS.
3. List and discuss at least three elements in the preparedness cycle.
4. List three response agencies in your community or jurisdiction and describe their roles in the NRF.
5. Select a major local disaster or attack and list five or more emergency support functions and describe their functions in the event.

Chapter Project

Develop an outline of a local preparedness plan based on the NRF preparedness cycle.

Vital Vocabulary

Emergency support function annexes Areas in the NRF that explain and outline emergency support functions.

Emergency support functions (ESFs) A defined set of actions and responsibilities for fifteen federal disaster support functions including lead federal agencies and secondary support agencies for each function.

Federal coordinating officer The focal point of coordination in the unified coordination group for Stafford Act incidents, ensuring integration of federal emergency management activities.

Forward-leaning posture A preparedness and response philosophy that advances from citizens/households upward through governments to the federal level because incidents can rapidly expand and escalate.

Incident annexes The description of the response aspects for broad incident categories (e.g., biological, nuclear/radiological, cyber, mass evacuation).

Incident management teams The incident command organizations composed of the command and general staff members with appropriate functional units of an incident command system organized as regionally based interagency special response teams.

Joint field office (JFO) A temporary federal facility that provides a central location for the coordination of response and recovery activities of federal, state, tribal, and local governments. The JFO is structured and operated using NIMS and ICS as a management template. The JFO does not manage on-scene activities.

Joint task force commander Person designated by the Department of Defense to command federal military activities to support an incident.

National Counterterrorism Center The primary federal organization for integrating and analyzing all intelligence pertaining to terrorism and counterterrorism and for conducting strategic operational planning by integrating all instruments of national power.

National Infrastructure Coordinating Center (NICC) Center that monitors the nation's critical infrastructure and key resources on an ongoing basis and provides a coordinating forum to share information across infrastructure and key resources sectors through appropriate information-sharing entities such as the information sharing and analysis centers and the sector coordinating councils.

National Military Command Center The nation's local point for continuous monitoring and coordination of worldwide military operations.

National Operations Center (NOC) The primary national hub for situational awareness and operations coordination across the federal government for incident management.

National Response Coordination Center (NRCC) A 24/7 operations center that monitors potential or developing incidents and supports the efforts of regional and field components.

National response doctrine The five key principles that support national response operations that are engaged partnerships, tiered response, scalable/flexible/adaptable capabilities, unity of effort through unified command, and readiness to act.

National Response Framework A document outlining a coherent strategic framework for senior emergency response chiefs, emergency management practitioners, and senior executives in the private sector.

Preparedness cycle The cycle of planning, organizing, training, equipping, exercising, and evaluating for im-

44

Acknowledgments

Authors

Paul M. Maniscalco, PhD(c), MPA, MS, EMT/P

Paul M. Maniscalco is a Senior Research Scientist and Principal Investigator with The George Washington University and a member of the GWU Emergency/Crisis Management Senior Leadership team. Paul presently serves as the president of the International Association of Emergency Medical Service Chiefs (IAEMSC) and is a former president of the National Association of Emergency Medical Technicians (NAEMT).

Chief Maniscalco retired from the City of New York as a Deputy Chief/Paramedic after completing almost 23 years of service. He has over 30 years of public safety response experience including supervisory, management, and executive service, during which he has had the responsibilities of planning for, responding to, and managing a wide array of emergencies and significant events, including aviation and rapid transit emergencies, natural and technological disasters, civil disturbances, and acts of terrorism. Chief Maniscalco has been engaged in command roles for planning and managing large, high-profile special events such as dignitary visits, national political conventions, sport championships, and a wide variety of mass gatherings.

Additionally, he has participated in capacity-building projects for public safety, domestic security, and disaster response in Tanzania, Kenya, India, China, Turkey, Portugal, and the Caribbean. Chief Maniscalco has also been the executive lead on crisis/disaster management policy development and corporate response capacity assessment projects for large private sector entities within the Fortune 100. In this role, he designed, implemented, and managed comprehensive review and assessment programs examining resiliency and response capacity. One recent project involved coordination of twelve "tiger teams" concurrently traveling four continents—conducting policy reviews, testing operational response effectiveness, and evaluating executive readiness for crisis management with the formal presentation of investigation findings to the corporate board in 45 days.

Chief Maniscalco is widely published in academic and professional journals on disaster/crisis management, emergency medical services, special operations, fire service, public safety, and national security issues. He has co-authored ten textbooks and has also served as a contributing author on another ten books. Some of these publications include *The EMS Incident Management System: EMS Operations for Mass Casualty and High Impact Incidents; Hype or Reality? The 'New Terrorism' and Mass Casualty Attacks; Model Procedures Guide for Emergency Medical Incidents, 1st Edition; Understanding Terrorism and Managing the Consequences; Mass Casualty and High Impact Incidents: An Operations Management Guide*; and the IFRC/RC Societies and Johns Hopkins School of Hygiene and Public Health Center for Disaster and Refugee Studies *Public Health Guide for Emergencies*.

Chief Maniscalco is an appointee to the President's Homeland Security Advisory Council—Senior Advisory Committee for Emergency Services, Law Enforcement, and Public Health and Hospitals and a charter member of the Inter-Agency Board (IAB). He has served as a member of the Department of Defense, Defense Science Board (DSB), Transnational Threat Study and the DSB—Homeland Defense—Chemical Weapons Task Force; an Advisor to the DARPA; and a member of the Board of Advisors for the Oklahoma City National Memorial Institute for the Prevention of Terrorism. Paul M. Maniscalco was also an appointee to the congressionally mandated National Panel to Assess Domestic Preparedness (Gilmore National Terrorism Commission), where he served as the chairman of the Threat Reassessment Panel, State and Local Response Panel, and the Commission Research Panel. In addition, he served on the Cyber-terrorism and the Critical Infrastructure Protection Panels during this five year commission.

In December of 1999, Paul M. Maniscalco received an appointment to the Harvard University, John F. Kennedy School of Government and U.S. Department of Justice (DOJ)—Executive Session on Domestic Preparedness, a 3-year fellowship sponsored by DOJ.

Maniscalco has earned numerous awards and honors for professional achievement and service from government, corporate, and professional organizations. Chief Maniscalco was awarded over 100 commendations from the City of New York, including the Medal of Honor. In 2003, he received the NREMT and National Association of EMTs' Rocco V. Morando Life Time Achievement Award for significant professional achievement and sustained contributions of national impact to the profession.

Paul M. Maniscalco earned his baccalaureate degree in Public Administration–Public Health and Safety from the City University of New York, a Master of Public Administration–Foreign Policy and National Security from the New York University Wagner Graduate School of Public Service, and a Master of Science degree in Emergency Services Management from The George Washington University. He is presently completing doctoral studies in homeland security leadership and policy focusing on organizational behavior/response to crisis.

Dr. Hank T. Christen, EdD, MPA

Dr. Hank Christen has been a consultant in the fields of emergency response and counter-terrorism for Department of Defense agencies, federal response agencies, and local government public safety agencies since 2000.

He was previously a battalion chief for the Atlanta Fire Department, Director of Emergency Services for Okaloosa County, Florida, and Director of Emergency Response Operations for Unconventional Concepts, Inc. He served as unit commander for the Gulf Coast Disaster Medical Assistance Team (DMAT) and has responded to twelve national level disasters, including the 2001 World Trade Center attack.

Hank Christen is a contributing editor for *Firehouse Magazine* and has published over thirty articles in technical journals. He has co-authored eight books in the emergency response field, speaks at national level conferences, and is the lead researcher for Fullyinvolvedfire.com. He was a member of the Department of Defense, Defense Science Board (Transnational Threats, 1997) and the U.S. Army Interagency Board for Medical Logistics. He participated in the Executive Session on Domestic Preparedness, John F. Kennedy School of Government, Harvard University, and is currently an affiliate faculty member with The George Washington University Department of Health Sciences; Capella University School of Public Service Leadership; Auburn University; and the Gordon Center for Research in Medical Education, University of Miami.

Hank Christen is a Miami native; he completed his undergraduate studies at the University of Florida and graduated as a Doctor of Education in 2009 from the University of West Florida. His doctoral specialty is Human Performance Technology.

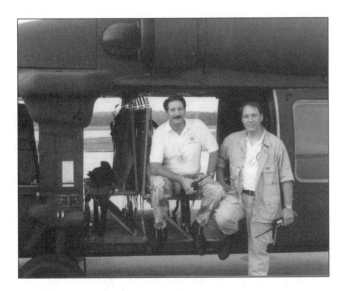

From the Authors

Paul M. Maniscalco, PhD(c), MPA, MS, EMT/P

To my wife Connie Patton, whose love, patience (most times), and encouragement are a constant source of inspiration and motivation. She continues to be my best friend and the best thing that has ever happened in my life! To my father and role model, Anthony S. Maniscalco, whose positive lifelong influence has played an instrumental and critical role in my life and public service career; you left us way too early. To my mother, Patricia O'Brien Maniscalco, her guidance and constant reinforcement of helping others as a noble calling has brought me to appreciate my chosen career even more. To my brothers, Peter, Mark, John, and Matthew, whose invaluable support is constant and greatly appreciated (*even if they still believe that each of them is the "favorite son" . . .*).

To Dr. Gregory Saathoff, UVA CIAG; Dr. Bruce Hoffman, RAND; Dr. Chris Holstege, UVA; Dr. Brad Roberts, Institute for Defense Analysis, Lt.Gen. (USAF ret.) and Under Secretary of Defense James Clapper; Lt. Gen. (USA ret.) William Garrison; Lt. Gen. (USA ret.) William Reno; FBI Asst. Director (ret.) James Greenleaf; John Flood, FBI CIRG; Dr. Richard Falkenrath, NYPD; Secretary of the Army (ret.) and Congressman (VA-ret.) John O. Marsh; Mr. Giandomenico Picco, UN Chief Hostage Negotiator (ret.); Mr. Michael Wermuth, RAND; Dr. Roy Sparrow, NYU-Wagner School of Public Service; Dr. Jean Johnson GWU SMHS. The valuable guidance, assistance, and knowledge each of you have provided me over the years is greatly appreciated and applied daily.

For the immeasurable long time support and assistance provided to me by my many peers I would like to thank: MacNeil C. Cross, Dr. Paul Kim, Judson Fuller, Neal Dolan, Donald Hiett, Dr. Keith Holtermann, Daniel Gerard, Jeff Abraham, Michael Newburger, Frank Cilluffo, Mark Steffens, James Denney, Don Lee, Erik Gaull, John Sinclair, X234, Robert Sudol, Eugene J. O'Neill, Dean Wilkinson, Geoffrey T. Miller, Christopher Kozlow, Edward Sawicki, Richard Serino, Diane Cavaleri, Lawrence Tan, Christian Callsen, Dr. Donald Walsh; Donald M. Gilberg, and Graydon Lord. Each of you has been a great friend and confidant.

To Hank Christen, without whom my writing would be laborious and boring, thanks for being a great friend, partner, and contributor. You are truly a gentleman and a scholar.

Dr. Hank T. Christen, EdD, MPA

The foundation of my personal and professional success comes from my father, the late Henry T. Christen Sr., District Chief, City of Miami Fire Department, and my mother, Louisa Worth Christen, who set the bar for education in our family. My wife Lynne, a successful travel writer, offered support, patience, candid insights, and editing suggestions during this endeavor. More importantly, Lynne is my closest friend and confidant. I am very proud of my sons, Eric and Ryan, who are professionals in their milieu and set examples for me to follow.

During my emergency response career, many people in the Atlanta Fire Department and Okaloosa County Emergency Services taught, encouraged, and befriended me. I appreciate Lou Cuneo, David Chamberlin, Claude Lemke, Phil Chovan, Elmo McDonnell, Ron Weed, Mike Blakely, George Collins, John Hodgkinson, and Marc Steinman. My apologies for the names I left out.

My private sector experience at Unconventional Concepts, Inc. was enlightening and revealed a new world in the national defense and terrorism response arena. I offer my thanks to Mike Malone, Chuck Linden, Patty Hazlewood, and Dean Preston.

My academic life includes myriad friends and colleagues, including Bill and Sandy Hartley, Geoff Miller, Gregg Lord, Dr. Lisa Powell, Dr. Charles Tippin, Dr. Jeff Lindsey, Dr. Daved van Stralen, and Dr. Don Walsh. It is a pleasure to be affiliated with outstanding institutions, including The George Washington University, the John F. Kennedy School of Government at Harvard University, the Gordon Center for Medical Research and Education at the University of Miami (Dr. S. Barry Issenberg), Auburn University, the Joint Special Operations University, and the School of Public Service Leadership at Capella University. The University of West Florida deserves recognition for molding me into a Doctor of Education. Special thanks to Mike Barry, Janet Pilcher, Wilbur Hugli, David Goetsch, Mary Rogers, and Robin Largue.

I conclude with thanks to my friend and co-author, Paul Maniscalco. We began as co-writers in the 90s and have maintained a professional relationship and personal friendship that is deeply meaningful to me. Whenever I have a question in the emergency response business that I cannot answer, I call Paul.

Contributors

Benjamin T. Delp, MPA
Assistant Director for Administration and Policy
Institute for Infrastructure and Information Assurance
James Madison University
Harrisonburg, Virginia

James P. Denney, MA
Captain, EMS Bureau (ret.)
Los Angeles City Fire Department
Faculty, EMS Baccalaureate Program
Loma Linda University
Los Angeles, California
1947–2006

Neal J. Dolan, MCJ
Deputy Director
South Carolina Law Enforcement Division (SLED)
Columbia, South Carolina
Special Agent In Charge (ret.)
United States Secret Service
Columbia, South Carolina

Dr. Christopher Holstege, MD, FACEP, FAAEM, FACMT
Director, University of Virginia Division of Medical Toxicology
Professor of Integrated Science and Strategic Leadership
Medical Director, Blue Ridge Poison Center
Charlottesville, Virginia

Harold W. Neal III, MS, EMT/B
Senior Research Associate
The George Washington University
Office of Homeland Security
Washington, DC

Kenneth F. Newbold, Jr., MPA
Director of Research Development
Administrative Director—Institute for Infrastructure and Information Assurance
James Madison University
Harrisonburg, Virginia

Dr. John B. Noftsinger, Jr.
Vice Provost and Professor of Integrated Science and Strategic Leadership
James Madison University
Harrisonburg, Virginia

Dr. Frederick R. Sidell, MD
Physician, Scientist, Mentor, & Friend
Institute of Chemical Defense
Aberdeen Proving Ground, Maryland
1934–2006

Dr. Charles Stewart, MD, FACEP, FAAEM
Director, Oklahoma Institute for Disaster and Emergency Medicine
Director of Research and Professor of Emergency Medicine
Oklahoma University Department of Emergency Medicine
Tulsa, Oklahoma

Andrew Wordin, BS, MICP
Captain II, Paramedic
Los Angeles City Fire Department
Los Angeles, California

Reviewers

Neil P. Blackington, EMT-T
Deputy Superintendent
Commander, Support Services Division
Boston Emergency Medical Services
Boston, Massachusetts

Eric Thomas Dotten, REMT-P
Clinical Programs Coordinator
Emergency Medicine Learning Resource Center
Orlando, Florida

Greggory J. Favre, MS, BS, BS, SME
Member, St. Louis Fire Department
Bureau of Suppression, 6th Battalion
St. Louis, Missouri

Donell Harvin, MPA, MPH, EMT-P
Adjunct Professor, Advisory Board Member
Reganhard Center for Emergency Response Studies
John Jay College of Criminal Justice
New York, New York

Gregg Lord, MS, NREMT-P
Associate Director, George Washington University Medical
  Center Office of Homeland Security
Commissioner, National Commission on Children
  & Disasters
Washington, DC

John L. Morrissey, NREMT-P
New York State Department of Health
NYS Incident Management Team
Liverpool, New York

Edward Piper
Director of Public Safety and Emergency Management,
  Georgetown Law
Dean of Homeland Security Studies, Canyon College
Adjunct Professor, Security Management, Johns
  Hopkins University
Doctoral Student, Georgetown University
Baltimore, Maryland

Nelson Tang, MD, FACEP
Chief Medical Officer
Center for Law Enforcement Medicine
Director of Special Operations
Johns Hopkins Emergency Medicine
Baltimore, Maryland

Ricardo Tappan, CSHM, FF/NREMT-P
Training Coordinator, Center for Preparedness & Resilience
Office of Homeland Security
George Washington University
Washington, DC

Michael Tarantino, BA, MAS, NREMT-B
EMT Coordinator
Bergen County EMS Training Center
Paramus, New Jersey

Richard White, BS, MS
Retired USAF
Associate Director, Center for Homeland Security
University of Colorado
Colorado Springs, Colorado

Andrew J. Wordin, BS, EMT-P
Fire Captain
Los Angeles Fire Department
Los Angeles, California

Jason P. Zielewicz, MS, NREMT-P
Founding/Senior Partner, EMERGE Public Safety, LLC.
Plt. Chief, Susquehanna Regional EMS
EMERGE Public Safety, LLC. and Susquehanna
  Regional EMS
South Williamsport, Pennsylvania

Dedication

This book is dedicated to the "World's Front-Line of Defense," the men and women in emergency response, law enforcement, public safety, and emergency management.

Whether it was the events of Mumbai, London, Belfast, Moscow, Madrid, the World Trade Center in New York City, the Pentagon, the Murrah Building in Oklahoma City, Atlanta Centennial Park, the Embassies in Africa, or the myriad other terrorist-related events that have transpired around the world, in each instance we consistently witnessed extraordinary people rising to the occasion and answering the call for help. You have met the challenge head on to mitigate and remediate the horrific aftermath of these cowardly attacks, at times at great personal risk and peril.

All too often the people of the world discount the importance that members of emergency medical services, law enforcement, fire service, public health, security, emergency management, and medicine play in the preservation of civil society and national security. With the ever changing tactics and strategies of terror-related organizations, we now witness emergency responders being targeted for attack (such as the use of secondary devices focused on wreaking havoc and perhaps injuring or killing our peers operating at the scenes of these inci-

dents). These acts of cowardice have upped the personal threat ante to our fellow professionals. We developed this text to bring understanding, clarity, and sensibility to our fellow professionals so that when you respond to an act of terrorism you may be safer and more effective in helping those who need your assistance in their time of dire need.

While it is never our intention to discount the critical and vital role that the national defense forces play in protecting us, it is our belief that it is our nation's emergency response force, almost 4 million strong, that means the difference between life and death each and every day for our citizens. Unfortunately, we learned the terrible lessons of September 11, 2001, where in a few seconds we experienced the loss of hundreds of responders murdered in the line of duty. Moreover, due to their exposure to deadly fumes and particulate on that day—and the ensuing weeks afterward working at the site—we continue to witness associated line of duty deaths of friends and colleagues so many years after the initial incident. In our business, we have often said, "A good day is coming home… A great day is coming home in one piece!"

We pray and wish for each of you many days coming home to your family in one piece!

Introduction

This book is presented as an overview of strategic practices and serves as a basic and pragmatic guide for emergency response practitioners. In addition, our book is structured as a textbook for the academic community. Each chapter is preceded by a list of objectives based on Bloom's taxonomy of education. Chapters conclude with a wrap up including chapter questions and a chapter vocabulary. We also include one or more class projects at the end of each chapter. These projects are in-depth, graduate-level research assignments related to the chapter material.

There are two overarching perspectives that frame this book. First, we take an all-hazards approach. Granted, the core theme of our work is terrorism and homeland security, but our material addresses many of the threats and hazards confronting emergency responders and planners on a daily basis. Whether an incident is an attack, a crime, a natural disaster, or a technological accident, the principles of planning and response discussed in this book apply. Second, this book applies to all disciplines in the emergency response and emergency management arena. Our focus is on the traditional response agencies such as fire/rescue operations, emergency medical services, and law enforcement. However, the strategic planning and incident management principles that we elaborate on serve as a template for all public and private sector agencies, organizations, and not-for-profit political and private sector entities engaged in incidents or event planning/response.

We begin with an abridged history of terrorism that dates back to ancient times. The historical common thread is the use of violence and intimidation to accomplish political, religious, and economic goals. Throughout history, we have witnessed the development of new weapons followed by the violent application of these weapons to kill, injure, and terrorize populations. In the twenty-first century, some of the weapons are new, but the intent to terrify is not. Many of our historical perspectives were guided by insights from the late Captain James P. Denney.

An essential response tool that was lacking until the late twentieth century was a common incident management system that was effective for all disciplines and applicable to all hazards. In the United States we now employ the National Incident Management System

(NIMS) with an incident command system (ICS) as a core management element. We chose incident management as the first technical chapter because incident management is the supporting template for all further material. All of our planning, preparedness, response, and mitigation capabilities are grounded by a scalable and flexible NIMS.

The National Response Framework (NRF) follows our chapter on the NIMS because the NRF is a key component in America's homeland security strategy that complements the NIMS. The NRF is a framework (not a plan) that evolved from the original Federal Response Plan and National Response Plan. This framework begins with an in-depth preparedness cycle, starting with individual families, and progresses through the local, state, tribal, and federal levels. The NRF prescribes the roles of private sector, non-government, and federal government agencies, and includes emergency support functions, support annexes, and incident annexes.

We follow our NRF discussion with an insightful chapter about national infrastructure protection written by Dr. John Noftsinger, Kenneth Newbold, and Benjamin Delp. This chapter identifies the physical and cyber components of America's critical infrastructure and elaborates on key resources and key assets. Further, the chapter elaborates on the role of the Department of Homeland Security in critical infrastructure protection.

Next, we take a look at planning. Our approach to planning is balanced because we know that planning is critical, yet we experienced incidents during our days in the street where plans failed. We approach planning as a critical process that integrates with the NIMS and NRF. We emphasize that planning is anchored by a comprehensive emergency operations plan (EOP). The EOP is essentially a formal document with emphasis on incident support, including mutual aid, resource management, a multiagency coordination system (MACS), private sector assets, military coordination, and state/federal assistance.

An informal incident action plan (IAP) begins with the arrival of responders at an incident. The informal IAP becomes a formal IAP when practical. Our planning discussion concludes with a case study that demonstrates the effective integration of an EOP, informal IAP, and formal IAP.

Our chapter on response procedures is a tactical guide for safely operating at an attack or terrorism incident. We begin by defining convergent responders as civilians who render aid at an incident before official first responders arrive and discuss how convergent responders can play a positive role in the outcome of an incident. Further, we address the role of the first arriving unit at a chaotic incident. In addition, defensive and self-protection measures such as LACES (lookout, awareness, communications, escape, and safe zone) and the utilization of the buddy system (2 in and 2 out) are explained.

Operational security (OPSEC) is another defensive concept that is essential to protecting institutions, critical infrastructure, and responders. OPSEC is a military concept of protective countermeasures that morphed into the civilian response world after the attacks in 2001. OPSEC is a form of force protection that is new to many civilian responders and planners. It is an important concept because the threats to today's responders are significant. Our overview of OPSEC includes site security, operational security, critical components, and the intelligence cycle.

We use the term *weapons of mass effect* to identify threats or devices that cause mass fatalities/injuries or mass terror. These weapons fall into the general categories of chemical, biological, radiological, nuclear, and explosives (CBRNE). Each of these threats requires a lifetime of study and training to attain an expert proficiency level. We are indebted to contributions from Dr. Christopher Holstege, Dr. Fredrick Sidell, Dr. Charles Stewart, and Lt. Harold W. Neal. Clearly, these subjects cannot be addressed in a single chapter or book. Our intent is to provide a basic overview of CBRNE threats and to introduce critical factors and procedures that must be considered to ensure safe and effective incident operations.

CBRNE incidents require special personal protective equipment (PPE) that is often unavailable to first responders. Effective PPE must provide full protection, yet be lightweight, durable, simple to use, and low in cost. It must also allow complete mobility. No protective ensemble presently meets these criteria. Our effort centers on providing an exposure to basic PPE standards and a description of the four basic levels of protective ensembles presently addressed by National Fire Protection Association standards (NFPA 472). It is important to note that all responders operating in a CBRNE environment must be trained to an operations level. The operations level exceeds the awareness level that was previously mandated. This means that EMS and law enforcement responders must now be trained and certified at the operations level because they respond to and operate at CBRNE incidents.

CBRNE exposure also contaminates responders, victims, property, and the environment. Proper decontamination of all exposed individuals is essential to reduce further exposure to a CBRNE mechanism of injury and prevent contaminated individuals from spreading the mechanism of injury. The military has experience with many CBRNE exposures that are unknown to the civilian response community. For this reason, we have incorporated military and civilian decontamination protocols in our discussion. Captain II Andrew Wordin's expertise greatly enhanced this chapter.

Our final chapter provides an overview of evidence collection and crime scene procedures with guidance from Dep. Director Neal J. Dolan. Candidly, law enforcement readers will find this chapter very basic. However, many fire, emergency medical services providers, and emergency management responders, often fail to perceive an incident as a potential crime scene. Our intent is to provide basic steps of evidence preservation to convey a sense of responsibility to non–law enforcement responders for preserving vital evidence.

Hank T. Christen
Paul M. Maniscalco

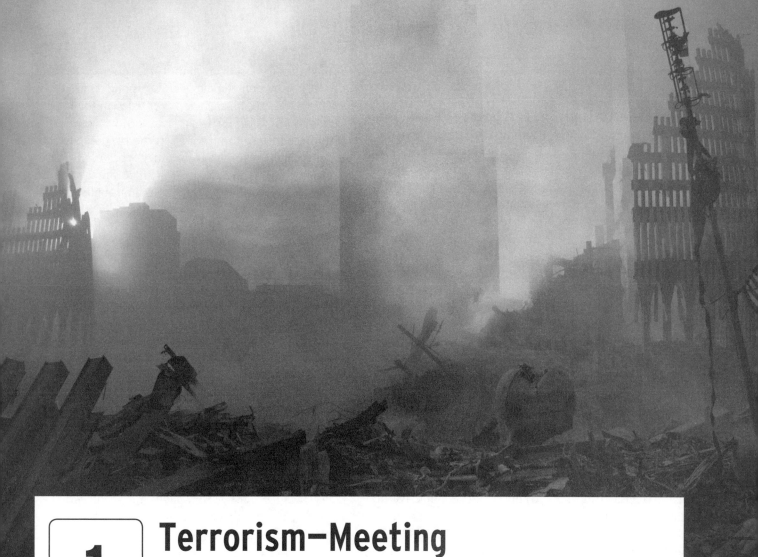

1

Terrorism–Meeting the Challenge

Paul M. Maniscalco
Hank T. Christen
James P. Denney

*While nothing is easier than to denounce
the evildoer, nothing is more difficult
than to understand him.*
— F. M. Dostoevsky

Objectives

- Discuss the differing definitions of terrorism.
- Describe the critical concept of local preparedness for terrorism/tactical violence response.
- List and describe the federal agencies in the national response spectrum.
- Recognize the changing history and threat evolution of terrorism.
- Discuss the capabilities and limitations of local response systems.
- List the risks to responders in the modern terrorism environment.
- Recognize the differences between advanced trauma life support protocols and casualty care in the urban combat environment.
- Outline the key concepts in a mass fatality management plan.

Introduction

What Is Terrorism? Why Is It Used?

Terrorism is not a new phenomenon for modern society. The threat of terrorism is present across the entire geographical and societal spectrum. Terrorism knows no jurisdictional boundaries, and it poses critical and complex challenges to the contemporary emergency response organization and leadership on how to effectively prevent, detect, deter, respond to, and recover from incidents. The use of terrorism as a tool ranges from individual acts of reckless destruction to property or person(s) to decidedly complicated events perpetrated by organizations with extreme social, environmental, religious, economic, or political agendas. These groups are domestic or international, centralized, and well organized with access to resources and finances. They might be a loose confederation of affiliated movements structured as a cellular type grouping with limited immediate capacity—but nevertheless, with dangerous motivation that feeds the creativity needed to acquire the support required to implement a plan and execute an attack.

History has demonstrated that all of these organizational constructs can be and have been effective in launching devastating attacks throughout the world. Terrorism threats range from organizations like al-Qaeda and affiliated cells with international, regional, and transnational capabilities to domestic groups and single issue movements centered on antigovernment, antitax, environmental, hate, and other extreme ideologies to homegrown, self-radicalized, unaffiliated terrorists with militant single-issue agendas and finite capabilities.

Irrespective of the historical context and the prescience of evolving terrorist threats, acts of terrorism are still often misunderstood and mislabeled. Subsequent to the existence of broadly deviating thoughts or opinions on what the proper adopted and applied definition for the term *terrorism* should be, this confusion contributes to obscuring a uniform, coherent grasp of the matter by policy makers and responders alike. An act of violence that is generally regarded in the United States as an act of terrorism may not be viewed the same in another country. The type of violence that distinguishes terrorism from other types of violence, such as ordinary crime or a wartime military action, can still be defined in terms that might qualify as reasonably objective.

Hudson notes in the research conducted for the Library of Congress, Federal Research Division, that:

> *Unable to achieve their unrealistic goals by conventional means, international terrorists attempt to send an ideological or religious message by terrorizing the general public. Through the choice of their targets, which are often symbolic or representative of the targeted nation, terrorists attempt to create a high-profile impact on the public of their targeted enemy or enemies with their act of violence, despite the limited material resources that are usually at their disposal. In doing so, they hope to demonstrate various points, such as that the targeted government(s) cannot protect its (their) own citizens, or that by assassinating a specific victim they can teach the general public a lesson about espousing viewpoints or policies antithetical to their own.* (Hudson, 1999, p. 11)

In the end, most emergency services leaders and responders still struggle with the technical definitions associated with terrorism—opting for the idea that it's easier to recognize the act than to define it. Yet, unquestionably, the ability to define terrorism in a somewhat uniform manner—or at least have the ability to identify the varying current definitions, why they vary, and whose definition it is—is an all-important issue for the contemporary emergency service leader and responder.

Terrorism is defined in a number of different ways using a variety of sources depending upon the need at hand. There is no single, universally accepted definition of terrorism presently in use. Definitions of terrorism created by government organizations such as the Federal Bureau of Investigation (FBI), the Department of Defense, and the State Department are all valid and relevant for their operational environments, but the elusive quest to define and adopt a single universal definition has been a daunting task confronting responders, military officers, intelligence and law enforcement officials, and researchers and legal scholars for years. Let's examine the definitions the Department of Defense, State Department, and the FBI use.

CRITICAL FACTOR ....

This chapter does not presume to present an exhaustive, comprehensive representation of terrorism events, groups, or methodologies; however, it does provide the learner with the opportunity to develop a fundamental analytical, biographical, historical, and theoretical understanding for further research on the general subject of terrorism as well as on particular terrorism groups or individuals.

The Department of Defense definition for terrorism is:

> The calculated use of unlawful violence to inculcate fear, intended to coerce or to intimidate governments or societies in the pursuit of goals that are generally political, religious, or ideological. (U.S. Department of Defense, 2003, p. 531)

The State Department utilizes a definition found in federal statute. Title 22 of the U.S. Code, § 2656f(d) defines terrorism as "premeditated, politically motivated violence perpetrated against noncombatant targets by subnational groups or clandestine agents, usually intended to influence an audience" (U.S. Department of State, 2007).

The FBI definition of terrorism is defined in the *Code of Federal Regulations* as ". . . the unlawful use of force and violence against persons or property to intimidate or coerce a government, the civilian population, or any segment thereof, in furtherance of political or social objectives" (U.S. Department of Justice, n.d.).

The FBI further describes terrorism as either domestic or international, depending on the origin, base, and objectives of the terrorist organization.

> • *Domestic terrorism is the unlawful use, or threatened use, of force or violence by a group or individual based and operating entirely within the United States or Puerto Rico without foreign direction committed against persons or property to intimidate or coerce a government, the civilian population, or any segment thereof in furtherance of political or social objectives.*
>
> • *International terrorism involves violent acts or acts dangerous to human life that are a violation of the criminal laws of the United States or any state, or that would be a criminal*

violation if committed within the jurisdiction of the United States or any state. These acts appear to be intended to intimidate or coerce a civilian population, influence the policy of a government by intimidation or coercion, or affect the conduct of a government by assassination or kidnapping. International terrorist acts occur outside the United States or transcend national boundaries in terms of the means by which they are accomplished, the persons they appear intended to coerce or intimidate, or the locale in which their perpetrators operate or seek asylum (U.S. Department of Justice, n.d.).

Both the State Department and the FBI definitions of terrorism share a common theme—the use of force intended to influence or bring about a course of action that furthers a political or social objective.

Organized Terrorism

In the past, what was referred to as an "international terrorist network" was attributed to the Tricontinental Congress held in Havana, Cuba, in January 1966. At that congress, 500 delegates proposed close cooperation among socialist countries and national liberation movements in order to forge a global strategy to counter American imperialism.

Meetings among terrorist organizations increased in the years that followed. Examples of networking include the American Black Panther leaders who toured North Korea, Vietnam, and China. In China, they had an opportunity to meet with Shirley Graham, wife of W.E.B. Du Bois, who was visiting with Zhou Enlai. The network advanced terrorism on global, national, and regional levels by providing economic support, training, specialty personnel, and advanced weaponry.

For example, in 1978, Argentine terrorists received Soviet-made rockets from Palestinian terrorists, and the Baader-Meinhof group supplied three sets of American night-vision binoculars to the Irish Republican Army (IRA) and American-made hand grenades to the Japanese Red Army. Terrorist training camps sprang up in Cuba, Algeria, Iraq, Jordan, Lebanon, Libya, and South Yemen, while Syria provided sites for advanced training.

Acts of terrorism prompted the Tokyo and Montreal counterterrorism conventions of 1963 and 1971 on hijacking and sabotage of civilian aircraft. This was followed by the 1973 convention to counter crimes against diplomats and the 1979 convention, sponsored by The Hague, against hostage taking. These conventions established categories of international crimes that were punishable by any state regardless of the nationality of the criminal, victim, or the location of the offense.

Following President Ronald Reagan's ordering of U.S. military forces to attack terrorist-related targets in Libya in 1986, seven Western industrial democracies pledged themselves to take joint action against terrorism. Those nations included the United States, Germany, Great Britain, Italy, Canada, France, and Japan. These nations agreed to deny terrorist suspects entry into their countries, to bring about better cooperation between police and security forces in their countries, to place restrictions on diplomatic missions suspected of involvement in terrorism, and to cooperate in a number of other ways.

The Cold War Ends; Threat Shifting Begins

The breakup of the former Soviet Union and the subsequent economic collapse significantly altered the global security landscape. At the time of the breakup, the Soviet Union was a superpower with well-developed nuclear, chemical, and biological warfare capabilities. Unfortunately, a more sinister threat began to emerge from the former Soviet Union—a thriving international black market in arms and weapons technology. At that time, the economic collapse of the Soviet Union manifested in the nations' inability to meet their fiscal obligations, including military and other payrolls. As a result, Russia suffered a tumultuous period with an ever-present threat of political unrest and organized crime emerging as a significant influencing factor within domestic and international affairs.

With available weapons ranging from nuclear devices to submarines and Mikoyan-i-Gurevich (MiG) aircraft to missiles, the former controlled threat was transformed into an uncontrolled threat market,

strongly influenced by the Russian organized crime syndicates, a market where unpaid government employees attempted to sell limited amounts of fissionable materiel and other materiel that was of great value to terrorist organizations.

In addition to the black market in weapons, there also exists a potential for weapon thefts, including those weapons stored at poorly guarded chemical and biological storage facilities located throughout the former Soviet Union and its satellite nations.

A New Threat Emerges

The region from the Middle East to South Asia is a central launching pad for many of the threats and challenges facing the United States in the new millennium. In the intelligence community, this collective geographic area is frequently referred to as the "Arc of Instability"— illustrative of the geospatial mapping curve that links the countries of concern and the associated activities that can be tied to terrorist activities. These regions have emerged as the primary contributor of personnel, funding, training, and arms for the current terrorist movement. Unlike the Marxist-Leninist groups of the 1960s and 1970s, who were motivated by political and social conditions, today's international terrorists are an amalgam consisting of anarchist-nihilist and Middle Eastern religious-based fundamentalists who despise American hegemony and the resulting influence on world policy. Bent specifically on the destruction of American values, influence, and economy, they have targeted U.S. interests worldwide.

The prevailing goals and objectives of terrorist organizations vary throughout the world. They can be domestic or international in origin and they can range from those of regional, single-issue terrorists to transnational terrorists. As a vibrant and robust democracy with significant global economic, military, and political influence, the United States is an appealing target of convenience for extremists and a desirable stage for terrorist organizations.

Dennis C. Blair, director of national intelligence, in his February 12, 2009, testimony before the Senate Select Committee on Intelligence, presented the annual threat assessment of the intelligence community. In this testimony, he presented two ominous observations/findings on what he called the *homegrown threat*:

. . . we remain concerned about the potential for homegrown extremists inspired by al-Qa'ida's militant ideology to plan attacks inside the United States, Europe, and elsewhere without operational direction from the group itself. In this regard, over the next year we will

remain focused on identifying any ties between US-based individuals and extremist networks overseas. Though difficult to measure, the spread of radical Salafi Internet sites that provide religious justification for attacks; aggressive and violent anti-Western rhetoric; and signs that self-generating cells in the US identify with [Osama] Bin Ladin's violent objectives all point to the likelihood that a small but violent number of cells may develop here.

Al-Qa'ida's propaganda efforts include messages in English and those aimed specifically at an American audience either in translated form or directly by al-Qa'ida's second-in command, Ayman al-Zawahiri, such as with his November 2008 video message following the US Presidential elections. US-born al-Qa'ida members such as Adam Gadahn, who was indicted by a US grand jury in October 2006 on charges of treason, providing material support to a designated foreign terrorist organization, and aiding and abetting terrorists, also participated in making these English-language propaganda messages (Blair, 2009, p. 7).

Continued threats by terrorist organizations against the United States and the West, continued intelligence analytical reports indicating a reasonable degree of validation for the threats, along with attack plots being interdicted raise the specter of concern for repeated attempts to launch additional terrorist attacks in the United States and against allies as well as our interests abroad. Moreover, in this testimony, Blair reported that:

. . . Over the coming years, we will continue to face a substantial threat, including in the US Homeland, from terrorists attempting to acquire biological, chemical, and possibly nuclear weapons and use them to conduct large-scale attacks. Conventional weapons and explosives will continue to be the most often used instruments of destruction in terrorist attacks; however, terrorists who are determined to develop CBRN [chemical, biological, radiological, and nuclear] capabilities will have increasing opportunities to do so, owing to the spread of relevant technological knowledge and the ability to work with CBRN materials and designs in safe havens.

- Most terrorist groups that have shown some interest, intent, or capability to conduct CBRN attacks have pursued only limited, technically simple approaches that have not yet caused large numbers of casualties.

In particular, we assess the terrorist use of biological agents represents a growing threat as the barriers to obtaining many suitable starter cultures are eroding and open source technical literature and basic laboratory equipment can facilitate production. Terrorist chemical attacks also represent a substantial threat. Small-scale chemical attacks using industrial toxins have been the most frequent type of CBRN attack to date. The chlorine attacks in Iraq from October 2006 through the summer of 2007 highlighted terrorist interest in using commercial and easily available toxic industrial chemicals as weapons.

Al-Qa'ida is the terrorist group that historically has sought the broadest range of CBRN attack capabilities, and we assess that it would use any CBRN capability it acquires in an anti-US attack, preferably against the Homeland. There also is a threat of biological or chemical attacks in the US Homeland by lone individuals (Blair, 2009, p. 21).

The compelling information being disseminated regarding the threat, combined with the historical experiences of terrorist incidents both in the United States and abroad are a clarion call for EMS, fire service, law enforcement, public health, and medical and emergency management leadership to no longer view terrorism as an exotic event and start to incorporate sustainable readiness strategies as a vital component of daily operations and standard operations procedures.

Terrorist threats vary from nonstate transnational networks with global reach capability such as al-Qaeda to terrorist cells affiliated with regional or international agendas and individual self-radicalized and unaffiliated terrorists with single-issue agendas. Each type of network or terrorist cell has criminal intentions limited by finite capability. Terrorists exist as a threat of the United States in the U.S. homeland and in U.S. presence throughout the world.

Globalization

Globalization is changing the context in which terrorists operate. **Globalization** is essentially a measure of the ease with which labor, ideas, capital, technology, and profits can move across borders with minimal government interference. Dr. Khan, in his work entitled *Terrorism and Globalization* (2001) further presents:

The world was rapidly moving to realizing the idea of a global village as commonalities in terms of economic aspirations and technological progress were emphasized by politicians and opinion makers, over differences such as religion, culture and *ethnicity. Globalization of the world was the ultimate celebration of the political, economic, and social homogenization of the global populations. On (the) political front there is a consensus that democracy was not only the best but also the only legitimate way of organizing modern polities. On the economic front, the globalization of the economy was a foregone conclusion as nations scrambled to liberalize their economies in order to live up to the new standards set by the World Trade Organization (Kahn, 2001).*

It is ironic that global terrorism, the phenomenon of terrorists operating in and against several nations simultaneously, was facilitated by globalization and is now the biggest challenge to globalization. Global terrorism depends on the success of globalization. Technological advances provided vis-à-vis globalization such as the Internet, satellite television and radio networks, 24-hour news networks, low-cost airlines, and open borders are exploitation opportunities for malevolent individuals and organizations bent on causing harm and societal disruption. U.S. Ambassador Henry Crumpton (2006), coordinator for counterterrorism for the U.S. State Department at the 2006 RUSI Conference on Transnational Terrorism, eloquently captured the essence of the threat society faces:

> *Our global interdependence makes us stronger, but also in some aspects, more vulnerable. There is also a backlash from those who view globalization as a threat to traditional culture and their vested interests. Some discontented, illiberal non-state actors perceive themselves under attack and, therefore, resort to offensive action. This is the case with al-Qaeda and affiliated organizations. Yet, these enemies face a strategic environment featuring nation states with an overwhelming dominance in conventional military forces. This includes but is not limited to the U.S. It's no surprise, then, that our actual and potential enemies have taken note of our conventional superiority and acted to dislocate it. State actors, such as North Korea and Iran, seek irregular means to engage their foes. Iran uses proxies such as Hezbollah. Non-state actors like al-Qaeda have also developed asymmetric approaches that allow them to side-step conventional military power. They embrace terror as a tactic, but on such a level as to provide them strategic impact. Toward that end, they seek to acquire capabilities that can pose catastrophic threats, such as CBRNE, disruptive technologies, or a combination of these measures (Crumpton, 2006).*

After the attacks of September 11, 2001, the capacity or commitment of a transnational terrorist organization, like an al-Qaeda, to create an intense level of fear in a society and inflict extensive damage/loss of life to a nation is no longer an academic argument. That attack, coupled with others such as the train attacks in Madrid, bus and train attacks in London, the Bali nightclub bombings, the Moscow theater attack, and the Beslan school attack in Russia are only a few past events illustrating that transnational terrorist groups have the resolve, capacity, and capability to plan, fund, and execute large-scale incidents to further advance their cause.

Advances in technology that have driven cost down and expanded performance capabilities of many products have leveled the technology field for nonstate actors while concurrently enhancing their operational capabilities. For instance, advances with information technology have effectively terminated the ability of countries to isolate themselves. Information and communication control is difficult, if not impossible to achieve because the information revolution has resulted in a democratic access to technology. Two important results are that the terrorists' recruiting prospect base has expanded exponentially and free speech and civil liberty have given them an inexpensive international medium with which to voice unfettered discontent.

The notional concept of centrally controlled international terrorist networks, previously investigated and vigorously debated during the 1960s and 1970s, was deemed unlikely due to conflicting ideologies, motivating factors, funding, and arming and training among global practitioners. However, networks with great geographic reach are feasible especially with the advent of public access to the Internet, the ability to transfer funds and conduct banking electronically, the international arms market, encrypted digital communication technology, and the emergence of stateless terrorism. An important result is that instant global communication between offensive action cells and their controllers is now possible. Controllers now have global reach and can run multiple independent cells from a single location with no interaction between the cells. They can also contract terrorism services utilizing mercenaries composed of local indigenous practitioners in a given target community.

The rapid expansion of technology also resulted in a reduced requirement for terrorist group infrastructure and has resulted in an asymmetry between cause and effect. The complexity of weapons acquisition, production, transportation, lethality, and delivery platform has been diminished.

Networks and Organizations

History documents many examples where terrorist organizations possessed and employed organizational traits that resemble military or modern corporate management structures. These constructs boasted robust hierarchical structures with a definitive chain of command that managed command and control responsibilities of the group. With these types of organizations, a more defined division of labor or functional specialization in subordinate cells/units was achieved by designating subunits to handle the finance, intelligence, operations, and logistics/support aspects of the group. Within the organization, generally only the cell leader possessed the full knowledge of what other components were charged with achieving and which individuals populated those units. Moreover, only the very senior leadership of the organization possessed the ability to comprehend the unified big strategic picture for the full organization.

Presently, many terrorist groups manage their affairs and operations by progressively employing an extensive system of smaller networks, integrating them into a decentralized network strategy. The creation of an operational strategy revolving around a network of networks lowers the risk profile of the traditional larger analogue terrorist group structure by remotely interconnecting smaller, discrete units—making it increasingly difficult to detect the group unless the opportunity for authorities to infiltrate the trusted smaller group presents and is successfully seized. Moreover, utility of this discrete configuration provides greater redundancy opportunities for the group.

Comprised in this manner, once operational goals, targeting objectives, and functional directions have been issued, terrorist groups can leverage the flexibility and independence of small affiliate groups and individual actors from a diverse member population and across geographic boundaries to conduct the designated operation with lesser chances of discovery.

John Arquilla and David Ronfeldt in their 2001 work entitled, *Networks and Netwars: The Future of Terror, Crime and Militancy*, present the work of William Evan to delineate types of networks. Evan posits that fundamentally there are three types of network topologies, which include:

- *The Chain or Line Network* (**FIGURE 1-1**)—Each cell links to the next node in the chain or line sequence.

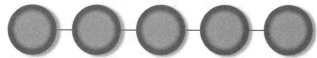

FIGURE 1-1 The chain or line network.

- *The Hub, Star, or Wheel Network* (**FIGURE 1-2**)— Each cell communicates with one central control element. The control element could be the leader or a designated proxy who has the delegated authority. A moderate deviation of the hub network is a wheel (network) design where the outer nodes communicate with one or two other outer cells in addition to the hub.

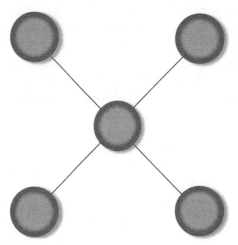

FIGURE 1-2 The hub, star, or wheel network.

- *The All-Channel or Full Matrix Network* (**FIGURE 1-3**)—All nodes connect to each other. Organizationally, the network is flat, indicating there is no hierarchical command with control distributed within the network. This format is communication intensive and can pose operational security threats if the linkages are compromised, identified, and tracked.

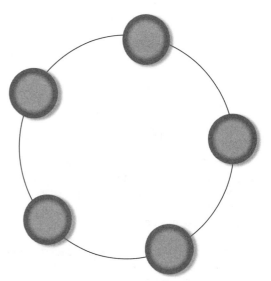

FIGURE 1-3 The all-channel or full matrix network.

The terrorist network distributes key function assignments and responsibility for planning, operations, and redundancy through the prescribed structure depending on the ways elements are linked to other elements of the structure. Individuals and cells have no contact with each other unless that contact is critical to the coordination of a specific task or executing the attack. By limiting interaction and diminishing potential for discovery, the leaders enhance group operational security and insulate themselves from accusations of involvement via the cellular layers involved in the implementation and execution phases of the attack.

Regardless of their differences, the three basic network types are leveraged together in hybrid organizations when their synergy is needed to accomplish the operational objective. A terrorist organization could employ chain networks for financing and money-laundering activities, attached to a wheel network handling logistics issues that is coupled with an all-channel network where leadership dictates the use of fiscal resources for operational activities of a hub network that is conducting pretargeting surveillance and reconnaissance activities for the attack.

Preparing for Threats Involving Weapons of Mass Destruction

The September 11, 2001, attacks of the New York City World Trade Center and the Pentagon in Washington, DC, the 1995 bombing of the Alfred P. Murrah Federal Building in Oklahoma City, and the 1993 bombing of the New York City World Trade Center, coupled with the myriad of attacks that have been interdicted clearly illustrate America's vulnerability to terrorism—not only abroad, but to the homeland as well. These acts demonstrate the willingness and ability of determined terrorists to carry out attacks against high-impact targets. The March 1995 sarin gas incident in the Tokyo subway demonstrated the terrorists' willingness to kill thousands

CRITICAL FACTOR ....

The historical, organizational, operational, and behavioral complexities posed by terrorist organizations are numerous. Although the previous section was designed to provide minimal clarity and foundation for the background material, it is only a snowflake on the tip of an iceberg. We encourage continued acquaintance with these issues by conducting in-depth research via any of the numerous comprehensive texts that were developed to address these topics.

in a single event. Attacks on mass transportation systems in Britain, Israel, Scotland, and Spain illustrate the continuing trend of commitment to use terrorism as a weapon against noncombatants.

Twenty-first century threat evolution requires public safety and emergency service organizations to reevaluate their priorities and consider their ability to address multiple new tasks. These tasks include support for new and emerging technologies; the increasing significance of establishing relationships with adjacent agencies and cooperation with specialized resources; and a better understanding of issues such as the threat environment including mass casualty terrorism, drugs, gangs, and crime. These changes, coupled with severe budgetary pressures to reduce costs and find more efficient ways to carry out their responsibilities, force these organizations to exercise greater care in matching available resources to priorities and to integrate political power with economic requirements.

To meet these challenges effectively, emergency service organizations must address flaws in their procedures for allocating personnel and financial resources to meet priorities and objectives, including training problems, staffing, and the inadequate integration of multifunction components. Unfortunately, these tasks are made more difficult by past management reforms such as decentralization and the devolution of decision making to lower level administrative units that have resulted in the development of new, multilevel policy systems. To summarize in the nicest way possible, local preparedness efforts to engender a greater level of community readiness for response to large-scale events is not solely waiting for the federal government to award a grant or send agency equipment. Enhancing community readiness also involves local elected officials and city/county managers investing in their public safety and health and law enforcement programs creating sustainable capacity that is augmented with federal program resources. Failure to do otherwise is irresponsible. Policy lacking resources is always rhetoric.

Emergency Medical Services

Prehospital health care no longer consists of a simple emergency transportation service. Since the early 1970s, new levels of training added to what was basically a first aid and transportation system. It is now known as the emergency medical service (EMS) system. The EMS system provides a sequential process including patient problem recognition, system access, basic and advanced intervention by first responders and bystanders, and transportation to the hospital, if necessary, by ambulance. The advent of this system completed the public safety management triad of law enforcement and crime prevention, fire prevention and suppression, and emergency medical care and transportation.

Prehospital health care changed significantly with the advent of specialized EMT and paramedic training. Capabilities now include responding to the public need with mobile intensive care units and providing specialized advanced life-support measures when necessary.

Public safety EMS is available nationwide and is provided by private and public agencies. The management and provision of the service provided by them represents a sizable investment in training, human resources, supplies, and equipment. The ability to utilize various system delivery models made it possible for agencies and communities of all sizes to participate in this vital public service.

Complex Organizational Capability

In the fire service, distribution of the workload is not characterized solely by volume, nor is it completely configuration dependent. In order for the fire service to maintain its robust capability, it vertically integrates multiple competencies, and each individual resource is configured for multitasking. Within the fire service, where consequence management is the fundamental imperative, high performance is measured by organizational effectiveness in the areas of preparedness levels, community loss prevention and reduction, and decreased mortality and morbidity.

Through integrated stability, the American fire service provides both high reliability and high trust to its constituency. High-reliability organizations are complex, and complexity mitigates risk. High reliability organizations use organizational structure to adapt and then mitigate events through processes such as risk awareness, decision migration, and process auditing.

As a result of budget corrections, operational adjustments, and technological advances beginning in the early 1990s, the 21st-century American fire service emerges as a complex, precision force that possesses the nation's dominant body of knowledge regarding emergency service consequence management.

Complex Interface Development

Interface complexities involving multiple interdependent agencies, external resources, and federal assets are mitigated through the implementation of a standard, multipurpose incident management system that conforms to the scope and type of incident and the capabilities of responding agencies. Although variations of this incident management system exist, it has not been fully implemented within the inclusive public safety–emergency service amalgam.

Unrealistic Expectation

Notional concepts, including the all-hazards capability, are unrealistic, unproven, and dangerous. The assumption that a local emergency resource is capable of managing an incident equivalent to that found in military warfare could potentially result in the loss of significant operational assets and personnel and place the community at catastrophic risk.

Contemporary training is invariably conducted in daylight, in good weather, and consistently results in a positive outcome. The ability to survive a given operation is not addressed, and casualties, if any, are attributed to the civilian population at risk. Training must now include an ability-to-survive-operation component and implementation measures when conventional practices fail.

Threat Issues

Since 1992, direct physical threats aimed at America's EMS, police, and fire responders began to emerge with increasing frequency. These threats specifically target first responders and public safety personnel. The tactics used appear similar to those espoused in the *Minimanual of the Urban Guerrilla*, written by Carlos Marighella in 1969, which states in part:

> *Thus, the armed struggle of the urban guerrilla points towards two essential objectives:*
>
> 1. *The physical elimination of the leaders and assistants of the armed forces and of the police;*
> 2. *The expropriation of government resources and the wealth belonging to the rich businessmen, the large landowners and the imperialists, with small expropriations used for the sustenance of the individual guerrillas and large ones for the maintenance of the revolutionary organization itself.*
>
> *It is clear that the armed struggle of the urban guerrilla also has other objectives. But here we are referring to the two basic objectives, above all expropriation. It is necessary for every urban guerrilla to always keep in mind that he can only maintain his existence if he is able to kill the police and those dedicated to repression, and if he is determined—truly determined—to expropriate the wealth of the rich businessmen, landowners and imperialists. (Marighella, 1969, p. 6)*

The threats are tactical violence and 911 target acquisition. These threats have four applications:

1. To control the criminal environment
2. To divert law enforcement attention
3. To kill or injure law enforcement personnel
4. To compel law enforcement–assisted suicide

Tactical Violence

Since the 1992 Los Angeles civil disturbance, a disturbing phenomenon that directly affects emergency service providers has surfaced. The phenomenon has been identified as **tactical violence**.

Tactical violence is primarily employed by criminals. It is defined as the predetermined use of maximum violence in order to achieve one's criminal goals, regardless of victim cooperation, level of environmental threat to the perpetrator, or the need to evade law enforcement or capture. This method also usually results in physical or psychological injury or death to the victim. The rationale for employing tactical violence is predatory control of the immediate criminal environment through the creation of chaos and the infliction of terror, trauma, and death on presenting targets.

911 Target Acquisition

One tactic utilized by the criminal and extremist elements (including but not limited to militias, white supremacists, environmentalists, animal rights activists, and antiabortionists) is 911 target acquisition. This tactic has been employed for the following purposes:

- To divert public safety resources prior to, during, or after the commission of criminal acts
- To draw resources into an ambush situation
- To draw resources into environments laced with improvised explosive antipersonnel devices
- To compel law enforcement–assisted suicide

Although these threats primarily target law enforcement organizations (crisis managers), fire and EMS first responders (consequence managers) have the highest exposure by virtue of their response configuration and resource staffing levels. Recovering from these events takes up to 1 year, during which time the community's vulnerability to all hazards is significantly increased.

Covert Intimidation

Local and federal law enforcement agencies are not the same as military units and rely to some extent on the intimidation factor. The primary goal of law enforcement is crime prevention/control. There are many subtle intimidation strategies incorporated into this function that have a psychological impact on the community, including vehicle color schemes and emergency lighting configuration, uniform design and color, the visible wearing of sidearms, and officer bearing and demeanor.

Overt Intimidation

Law enforcement special teams include special weapons and tactics (SWAT) and hostage response teams. These units are semimilitarized and affect quasimilitary status through the wearing of military-like/special operations/commando uniforms. They carry special weaponry and devices not seen in routine law enforcement operations. Their presence at an incident is an implied threat to targeted perpetrators and demonstrates the capacity to employ overwhelming force and special aggressive tactics if necessary.

Overt intimidation tactics have been adopted in other areas as well, such as the serving of high-risk warrants or drug raids. It is common to see various law enforcement agencies entering a suspect dwelling en masse, creating confusion, shouting commands, and displaying drawn weapons. Although intimidation plays a role in deterring terrorist activity, it will not be a factor once crisis management transitions into consequence management. Crisis management involves measures to identify, acquire, and plan the use of resources needed to anticipate, prevent, and/or resolve a threat or act of terrorism. Consequence management involves measures to protect public health and safety, restore essential government services, and provide emergency relief to governments, businesses, and individuals affected by the consequences of terrorism.

Outcome Training

Local law enforcement personnel are not trained to participate against sustained armed resistance with an opposing force without external support.

In all cases, law enforcement personnel are trained in a manner that results in a positive outcome for them on any given incident. Although vulnerability, danger, and personal risk are discussed, they are presented in general terms suggesting that, although they exist, it is unlikely they will occur to a particular individual if training is followed.

Special aggressor teams such as SWAT and hostage response teams are trained to conduct assaults if necessary in order to effect closure of a particular incident. However, this training implies that an assault is both inclusive and conclusive relative to a given criminal problem. This means inclusive of all threats and conclusive once the threat is neutralized. An example is to gain entry and subdue/arrest/kill perpetrators and/or rescue hostages.

Unlike the military, law enforcement agencies are not prepared to conduct an assault in the face of withering automatic weapons fire, rocket-propelled grenades, hand grenades, claymores, mortars, or other similar type weaponry. This is especially true if they incur substantial casualties among their personnel. They must rely instead on special teams for this type of activity. (England discovered this during an IRA assault against Parliament, as did the Los Angeles Police Department during a North Hollywood bank robbery.) Nor are law enforcement agencies, whose primary objective is the safety of its personnel, prepared to conduct operations against a sustained, widespread, or diffuse hostile faction operating from several venues simultaneously. These groups have no acceptable loss provisions.

Acts of terrorism perpetrated against society present many problems to those charged with crisis and consequence management response. An act of terrorism is similar to other man-made disasters because the main characteristic is sudden onset and the resultant effect is significant human injury and/or death. Because of the nature of the incident, in many cases, there is no opportunity for crisis management or intervention.

These incidents, by their nature, are not telegraphed in advance to the authorities, and therefore, the appropriate response may consist solely of consequence management and criminal investigation. To the consequence manager, these responses represent the greatest challenge faced by an emergency agency.

To begin with, the physical impact of a conventional terrorist incident is characterized by rapid onset. Unlike a common conventional response, where initial units are dispatched and the event accelerates or expands based on the observation and assessment of first-arriving units, conventional terrorist incidents require an immediate maximal response of appropriate resources in order to optimize the survivability of victims.

This may indicate that a new standard or ad hoc response configuration is necessary for terrorism incidents—one that combines emergency medical care providers, hazardous materials management, and search and rescue capability with conventional resources on the initial dispatch to specific types of incidents.

Federal Asset, First Responder Integration

The Marine Corps Chemical Biological Incident Response Force responds to incidents involving chemical, biological, radiological, nuclear, and explosive (CBRNE) hazards in support of local responders. Their mission is to deploy domestically or overseas to provide force protection and/or mitigation and to assist federal, state, and local responders in developing training programs to manage the consequences of a CBRNE event.

The National Guard originally commissioned 10 weapons of mass destruction (WMD) civil support teams (CSTs), formerly known as rapid assessment and initial detection teams. A CST is composed of 22 people, 7 officers and 15 enlisted personnel, from both the army and Air National Guard, with a variety of specialties. Assigned vehicles include a command vehicle, an operations van, a communications vehicle called the unified command suite (provides a broad range of communications capabilities including satellite communications), an analytical laboratory system van (contains a full suite of analysis equipment to support the medical team, and other general-purpose vehicles). The CST normally deploys using its assigned vehicles, but it can be airlifted if required. A deployment distance of up to 250 miles can usually be covered faster by surface travel, given the time required to recall an aircrew and stage an aircraft.

There are currently 55 CSTs (one per state/territory; but two in California).

The CST is on standby 24 hours a day, 7 days a week with an advanced echelon deploying within 90 minutes of notification and the rest of the team within 3 hours. This quick response gives the CST the ability to support the incident commander (IC) with critical information rapidly. The CST commander advises the IC as to the type and level of hazard present, possible courses of action, and additional National Guard assets that are available.

The communications capability of the unified command suite allows any member of the CST to contact a wide range of technical experts. It also allows the commander to pass information and situation reports up channel to keep the Joint Forces Headquarters, National Guard Bureau, and Northern Command apprised of the current status of events and actions.

Both of these response components integrate with local responders through implementation of the incident management system. With the establishment of a unified command, a fully capable civil-federal management team oversees management and operations of combined assets in WMD and other events impacting communities in the United States.

Although these external assets, along with other federal agencies (other divisions of the Department of Defense, Department of Health and Human Services, Centers for Disease Control and Prevention, Federal

Emergency Management Agency (FEMA), and Public Health Service), respond to assist after the primary impact, the response to the aftermath of an event remains the responsibility of local communities. It is critical that this facet is not lost in the planning process due to the reliance on federal response and capacity. Managers, chief officers, planners, and elected officials must remain cognizant of the critical factor that the arrival of these assets is time and distance limited. In many cases, depending on the proximity of federal resource stationing and/or the availability of aircraft with appropriate lift capacity, it can be many hours or perhaps days prior to arrival and full operational activity.

Physical Constraints

It is not unusual for terrorist incidents to involve structural collapse, multiple casualties, fire, and chemical release. Is there a difference between a terrorist act and a conventional incident? Aside from the possible psychological factors, there is no difference to the consequence manager, who must implement operations based on the present state of the event rather than the precipitating factors. Therefore, attribution is not a consequence priority. Regardless of motivation, both function as casualty generators that result in short-term resource commitment on a large scale. Both have the potential to cause collateral injury to responders, and, by their nature, generally do not afford an opportunity for crisis management or intervention prior to the incident.

However, because terrorism is a deliberate act, these incidents present unique hazards to response personnel. For example, it is not unusual for terrorists to plan secondary events that target emergency responders—events that are triggered once emergency operations begin and responders are most vulnerable to attack. The results of a terrorist act are different than a conventional incident; therefore, our approach to terrorism is different.

Aggressive response to these incidents must be curtailed. Courage, valor, honor, and integrity are not issues in these instances. Any response to suspected terrorist acts must be moderated and coupled with careful consideration of any potential secondary threats to responders and the general public. The events at the World Trade Center on September 11, 2001, taught us the hard lesson that emergency responders can and will be targeted as part of an attack.

Political Constraints

Terrorism is both a federal and a state crime. However, all incidents are manifested locally, and initial reaction to them is provided by local crisis and consequence orga-

nizations. As these incidents expand, they involve multiple organizations. Therefore, both at the planning and response level, local crisis and consequence managers must interact with external entities with, in some cases, broader authority over the incident and in other cases, with near equal power but radically different missions, perceptions, and value systems. They must also cooperate with political crisis managers and co-response organizations from within a unified command structure.

Political, strategic, operational, and tactical direction is necessary in every case of joint or combined force operations. Political direction sets political objectives, defines basic strategy to achieve these objectives, and provides basic guidance for operations. Strategic direction defines desired operational target conditions and sequencing. Operational direction will coordinate the efforts of multiple organizations to achieve a successful outcome. Tactical direction issues orders to the front-end operators actually engaged in problem resolution.

These unusual circumstances result in the consequence manager's inability to manage the incident effectively, particularly if the responding organizations do not have a familiar working relationship. It is therefore imperative that all responsible organizations plan, organize, and conduct training within a single national incident management system/incident command system (NIMS/ICS) and that individual organizational roles and responsibilities are clearly defined and agreed upon prior to an event and preferably during a comprehensive planning process.

Ethical Constraints

In unconventional terrorist incidents involving CBRNE, local agency limitations may preclude response into an impacted area. Therefore, the interval to intervention time increases. This is one of the more difficult concepts for emergency managers to instill in their personnel.

However, the current response capability of specialized federal resources is limited by geographic/regional time constraints and may not be available for the better part of a day. Additionally, the medical community currently has limited to no capability to effectively manage mass care for local populations, especially for extended periods of time. This is further complicated when one calculates the limitations of logistics in the medical community, particularly in systems where just-in-time restock strategies are in place. In these scenarios, the lack of supply depth combined with an event that consumes vast quantities of resources quickly could result in an ill-equipped and -prepared medical system collapsing.

Under these circumstances, the function of emergency response organizations is to limit environmental expansion of the incident if possible, protect the unaffected population through supporting the implementation of community shielding strategies or initiating evacuations and establishing shelters or safe havens capable of providing for basic human needs due to the magnitude of the event and the loss of infrastructure and residences.

Because of potential delays in access to unconventional incident sites involving CBRNE, the critical interval to intervention time may be protracted. Therefore, the survivability potential for victims diminishes. Prolonged waiting times increase mortality, and the consequence manager has to consider the implementation of disaster mortuary plans a priority once the site becomes accessible.

Unconventional incidents involving CBRNE are likely to convert from EMS/fire/rescue incidents to body recovery, identification, and disposal operations in co-operation with criminal investigative organizations. This final fact, as observed in the Oklahoma City bombing and the September 11, 2001, events, has a tremendous psychological impact on emergency response personnel who are neither trained nor experienced in mass fatality management.

Evolution and Application of the ICS

The ICS began as a firefighting system for managing California wildfires. The system has expanded into an all-hazard (all-risk) system and is employed at routine emergencies as well as natural disasters, technological disasters, and mass casualty incidents.

The ICS is designed to manage operations and co-ordinate resources. It is a functionally based system structured on the principles of common terminology, resource allocation, support functions, span of control, and chain of command. The ICS structure is based on a management staff that directs and supports four major sections. The staff is broken down into two groups—the command staff and the general staff. The command staff consists of an IC, a liaison officer, a safety officer, and a public information officer. The general staff is made of four section leaders (chiefs) breaking down the incident into operations, logistics, planning, and administration/finance.

The ICS is very similar to the military organization of North Atlantic Treaty Organization countries. The military staff positions of intelligence, logistics, and plans/operations closely parallel the four civilian ICS sections. The civilian system also utilizes a liaison officer and the concept of unified command to integrate with a military counterpart. This is an effective boilerplate for defense support to civil authorities and coordination during a terrorism/tactical violence incident.

The mass casualty aspect of ICS makes it effective for managing terrorism/tactical violence incidents. For mass casualties, a medical branch is assigned to the operations section and manages a triage unit, a treatment unit, and a transportation unit. The system stresses early triage and transport of critical patients and scene safety for the rescuers.

In the terrorism/tactical violence arena, the common weapons are still automatic weapons and improvised explosive devices. A chemical attack is managed by an extension of the hazardous materials ICS, with emphasis on detection, personal protective equipment, and patient decontamination. A biological attack has a delayed onset and presents special problems relating to recognition, pathogen identification, treatment protocols, and personal protection. The overwhelming requirement in the biological attack is for EMS, public health, hospital, and medical leadership to provide leadership and coherent management utilizing their lead agency obligations as command under ICS or a unified command dependent upon local protocol and statutory authorities.

Hospital Emergency Incident Command System

The hospital emergency incident command system (HEICS) is a management tool modeled after the ICS. The core of the HEICS comprises the following two main elements: (1) an organizational chart with a clearly delineated chain of command and position function titles indicating scope of responsibility, and (2) a prioritized job action sheet (job description) that assists the designated individual in focusing upon an assignment.

The benefits of a medical facility using HEICS are seen not only in a more organized response, but also in the ability of that institution to relate to other healthcare entities and public/private organizations in the event of an emergency incident. The value of the common communication language in HEICS becomes apparent when mutual aid is requested from or for that facility.

The California earthquake preparedness guidelines for hospitals served as a cornerstone in the development of the HEICS. The HEICS embodied those same characteristics that make the ICS so appealing. Those attributes include the following:

1. Responsibility-oriented chain of command
2. Wide acceptance through commonality of mission and language
3. Applicability to varying types and magnitudes of emergency events
4. Expeditious transfer of resources within a system or between facilities

5. Flexibility in implementation of individual sections or branches of the HEICS
6. Minimal disruption to existing hospital departments

The HEICS includes an organizational chart showing a chain of command, which incorporates four sections under the overall leadership of an emergency IC. Each of the four sections—logistics, planning, finance, and operations—has a chief appointed by the IC responsible for the section. The chiefs in turn designate officers for subfunctions, with managers and coordinators filling other crucial roles.

Each of the 36 roles has prioritized job action sheets describing the important assignments of each person. Each job action sheet also includes a mission statement to define the position responsibility. The end product is a management system with personnel who know what they should do, when they should do it, and who to report it to during a time of emergency.

Federal Emergency Management Agency First Responder CBRNE Training

As a result of the changing nature of global politics, the aftermath of September 11, 2001, and the continuing threat of terrorism, new information, training, and technology have emerged and continue to evolve, providing responders with the latest science, technology, and tactical advances to keep us safe and our operational responses sustainably effective during times of incredible demands. The ability of first responders to recognize and manage acts of terrorism has become essential. The Department of Homeland Security (DHS)/FEMA terrorism training programs are an integral component of national preparedness. Classes were developed for and directed to emergency service first responders, law enforcement personnel, emergency management, public health workers, medical personnel, government officials, and nongovernmental organizations through the National Domestic Preparedness Consortium and their training partners via funding provided by Congress through DHS—specifically fire fighters, hazardous materials personnel, and EMS providers. The programs are highly effective, relevant, and free of charge. This opportunity is well worth your individual and agency participation—especially when the team comes to your agency and says, "We're with the government, and we are here to help." It is a genuinely honest statement and they mean it!

Metropolitan Medical Response System

Most CBRNE events present a relatively limited opportunity for the successful rescue of viable victims (usually no more than 3 hours). However, the more expeditious and aggressive the actions taken in the initial stages of the event, the more victims will be recovered and decontaminated, treated, and provided access to advanced medical interventions.

The metropolitan medical response system (MMRS) was developed to provide support for, and assistance to, local jurisdiction first responders in nuclear, biological, or chemical (NBC) terrorist incidents. The MMRS has a strong emergency medical care focus and has the capability to provide rapid and comprehensive medical intervention to casualties of NBC events.

MMRS development was based upon providing a coordinated response to CBRNE incidents in a metropolitan environment. Special emphasis is placed on the ability to identify the specific agent involved and provide the earliest possible correct medical intervention for victims of these situations.

The MMRS is a specially trained and locally available CBRNE incident response team. MMRS provides the platform for rapid and efficient integration of state and federal medical resources into the local incident management system. Through its established multiagency, collaborative planning framework, the MMRS program also promotes effective regional coordination of mutual aid with neighboring localities. The MMRS is organized, staffed, and equipped to provide the best possible prehospital and emergency medical care throughout the course of an incident, and especially while on the scene. Medical personnel are responsible for providing the earliest possible medical intervention for the responders and civilian victims of NBC incidents through early identification of the agent type and proper administration of the appropriate antidote(s) and other pharmaceuticals as necessary.

Additional response assets that augment and support the MMRS strategy include not only traditional local, regional, and state emergency response organizations but response elements such as disaster medical assistance teams, disaster mortuary operational response teams, and other response assets that become federalized in time of disaster declarations such as urban search and rescue teams. These assets are staffed by local response professionals and become part of the national response architecture when they are activated by the national government and issued a mission order.

Casualty Care in the Combat Environment

Unlike the military, civil first responders are not trained with consideration for the ability to survive a given operation. Civil mission priority does not prospectively accept personnel losses, and no first responder organization includes an acceptable loss ratio as part of its mission goal or planning efforts.

First responders are currently trained to manage trauma-based incidents on the principles of a standardized approach to trauma care. However, there are issues inherent in the training programs relative to appropriateness and application in the combat environment, including:

- The assumption that hospital diagnostics and therapeutics can be accessed rapidly
- No presupposition of delayed transportation
- No tactical context

Most trauma training programs do not take into consideration the issues of care under fire, in complete darkness, various environmental factors, and delays to definitive care or command decisions.

Tactical care objectives include turning casualties into patients, preventing additional casualties, and preventing response personnel from becoming casualties. Under these circumstances, basic protocols should be considered a starting point; ad hoc protocol modification may have to occur in response to a specific situation. In tactical situations, medics must be prepared and permitted to adapt and improvise within their scope of practice as conditions dictate.

The following new terminology and definitions appropriate to tactical field care must be added to the trauma training programs and incorporated into the various syllabi in order to reflect the care rendered in the tactical environment:

I. **Care Under Fire**
   A. Care under fire is the care rendered by a medic at the scene of an injury, in a hostile environment, while at risk.
   B. Available medical equipment and supplies are limited to those carried by the individual medic.
   C. Aseptic technique is not a consideration.
   D. Control of hemorrhage is the top priority because exsanguination (severe blood loss) from extremity wounds is the number one cause of preventable death in the combat environment.
   E. Patient extraction is delayed due to the threat potential.

II. **Tactical Field Care**
   A. Tactical field care is the care rendered by a medic at the scene of an injury, in a hostile environment, when not at risk.
   B. Available medical equipment and supplies are limited to those carried in the field.
   C. There is more time to render care.

   D. Care is rendered under nonsterile conditions.
   E. Patient extraction is possible.

Mass Fatality Management

When planning for CBRNE incidents or other acts of terrorism, the plan must include provisions for the management of mass fatalities. Evolving terrorist capabilities, coupled with the availability of CBRNE materiel, lead to consideration of the potential for mass fatalities. Many chemical agents result in fatal injuries to those exposed within a short period of time. In a similar manner, large, improvised explosive devices placed strategically within a high-rise building, apartment, or other large public gathering place can result in hundreds, if not thousands of deaths. Unlike the military, civil authority rarely finds itself in the position of managing, processing, and disposing of contaminated human remains. But events such as the World Trade Center attacks on September 11, 2001, and the Oklahoma City bombing unfortunately illustrate the need for such plans and capabilities.

A mass fatality management plan providing organization, mobilization, and coordination of all provider agencies for emergency mortuary services is an imperative. It is important to delineate the authority, responsibility, functions, and operations of providers by agreement prior to an event of magnitude.

Mass fatality plans should be regional and come under the auspices and management of the local coroner or medical examiner. The operational concept of the mass fatality management system is exclusive of cultural, religious, and ethnic beliefs and practices but may be modified as conditions permit. It is a utility system based on the following three levels of response:

- **Level I**—A minor to moderate incident wherein local resources appear to be adequate and available. A local emergency may or may not be proclaimed and fatalities may range from 50 to 100.
- **Level II**—A moderate to severe incident wherein local resources are not adequate and assistance is requested from other jurisdictions or regions. A local emergency declaration is imminent. Fatalities may exceed 100.
- **Level III**—A major incident wherein resources in or near the impacted area are overwhelmed and extensive state and/or federal resources are required. A local and state emergency is proclaimed and a principal declaration of an emergency or major disaster is requested. Fatalities may be in the thousands.

Mass Casualty Target Management

Many population centers include high-rise building complexes that commonly have transient censuses exceeding 10,000 people. The complexities involved in planning a response to these edifices are a daunting task. These buildings exist globally, and because of their accessibility, they represent attractive targets to terrorists.

For example, the New York City World Trade Center represented a target of colossal proportions and an unprecedented opportunity to strike at the symbol of Western international commerce. In a single act of terrorism in 1993, over 150,000 individuals were placed at risk when an improvised explosive device detonated in a subterranean parking complex. With the 2001 attack, that same size population was placed at risk again. In the aftermath of the attack and the collapse of the towers, almost 3,000 were killed. At the Pentagon attack, almost 200 were killed.

Fortunately, high reliability organizations such as EMS, fire, and law enforcement agencies use organizational structure to adapt to, and then mitigate the uncommon yet catastrophic event. This emergency was mitigated by a diverse public safety system, a convergent volunteer effort, and a systematic approach to disaster service operations. The adherence to an ICS provided the impetus for a unified command structure and an unprecedented level of cooperation between local and regional resources and state and federal assets. Through the application of this management process, a catastrophe was averted.

Mitigation of Individual Performance Degradation in Terrorism

Domestic CBRNE terrorist events are rare and catastrophic events. The unknowns are when and where these events will occur. The type and material used are also unknown.

The basis of system function is performance of the individual, yet how citizens and first responders will perform is unknown. Algorithms developed to assist in responding are based on a reductionist approach that most problems can be identified, separated from the larger response, and prepared for. Algorithms for response are best guesses in a totally unknown arena where human and environmental pathology merge.

Latent system error, human performance error—slips and mistakes as well as shortcomings caused by limitations of normal human physiology—interfere with well-planned algorithms, policies, and procedures. Organizational structure and decision-making methods for emergency events that mitigate performance degradation already exist. Use of high-reliability organizational techniques and decision-making methodology adapted from the military can mitigate CBRNE terrorist events in real time as an event evolves.

Latent error occurs when the system sets up the error, but the individual commits the act. On later review, a long train of events tied together by ineffective policies and procedures can be identified as the actual cause of the error. Though latent error is sometimes identified or prevented by review of the system as a whole, the more deeply enmeshed latent errors cannot. They appear only when the system is strained under the conditions of a catastrophe. The perceptions and actions of individuals help to identify and mitigate latent error early in the period of disorder or dysfunction.

Error is a part of human performance, despite a commonly held view that error cannot exist without negligence. Some consider complications as errors, when they are actually expected but unwanted results of interventions. Errors can be unconscious slips or conscious mistakes. Slips are rule-based or skill-based errors that easily occur when an incident evolves in unexpected ways or human performance cannot or does not match environmental demands. Mistakes are more complex, knowledge-based errors where the decision-making process is at fault. Interference with effective decision making comes from a number of heuristics and biases such as representativeness, availability, confirmation bias, reversion under stress, or coning of attention.

Fear, as fight or flight, is a well-known, expected, and natural physiologic response to life threats. Less well known is how these responses present themselves during the threat. Fight manifests itself as anger, particularly when focused on an individual or tool. It is made plausible by the presentation that an individual's performance is inadequate, causing the anger, when, in actuality, it is the angry individual's response that leads to performance decrements. Flight manifests as avoidance and is made plausible by redirection of attention to a seemingly more important but safer task. Freeze is an often-unrecognized fear response mediated by cortisol and leads to confusion, inaction, or even paralysis (as in paralysis by analysis).

Decision-making techniques modified from the military, such as the closed-loop decision cycles, allow individuals to learn what works through action. They permit response when the nature of the threat is fuzzy and ill defined or ill identified. In fact, closed-loop cycles allow identification of the structure of the threat and success of the response. They provide a margin of safety by self-monitoring responses to actions for early warning of dangers created by actions of the response team. They are rapid and adaptable to those situations where unintended or unexpected outcomes occur.

Roberts and Libuser's high reliability theory, also developed from military studies, states that complexity will mitigate rare but catastrophic events. This apparent paradox occurs because disasters and terrorist events are nonlinear systems. Linear, reductionist approaches such as response algorithms and prearranged ICSs do not apply. High-reliability organizations can learn and have a culture of both safety and reliability. They allow decision migration and diminish authority gradients that will permit the necessary free flow of information during the terrorist event. They allow effective action before implementation of algorithms, policies, and procedures can be instituted in a rapidly evolving terrorist threat. These organizations will respond to a catastrophic event in the same manner they respond to routine events.

Chapter Summary

The complexities posed by the multiple challenges created by planning for, responding to, operating at, and recovering from a terrorist attack are numerous. The ability to respond effectively in the safest possible manner is dependent upon coherently understanding the response system framework and players at the national, state, territorial, state, tribal, and local community level.

Identification of vulnerabilities prior to an incident and working to fill those planning and operational gaps is integral to possessing response readiness. Accomplishing this daunting, and sometimes lofty, expectation requires that the contemporary leader recognize the historical trending of terrorist incidents as well as the evolving tactics being employed by the actors. Additionally, implementing strategies that work toward mitigating risks to responders to the lowest possible levels when managing the modern terrorism environment cannot be overstated. Such strategies include but are not limited to the identification training gaps and provision of the requisite training, education, and equipment to satisfy these requirements.

Wrap Up

Chapter Questions

1. List and discuss the definitions of terrorism from the Department of Defense, FBI, and State Department.
2. List and describe the three types of terrorist group networks.
3. List and discuss at least three major response agencies at the local level. What are the limitations of these agencies in terrorism response?
4. Discuss the evolving threats of 911 target acquisition and tactical violence.
5. What are the basic functions of the following special units?
   - U.S. Marine Corps Chemical Biological Incident Response Force
   - National Guard Civilian Support Teams (CSTs)
   - Metropolitan Medical Response System (MMRS)
6. Discuss how mass casualty care in the combat environment differs from standard advanced trauma life support protocols.
7. Outline the major elements in a mass fatality management plan.

Chapter Projects

- Identify and discuss the various definitions of terrorism, examining the rationale used to obtain each definition by the adopting agency.
- Discuss the components of the MMRS and how the various elements fit into the MMRS system. Further examine the mechanisms for requesting and integrating these resources into an emergency response strategy in your community.

Vital Vocabulary

Globalization A measure of the ease with which labor, ideas, capital, technology, and profits can move across borders with minimal government interference.

Tactical violence The predetermined use of maximum violence to achieve one's criminal goals, regardless of victim cooperation, level of environmental threat to the perpetrator, or the need to evade law enforcement or capture.

Terrorism Individual act(s) of reckless destruction to property or person(s) or decidedly complicated events perpetrated by organizations with extreme social, environmental, religious, economic, or political agendas.

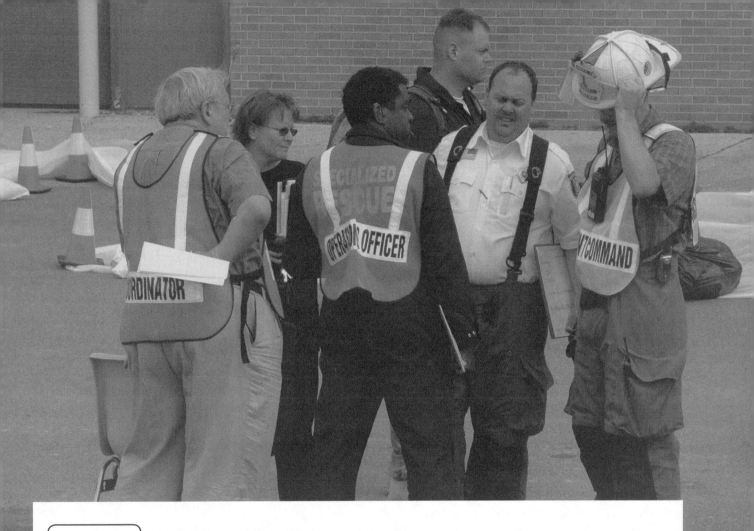

2 National Incident Management System

Hank T. Christen
Paul M. Maniscalco

Objectives

- Describe the evolution of the 1970s incident command system (ICS) to the modern national incident management system (NIMS).
- Diagram and define the key positions in the command staff.
- Compare and contrast incident command (IC) with unified command (UC).
- Define the key principles of ICS.
- Define the five key functions in ICS.
- Diagram the general staff and command staff in ICS.
- List and define the components in the NIMS structure that complement ICS.

Introduction

The **national incident management system (NIMS)** is the template for preparedness, planning, and response to emergency incidents and is an all-hazard incident management system, meaning that it is a framework for responding to all types of incidents including terrorism and tactical violence events. NIMS is the model for all government levels beginning at the local level and expanding to state and federal levels as well as tribal governments and private-sector entities. The emphasis is on the local level because all incidents begin with a local response. The system is scalable to all types of responses. All disciplines including law enforcement, fire/rescue departments, emergency medical services (EMS), public works, emergency management, and public health are mandated to use the NIMS as a planning and response model. This includes the Department of Defense when military agencies act to support incidents within the United States or its territories. NIMS is significant because response and support agencies at all levels and disciplines now have a common template for the first time in history.

The authorization for the establishment of a NIMS is found within Homeland Security Presidential Directive 5 (HSPD-5), which was issued on February 28, 2003. This directive establishes that the Secretary of Homeland Security shall develop and administer a NIMS. Specifically, HSPD-5 states:

This system will provide a consistent nationwide approach for Federal, State, and local governments to work effectively and efficiently together to prepare for, respond to, and recover from domestic incidents, regardless of cause, size, or complexity. To provide for interoperability and compatibility among Federal, State, and local capabilities, the NIMS will include a core set of concepts, principles, terminology, and technologies covering the incident command system; multiagency coordination systems; unified command; training; identification and management of resources (including systems for classifying types of resources); qualifications and certification; and the collection,

tracking, and reporting of incident information and incident resources (Homeland Security Presidential Directive-5, 15).

The focus of this is chapter is the **incident command system (ICS)** in NIMS because ICS is the overarching tactical and strategic framework for terrorism response. Other components of NIMS include preparedness, resource management, communications and information management, supporting technologies, and ongoing management and maintenance. These components are critical support entities and are discussed as an overview.

Incident Command History

In the 1970s, a series of catastrophic wildland fires in California destroyed thousands of structures. Large numbers of local and state fire agencies responded, but their efforts often lacked coordination. Effective incident response and management were plagued by incompatible radio frequencies, lack of priority resource allocation, and poor coordination/control among a myriad of federal, state, and local agencies. California's FIRESCOPE (Fire Fighting Resources of Southern California Organized Against Potential Emergency) program was developed to respond to IC issues. Key agencies and planners agreed on several objectives. They agreed to establish the following:

1. A system of command, where a single individual (or UC team) is responsible for the ultimate outcome of the incident.
2. A system of common terminology to allow all agencies to understand each other.
3. A system of coordination between diversified disciplines.
4. A communications system with shared frequencies and common language.
5. A system for resource allocation including typing, prioritizing, and tracking.
6. A system that applies to all hazards and disciplines.

A functionally based national ICS evolved based on the functions of command, operations, logistics, plans, and administration. The initial ICS was oriented to wildland firefighting (**FIGURE 2-1**) and eventually modified for all hazard incident management. ICS further evolved into models for EMS, law enforcement, public works, emergency management, and hospital management.

After the terrorist attacks on September 11, 2001, HSPD-5 became the impetus for NIMS, based on the initial ICS template and developed by the Secretary of

---

CRITICAL FACTOR ....

NIMS is scalable to all types of responses and all disciplines including law enforcement, fire/rescue departments, emergency medical services, public works, emergency management, and public health.

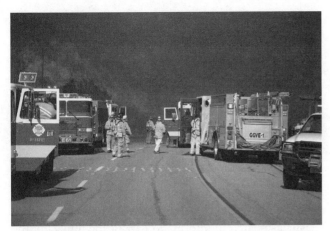

FIGURE 2-1 Brea, Calif. November 15, 2008. Devastating California wild-land fires of the 1970s, much like this fast-moving wildfire of 2008, triggered the development of FIRESCOPE, which eventually evolved into ICS.

Homeland Security. NIMS has been best described as "ICS on steroids" because NIMS expands the original ICS model to include support components. These components ensure that NIMS is a flexible and scalable framework applicable to all disciplines and levels of government.

The Incident Command System

The ICS is defined and diagrammed in the command and management component of NIMS. ICS specifies the operating characteristics, interactive management components, and structure of incident management and emergency response organizations engaged throughout the life cycle of an incident. ICS is used routinely by all response disciplines throughout the country to manage incidents as simple as a minor traffic accident or as complex as a terrorist attack or hurricane. ICS is designed using proven management principles such as command and control, unity of command, chain of command, span of control, resource management, accountability, and planning. ICS is also a functionality-based system rather than a hierarchy or rank structure. This means that the ICS template is framed by a series of functions rather than a top-to-bottom rank system. The five major functions of ICS are IC/UC, operations, logistics, planning/intelligence, and administration/finance. In incidents involving national security, the intelligence function may be separated from planning and be assigned as a sixth function (**FIGURE 2-2**).

Command and Unified Command

The principle of command means that a single person or UC team is responsible for the management of every incident regardless of size or scale. Command begins with the first unit to arrive on a scene by an individual formally assuming command and notifying the dispatch center that he or she has command. This position is called the **incident commander (IC or Command)**. The IC becomes immediately responsible for all functions related to the incident. As an incident escalates, command is formally transferred to other individuals as appropriate. Every transfer of command is announced by radio to keep all units and entities aware of the command structure.

Many incidents involve the overlap of jurisdictional authority due to functional areas, legal authority, geography, or other factors. This realization is addressed by the development of the UC concept. UC should be used in incidents involving multiple jurisdictions, a single jurisdiction with multiagency involvement, or multiple jurisdictions with multiagency involvement. Terrorism

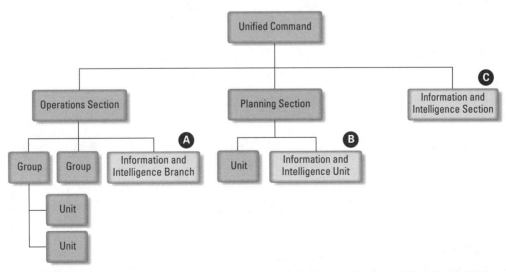

FIGURE 2-2 During an incident where there is a need for tactical or classified intelligence, the information and intelligence function can be organized as follows: **A.** a branch within the Operations Section; **B.** a unit within the Planning Section; and **C.** a separate General Staff Section. The type of organization used depends on the nature of the incident and the operational scope.

incidents meet one or more of these criteria. For example, a terrorist attack may involve local, state, and federal agencies, along with multiple disciplines such as EMS, fire/rescue, law enforcement, and public works. The strength of UC is that it allows agencies with different legal, geographic, and functional authorities and responsibilities to work together effectively without affecting individual agency authority, responsibility, or accountability. The effective use of UC depends on its routine use, training, formal planning, and an established relationship between personnel likely to assume UC roles.

For example, consider a bombing at a crowded shopping mall. The first due engine officer formally assumes the IC role. Command is later formally transferred to the fire battalion chief. It becomes apparent that this is a mass casualty incident with firefighting and rescue challenges. It is also a major crime scene. The IC transfers the command role to a UC team that includes a law enforcement chief, a fire chief, and an EMS chief. Later, state and federal law enforcement officials become part of the UC team.

The Command Staff

The IC or UC is supported by the command staff (**FIGURE 2-3**). The positions on the command staff are safety officer (SO), the public information officer (PIO), and the liaison officer. The IC or UC assumes the roles of any command staff position that is not delegated.

Public Information Officer

The **public information officer (PIO)** is responsible for providing understandable and clear information to the public and media. The PIO routinely provides information to or collects information from other agencies with incident-related information (such as casualty status information from hospitals or transportation information related to the incident and its impact on the local community). The PIO develops accurate and complete information on the incident's cause, size, and current situation, the resources committed, and other matters of general interest for both internal and external use. The PIO also drafts key messages related to information about the impact of the incident on the community and educating the community about the event as it relates to mitigation and recovery activities. In addition to providing information, the PIO also serves as a valuable tool for monitoring the media's coverage of an incident. In today's age of immediate access to satellite imagery, it is not unusual for local and national news sources to have information that is not available to the incident management team. This function requires the on-scene PIO to closely monitor media information.

Whether the command structure is single or unified, only one official incident PIO should be designated. PIOs from other agencies or departments may be available to assist the incident PIO or disseminate information specific to their agencies. For example, a fire department PIO may defer to a police department PIO for comments

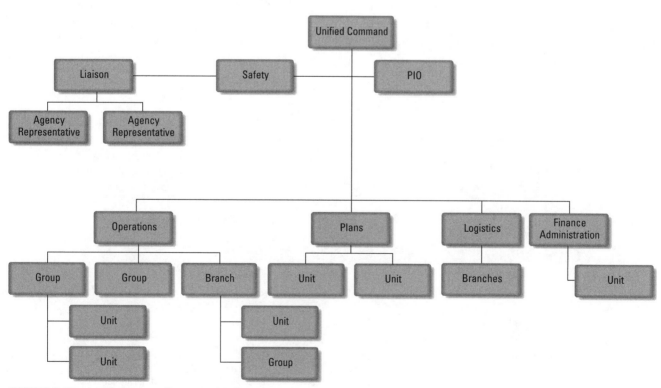

FIGURE 2-3 Complex ICS structure with command staff.

about police bomb squad operations. The IC/UC must approve the release of all incident-related information. Following major incidents, the on-scene PIO is part of the joint information system and must coordinate with other public information entities that may be located in various locations. Based on the type of incident, public information may be reviewed by the intelligence personnel within the joint information center to ensure that sensitive information is not inadvertently released.

Safety Officer

The **safety officer (SO)** monitors incident operations and advises the IC/UC on all matters relating to operational safety, including the health and safety of emergency responder personnel. The SO also has the authority to terminate any operation that threatens the safety of responders, victims, or bystanders. SO responsibilities include establishing ongoing assessments of hazardous environments. It is important to remember that responsibility for incident safety is clearly assigned to the IC/UC and supervisors at all levels of incident management. This is done in cooperation with environmental management agencies and hazardous materials specialists. The SO is also responsible for coordinating multiagency safety efforts through the use of deputies who are qualified to assess specific activities in various disciplines. Special units such as special weapons and tactics (SWAT) units, hazardous materials teams, or bomb squads will also have an SO. Additionally, high-risk operations may require deputies with detailed technical knowledge associated with the operation (e.g., heavy equipment operations, law enforcement tactical operations, etc.). The responsibilities of the SO also extend to victims and bystanders in the incident area.

In order to ensure that safety is a key component of incident operations, the SO, operations section chief, and planning section chief must coordinate closely regarding operational safety and emergency responder health and safety issues. The SO also must ensure the coordination of safety management functions and issues across jurisdictions, across functional agencies, and with private sector and nongovernment organizations. It is important to note that the agencies, organizations, or jurisdictions contributing to joint safety management efforts do not lose their individual identities or responsibility for their own programs, policies, and personnel. Rather, each entity contributes to the overall effort to protect all responder personnel involved in incident operations.

Liaison Officer

The **liaison officer** is the point of contact for representatives of other government agencies, nongovernment organizations, and/or private entities. In an IC/ UC structure, representatives from assisting or cooperating agencies and organizations (defined as those not represented in the UC group) coordinate through the liaison officer. The liaison provides a conduit to the IC/ UC from these supporting organizations. This structure eliminates confusion because support and service agency representatives are not at the command post. In essence, organizations not represented in the IC/UC access the IC/UC through the liaison.

A key functional component of the liaison concept is that agency and/or organizational representatives assigned to an incident must have the authority to speak for their parent agencies and/or organizations on all matters, following appropriate consultations with their agency leadership. Assistants and personnel from other agencies or organizations (public or private) involved in incident management activities may be assigned to the liaison to facilitate coordination.

ICS Management Principles

The foundation of ICS is sound management principles from business, military, and emergency response arenas. These principles include chain of command, unity of command, span of control, resource management, planning, and accountability.

Chain of command means that there is a clear line of authority within the structure of the ICS organization. Operations reports to command, the medical branch reports to operations, and the triage group reports to the medical branch. Each supervisory member of the ICS organization clearly understands who provides them with their tactical objectives and who they supervise. Chain of command does not imply that information flows downward only. It is explicit in ICS that information also flows upward and laterally.

Unity of command means that every individual, unit, function, or entity has only one supervisor at the scene of the incident. Every player and manager understands his or her relationship to his or her superior, peers, and subordinates.

Span of control is a key concept within the structure of the ICS. Span of control means that each ICS supervisor or manager has a limit as to how many personnel he or she can effectively manage. Based on general business management concepts, this number has been set at five to seven direct subordinates to one manager. A *span of control of three or four* is appropriate for emergency operations (**FIGURE 2-4**). The expansion of the ICS allows IC/UC to maintain these numbers throughout the organization. Although this number is generally accepted, each situation is unique, and a specific supervisor may be responsible for

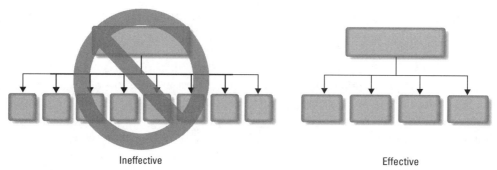

Ineffective   Effective

FIGURE 2-4 Ineffective versus effective span of control.

a greater number of individuals when similar resources are performing similar functions (e.g., police officers managing the perimeter of a large crime scene). It is important to remember that in ICS, span of control is flexible and adjusts to the specific type of incident, the nature of the task, hazards, and safety factors. All of these factors substantially influence span-of-control considerations.

Resource management is a comprehensive system for prioritizing and managing personnel, vehicles, equipment, supplies, and facilities that are available or potentially available for assignment to support of IC and response activities. A comprehensive plan to prioritize resource allocation is important because most major incidents quickly deplete response resources and create a resource-scarce environment. During on-scene operations, the ICS logistics section chief is responsible for resource management functions. The logistics section chief also utilizes processes for requesting, staging, deploying, demobilizing, and accounting for incident resources. These activities often require coordination with a multiagency coordination system (MACS), which is a system of off-scene resource processes and entities. The purpose of the MACS is to organize and operate a full-scale logistics system to support the resource requirements of single or multiple incidents in a local area or region. Entities in the MACS include government agencies, nongovernment agencies, volunteer organizations, and private-sector resources. The MACS is usually located in a local or regional emergency operations center, because these centers have the staff and communications capability to support MACS efforts. Remember that a MACS is a *system* of coordinated entities, not a specific location.

An **incident action plan (IAP)** is an oral or written plan containing general objectives reflecting the overall strategy for managing an incident. IAPs provide a coherent means of communicating the overall incident objectives for operational and support activities. In the early stages of a dynamic incident, the IC quickly develops a verbal IAP. As the incident escalates, the ICS expands with the addition of a planning section chief. The IAP becomes a written plan

that is presented to incident managers via periodic briefing cycles. The IAP is discussed in detail in Chapter 5.

Accountability is the process of tracking and accounting for personnel and equipment resources on the incident scene. Incident safety depends on the use of an effective personnel and resource accountability system. In order to achieve and implement an accountability system, several key components and processes are incorporated into the ICS. First, resources are checked in when they arrive in the staging area and deployed only after they are assigned to a specific function. Second, resources are deployed in coordination with specific tactical objectives or tasks associated with the IAP. To ensure unity of command, each resource is assigned to a specific supervisor. Personnel or units must know to whom they report. In addition, resources must be deployed within a span of control that allows supervisory personnel to maintain knowledge of resource location and operations.

ICS Operations

The operations function in ICS is managed by the **operations section chief (operations chief)** who reports directly to the IC/UC (**FIGURE 2-5**). The operations chief is responsible for accomplishing the incident objectives established by the IC/UC in the IAP. The operations chief is an individual with technical knowledge and experience related to the tactical problems at the incident. In major terrorism incidents, the operations section may expand to a unified operations section encompassing specialists from several agencies or disciplines. Operations units are the most visible entities on an incident scene and include multiple disciplines such as EMS, fire/rescue, law enforcement, public health, and public works. Terrorism incidents require multiple operations disciplines. To ensure adherence to ICS management principles, the operations section is divided into **branches** for each operational discipline. A branch is managed by a branch director (example, law enforcement branch director) who uses an ICS template for an attack with casualties that requires law enforcement, fire/rescue, and EMS branches.

The branching tools in the ICS provide management tools that accommodate air and water operations. Complex terrorism incidents, transportation accidents, fires, and natural disasters may require an air operations branch and/or a water operations branch. The most common type of air operations involves law enforcement aircraft or helicopters operating in the same airspace with medical helicopters. Air operations require special communications along with the establishment of medical helicopter landing zones. Water operations provide similar challenges. Coordination with marine units require marine radio frequencies and appropriate communications protocols.

Groups and Divisions

Divisions are used to divide an incident geographically. The manager of a division is designated as a division supervisor. The geographical division of the incident scene is usually determined by the needs of the incident, natural geographic barriers (e.g., rivers, mountains, lakes, shorelines, valleys), or man-made obstacles (e.g., buildings, roadways, walls). When geographic features are used to determine boundaries, the size of the division should correspond to appropriate span-of-control guidelines.

The most common method for identifying or labeling divisions is by using letters (A, B, C, etc.). Other identifiers ("city park," "west city," etc.) may be used as long as the division identifier is known to all assigned responders. The important thing to remember about ICS divisions is they are established to divide the incident into geographic areas of operation.

Groups are used to describe functional areas of an operation. Like divisions, the individual assigned to be in charge of each group is designated as a *group supervisor*. The type of groups established is determined by the needs caused by the incident. Groups are usually labeled according to the job that they are assigned (e.g., decontamination group, traffic control group, etc.). Groups work within the incident wherever their assigned task is needed and are not limited by geographic boundaries.

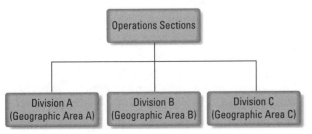

FIGURE 2-5 Dividing an incident geographically.

Task Forces and Strike Teams

Task forces are any combination of resources assembled by operations to accomplish a specific mission and are usually operations units. Task forces have a designated *task force leader* and operate with common communications between units. Combining resources into task forces allows several key resource units to be managed under one individual's supervision, thus aiding in span of control. When the mission is completed, the task force is assigned a new mission or demobilized. Examples of task forces are as follows:

- Law enforcement task force—bomb unit and three patrol units
- Fire/rescue task force—three engines, two ladder trucks, and a rescue unit
- EMS task force—three ambulances and a mass casualty bus unit
- Public works task force—three dump trucks and two front loaders

Strike teams are a set number of resources of the same kind and type operating under a designated strike team leader with common communications between units. Strike teams represent known capabilities and are highly effective operations teams. Examples of strike teams are as follows:

- Law enforcement strike team—four patrol units
- Fire/rescue strike team—five engines
- EMS strike team—three ambulances
- Public works strike team—four front loaders

Logistics

The **logistics section** is responsible for all support requirements needed to facilitate effective and efficient incident management, including ordering resources from a MACS. The logistics section provides facilities, transportation, supplies, equipment maintenance and fuel, food services, communications, and information technology support.

The logistics section supports the incident by ordering resources through appropriate procurement authorities from outside locations. The logistics section also provides facilities, transportation, supplies, equipment maintenance and fueling, food service, communications, and medical services for incident personnel.

The logistics section is led by the logistics section chief. A deputy may also be assigned to logistics on major incidents. In terrorism attacks or natural disasters requiring a number of facilities and large numbers of equipment, the logistics section is divided into support and service branches to maintain a narrow span of control (**FIGURE 2-6**).

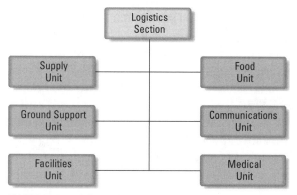

FIGURE 2-6 Logistics section branch organization.

Unified Logistics

The concept of unified logistics is similar to UC. Unified logistics is the utilization and coordination of two or more agencies or jurisdictions in the logistics section.

Unified logistics applies to high-impact, long-duration incidents where several diverse agencies have specialized logistics requirements. In these cases, a single logistics section chief may not have the skills and proficiency to support multiple agencies with differing support needs. Consider the Oklahoma City bombing, the Pentagon attack, major hurricanes, and earthquakes. In each case, fire, law enforcement, and medical agencies have demanding but diverse logistics requirements. Fire fighters need air cylinders, chemical suits, and respirators. EMS personnel need medications, oxygen, and cardiac monitors. Law enforcement agencies need barricades, body armor, and evidence-collection kits. It is unlikely that a single logistics chief can support such a diverse shopping list.

Unified logistics is implemented by assigning two or more logistics specialists from different agencies or jurisdictions to a unified logistics section. Private sector logistics managers also may be assigned. For example, fire, law enforcement, and private provider EMS logistics officers may be assigned to manage a unified logistics section in a terrorist attack.

Unified logistics is also accomplished by assigning appropriate specialists to units within the logistics section. For example, an EMS specialist might be assigned to the supply unit to manage orders for medications and specialized medical devices or equipment, or fire maintenance personnel and public works maintenance personnel might be assigned to the ground support unit. Because of the flexibility of the ICS, a unified logistics section can be implemented in a number of different ways. The desired end state is a logistics section that supports a wide range of supplies, tools, vehicles, equipment, and personnel needs.

Support Branch

The **support branch** provides services that assist incident operations by providing supplies, facilities, trans-

port, and equipment maintenance. The support branch consists of the supply unit, the facilities unit, and the ground support unit.

Supply Unit

The **supply unit** orders, receives, stores, and processes all incident resources. Once established, the supply unit orders all resources, including tactical and support resources, personnel, and expendable and nonexpendable supplies required for incident support. Tactical resources include tools, helicopters, fire units, ambulances, and equipment such as chain saws or generators. Support resources include fuel, tents, water, and food. Personnel resources include fire fighters, paramedics, police officers, special teams, and medical teams. Expendable supplies are materials that are consumed and cannot be reused and include oxygen, medications, bandages, and water. Nonexpendable supplies can be reused. Nonexpendable supplies include backboards, fire hoses, and body armor.

The supply unit provides the support required to receive, process, store, and distribute all supply orders. The supply unit also handles equipment operations, which includes storing, disbursing, and servicing all tools and portable, nonexpendable equipment.

Facilities Unit

The **facilities unit** establishes, maintains, and demobilizes all facilities used in support of incident operations. The unit also provides facility maintenance and security services required to support incident operations. The facilities unit sets up area commands, the command post, incident base, and camps, as well as trailers and/or other forms of shelter for use in and around the incident area. The incident base and camps often may be established in areas having existing structures, which may be used in their entirety or in part. The facilities unit also provides and sets up necessary personnel support facilities, including areas for food and water services, sleeping, sanitation, and showers. This unit also orders, through the supply unit, additional support items such as portable toilets, shower facilities, and lighting units.

Ground Support Unit

The **ground support unit** maintains and repairs primary tactical equipment, vehicles, and mobile ground support equipment; records usage time for all ground equipment assigned to the incident; supplies fuel for all mobile equipment; provides transportation in support of incident operations (except aircraft); and develops and implements the incident traffic plan. The incident traffic plan specifies traffic routes and procedures for vehicles entering and departing an incident site, command post, or support area.

In addition to its primary functions of maintaining and servicing vehicles and mobile equipment, the ground support unit also maintains a transportation pool for major incidents. This pool consists of vehicles that are suitable for transporting personnel. A vehicle pool may require coordination with mass transit authorities, school transportation services, or contracted transportation companies. The ground support unit also provides up-to-date information on the location and status of transportation vehicles to the resources unit.

Service Branch

The **service branch** provides communications, food, water, and medical services. The service branch consists of the communications unit, food unit, and a medical unit.

Communications Unit

The **communications unit** develops the communications plan (ICS form 205) to ensure effective use of the communications equipment and facilities assigned to the incident, installs and tests all communications equipment, supervises and operates the incident communications center, distributes and recovers communications equipment assigned to incident personnel, and maintains and repairs communications equipment on site. The communications unit must coordinate with dispatch centers, department operations centers, and the emergency operations center during major incidents.

The communications unit's major responsibility is effective communications planning for the ICS, especially in a multiagency incident. Planning is critical for determining required radio nets, establishing interagency frequency assignments, and ensuring the interoperability and the optimal use of all assigned communications capabilities. A radio net is a network of like functions or units assigned to a specific radio frequency for coordination purposes. For example, all units in the EMS transport sector are assigned to communicate on the Med 8 frequency.

The communications unit leader should attend all incident planning meetings to ensure that the communications systems available for the incident can support the tactical operations planned for the next operational period. Incident communications are managed through the use of a common communications plan and an incident-based communications center established solely for the use of tactical and support resources assigned to the incident. Advance planning is required to ensure that an appropriate communications system is available to sup-port incident operations requirements. This element is critical for interoperability and is often lacking in many communities. This planning includes the development of frequency inventories, frequency-use agreements, and interagency radio caches.

Complex incidents require an incident communications plan. The communications unit is responsible for planning the use of radio frequencies; establishing networks for command, tactical, support, and air units; setting up on-site telephone and public address equipment; and providing any required off-incident communication links. Codes should not be used for radio communication; a clear spoken message based on common terminology that avoids misunderstanding in complex and noisy situations reduces the chances for error. Radio networks for large incidents include command, tactical, support, ground-to-air, air-to-air, and marine networks.

Command Net

The **command net** links together command staff, section chiefs, branch directors, and division and group supervisors. The command net must be interoperable with Department of Defense and other federal agencies. Federal Communications Commission requirements prohibit local and state agencies from installing and using federal radio frequencies.

Tactical Nets

Several **tactical nets** may be established to connect agencies, departments, geographical areas, or specific functional units. The determination of how nets are set up should be a joint planning, operations, and logistics function. The communications unit leader will develop the overall plan.

Support Net

A **support net** may be established to track changes in resource status and process logistical requests and other nontactical functions. This net is a key coordination element between the supply unit and the resource status unit (planning section).

Ground-to-Air Net

The **ground-to-air net** is utilized for communications and coordination between ground and aviation units. To coordinate ground-to-air traffic, either a specific tactical frequency may be designated or regular tactical nets may be used.

Air-to-Air Nets

Air-to-air nets will normally be planned and assigned for use at the incident. Aircraft crews use approved Federal Aviation Administration frequencies. These nets become more complex when coordinating civilian and military aviation assets due to incompatible military and civilian frequencies.

Marine Nets

Many incidents occur in coastal areas where federal and local marine units have operational assignments. **Marine nets** are used for communications between marine patrol/rescue boats and land-based agencies. Land-based command posts need marine frequencies to ensure coordination between marine and land units.

Planning

In an on-scene ICS structure, the **planning section** has the responsibility of incident planning and is managed by the **planning section chief (plans)**. The planning section includes four functional entities called the resource unit, situation unit, documentation unit, and the demobilization unit (**FIGURE 2-7**). Comprehensive terrorism and disaster planning, beyond on-scene activities, is addressed in Chapter 5.

The planning section collects, evaluates, and disseminates incident situation information and intelligence to the IC/UC and incident management personnel, prepares status reports, displays situation information, maintains the status of resources assigned to the incident, and develops and documents the IAP based on guidance from the IC/UC.

Unified planning is the utilization of two or more planners from different disciplines functioning in a coordinated planning environment. It is unlikely that a single individual has the skills to develop an effective plan when multiple disciplines are functioning at a complex event. An example is an EMS, law enforcement, and fire planner managing a unified planning section in a terrorist attack. Other major incidents may require planning expertise from public works, utilities, transportation, or public health agencies.

The Planning Section Chief

The planning section chief (plans) oversees all incident-related data gathering and analysis regarding incident operations and assigned resources, develops alternatives for tactical operations, conducts planning meetings, and prepares the IAP for each operational period. This individual will normally come from the jurisdiction with primary incident responsibility and may have one or more deputies from other participating jurisdictions. Chapter 5 includes a detailed discussion of the elements in an effective IAP.

It is critical for plans to stay in constant contact with the IC/UC and the operations section. ICs should consider the appointment of the planning section chief as a critical priority. Events involving multiple agencies and/or jurisdictions can quickly overwhelm a single planning section chief because of the complexities inherent in crafting strategic and tactical IAP objectives.

Plans developed by a unified IAP with the assistance of personnel from organizations represented in the UC as well as other personnel whose skills and/or knowledge are utilized to achieve the tactical objectives of the incident during the next operational period. This unified approach also extends to units within the planning section, especially the resource unit and the situation status unit. The intelligence unit is an optional component. It can be established within the planning section or as a separate intelligence section.

Resources Unit

The **resources unit** ensures that all assigned personnel and other resources have checked in or been checked in at the incident. Physical resources consist of personnel, teams, facilities, supplies, and major items of equipment available for assignment to or employment during incidents. This unit has a system for keeping track of the incident location and status of all assigned resources and maintains a master list of all resources committed to incident operations.

Each resource must be categorized by capability and capacity across disciplines with continuous status tracking for the resources unit to effectively manage and deploy resources. Resource status is categorized as available resources, assigned resources, or out-of-service resources. Tracking the status condition of each resource

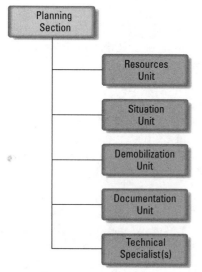

FIGURE 2-7 ICS planning section.

is essential for maintaining an up-to-date and accurate picture of resource utilization.

Situation Unit

The **situation unit** collects, processes, and organizes ongoing situation information including weather reports, prepares situation summaries, and develops projections and forecasts of future incident events. The situation unit also prepares maps and gathers and disseminates information and intelligence for use in the IAP.

Documentation Unit

The **documentation unit** maintains accurate and complete incident files, including a complete record of the major steps taken to resolve the incident, provides duplication services to incident personnel, and stores incident files for legal, analytical, and historical purposes. Documentation is part of the planning section primarily because this unit writes the IAP and maintains files and records developed as part of the IAP and planning function.

Demobilization Unit

The **demobilization unit** develops an incident demobilization plan that includes specific instructions for all personnel and resources that will require demobilization. This unit begins its work early in the incident by creating rosters of personnel and resources and obtains missing information as check-in proceeds.

Technical Specialists

Because the ICS functions effectively for **all hazards**, **technical specialists** with a myriad of skills are often needed to assist the planning section. Technical specialists can serve any function in the ICS organization; however, they are critical to the planning section, especially during the development of the tactical objectives in the IAP. Technical specialists are frequently maintained on resource lists by response organizations and are activated when needed to address specific situations. Examples of technical specialties needed during terrorism attacks are explosives experts, meteorologists, structural engineers, radiation physicists, legal counsel, toxicologists, industrial hygienists, safety engineers, and epidemiologists.

Administration/Finance

The administration/finance section is managed by the administration/finance section chief. This section is responsible for monitoring costs and expenditures, procurement, compensation/claims, and employee time keeping. Finance and administration is important because cost recovery is a critical fiscal issue, especially for financially stressed local and state governments. Proper financial tracking and record keeping can result in millions of dollars being reimbursed to local and state agencies by the federal government. In essence, poor documentation often means low reimbursement. There are also important legal considerations related to the documentation of workmen's compensation issues and employee compensation. On routine incidents, agencies and jurisdictions perform administration and finance functions at facilities separate from the incident scene. An administration/finance section may be established at an emergency operations center on long-term incidents. An administration/finance section is commonly established on an incident scene. **FIGURE 2-8** shows a diagram of the administration/finance section. An in-depth discussion of administrative and financial responsibilities is not within the scope of this text.

Other Components of NIMS

The focus of this chapter has been the ICS, which is part of the command and management component of NIMS. It important to note that NIMS consists of five additional components (**FIGURE 2-9**) that support IC and complement the entire spectrum of terrorism response, preparedness, and planning; NIMS is not just IC.

Preparedness

Effective incident management begins with a host of preparedness activities conducted on a steady-state basis, well in advance of any potential incident. Preparedness involves an integrated combination of planning, training, exercises, personnel qualification and certification standards, equipment acquisition and certification standards, mutual aid, and publication management.

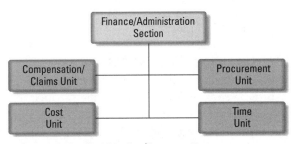

FIGURE 2-8 The administration/finance section.

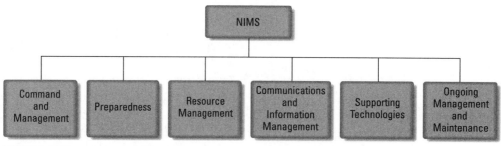

FIGURE 2-9 The central components of NIMS.

Resource Management

The NIMS defines standardized mechanisms and establishes requirements for processes to describe, inventory, mobilize, dispatch, track, and recover resources over the life cycle of an incident. Recently, the Department of Homeland Security has released, through the Federal Emergency Management Agency (FEMA), the resource classification tables for 120 different resource types. This tool enables incident management personnel to request the specific, defined resources they require in a manner that allows agencies in different parts of the country to provide the exact resources requested.

Communications and Information Management

The NIMS provides a standardized framework for communications, information management (collection, analysis, and dissemination), and information sharing at all levels of incident management. Developing technologies such as incident management software and communications like cross-band repeating that interconnect different radio systems are examples of technology currently being used by many ICS teams to improve incident management.

Supporting Technologies

Technology and technological systems provide support capabilities essential to implementing and refining NIMS. This includes voice and data systems, information management systems, and data display systems. Special technologies that facilitate terrorism response actions and incident management are included. An example of supporting technologies is chemical plume modeling software such as CAMEO.

Ongoing Management and Maintenance

The management and maintenance component of NIMS establishes the capability to provide strategic direction and oversight of NIMS, supporting both routine review and the continuous refinement of the system and its components. Organizations must continually update

and refine their internal NIMS-related processes. As threats change or new technology evolves, agencies and disciplines must review current plans and processes to ensure they are still appropriate. Implementing NIMS is not a one-time event but a commitment to ongoing development, review, and refinement.

Training

It is notable that HSPD-5 requires that all local, tribal, state, and federal response agencies that receive federal funding are trained and proficient in NIMS. It is imperative that response agencies and disciplines become proficient in using NIMS in all aspects of terrorism preparedness, planning, and response. Policy officials and support agencies require basic NIMS familiarization, whereas emergency response professionals require advanced training and experience verified by task books to attain and maintain NIMS certification in their area of expertise.

The NIMS integration center has developed the *Five-Year NIMS Training Plan* that is available as a PDF file at http://www.fema.gov/emergency/nims/nims_training.shtm. There is a multitude of NIMS courses available online. ICS 100 and 200 are basic courses. IS 700-level courses are also available online and include courses such as public information, resource management, communications and information management, preparedness, mutual aid, and resource typing. The online NIMS courses are available at https://training.fema.gov/IS/NIMS.asp. ICS 300 and 400 are advanced courses and available in a classroom setting as well as online.

Chapter Summary

The NIMS is an all-hazard and comprehensive incident management template developed by the Department of Homeland Security as mandated by HSPD-5. The six key components of NIMS are command and management, preparedness, resource management, communications and information management, supporting technologies, and ongoing management and maintenance. The ICS is part of the NIMS command and management component and is a functionally based system for IC at terrorism and disaster incidents.

The ICS model was initially designed to effectively manage catastrophic wildfires in California, but it has evolved into an all-hazards response template for all emergency response and support disciplines. The key planners of ICS designed the system to meet agreed-upon objectives including a system of command, common terminology, coordination between diversified agencies, shared communications with a common language, and a system of resource prioritizing and allocation.

The foundation of ICS is proven management principles such as chain of command, unity of command, span of control, resource management, incident management planning, and accountability. The five key functions in ICS are IC/UC, operations, logistics, planning, and administration/finance. An intelligence section is added to the planning section or established as a separate function when appropriate. Each section in ICS is managed by a section chief. The operations section includes branches for operational disciplines such as law enforcement, EMS, fire/rescue, public works, and public health.

The logistics section is responsible for allocating and tracking resources needed to accomplish incident objectives. The logistics section includes supply, facilities, ground support, communications, food, and medical units. The planning section is responsible for developing the IAP and includes resource, situation, documentation, and demobilization units. The administration/finance section is responsible for fiscal and administrative functions and includes claims/compensation, cost, procurement, and time units.

It is imperative that response and support agencies develop a proactive and continuous NIMS training program. Key ICS positions must be staffed by managers who are experienced and proficient in IC procedures. Support agencies and managers should at least have NIMS and ICS familiarization through online training courses.

Wrap Up

Chapter Questions

1. What are the six components of NIMS?
2. How does ICS differ from NIMS?
3. List the key management principles in ICS.
4. Diagram ICS including the command staff and the key functional sections.
5. Define divisions, groups, task forces, and strike teams.
6. List and describe the units in the logistics section.
7. Define the IAP. What factors determine if a verbal or formal IAP is appropriate?

Chapter Project I

Develop an outline for a comprehensive 5-year NIMS training program for the key response agencies in your community or jurisdiction. Consider which nongovernment and private-sector organizations should receive familiarization training.

Chapter Project II

Analyze after-action reports from a significant incident in your jurisdiction or region. Determine what ICS principles and functions were effectively utilized and what principles or functions were missing or ineffectively implemented.

Vital Vocabulary

Accountability The process of tracking and accounting for personnel and equipment resources on the incident scene.

Air-to-air nets Communications networks between aviation units using aviation radio frequencies.

All hazards A system that addresses a wide spectrum of threats including man-made hazards, natural disasters, and terrorist attacks.

Branch The ICS organizational level having functional, geographical, or jurisdictional branches that are responsible for major parts of incident operations. Branches are an effective tool for maintaining a narrow span of control.

Chain of command A clear line of authority within the structure of the ICS organization progressing from the command or unified command level to units or single resources.

Command net A communications network between the incident commander, command staff, and general staff.

Communications unit A unit in the logistics section responsible for the effective use and maintenance of communications equipment during an incident.

Demobilization unit A unit in the planning section responsible for the planning and execution of procedures for the release and return of incident resources.

Divisions An organizational level responsible for activities within a specified geographical area.

Documentation unit A unit in the planning section responsible for maintaining, administrating, and archiving all incident documents.

Facilities unit A unit in the logistics section responsible for the setup, maintenance, and demobilization of incident facilities.

Ground support unit A unit in the logistics section responsible for the maintenance, support, and fueling for vehicles and mobile equipment. This unit also provides transportation vehicles and support.

Ground-to-air net A communications network between ground functions and aviation units.

Groups An organizational tool in ICS used to divide the incident into functional areas of operation.

Incident action plan (IAP) A plan that contains objectives that reflect the incident strategy and specific control actions for the current or next operational period. An IAP is verbal in the early stages of an incident.

Incident command system (ICS) The combination of facilities, equipment, personnel, procedures, and communications under a standard organizational structure organized so as to manage assigned resources and effectively accomplish stated objectives for an incident.

Incident commander (IC or Command) Individual responsible for incident activities and functions including safety and the establishment of incident objectives and incident management.

Liaison officer The position within the incident command system that establishes a point of contact with the outside agency representatives.

Logistics section The section within the incident command system responsible for providing facilities, services, and materials for the incident.

Marine nets A communications system for marine units using maritime radio frequencies.

National incident management system (NIMS) A consistent, nationwide approach for federal, state, tribal, and local governments to effectively and efficiently prepare for, respond to, and recover from domestic incidents, regardless of the cause.

Operations section chief (operations chief) The general staff position responsible for managing all operations activities. It is usually assigned with complex incidents that involve more than 20 single resources or when command staff cannot be involved in all details of the tactical operation.

Planning section The section within the incident command system responsible for the collection, evaluation, and dissemination of tactical information related to the incident and for preparation and documentation of incident management plans.

Planning section chief (plans) The general staff position responsible for planning functions and for tracking and logging resources. It is assigned when command staff members need assistance in managing information.

Public information officer (PIO) The position within the incident command system responsible for providing information about the incident. The PIO functions as a point of contact for the media.

Resource management The coordination and management of assets that provide incident managers with timely and appropriate mechanisms to accomplish operational objectives during an incident.

Resources unit A unit in the logistics section responsible for the check-in and tracking of personnel, equipment, and major items on the incident site.

Safety officer (SO) The position responsible for monitoring incident operations and advising the IC/UC on all matters relating to operational safety, including the health and safety of emergency responder personnel.

Service branch A branch in the logistics section responsible for communications, food, and basic medical services. This branch contains the communications, food, and medical units.

Situation unit A unit in the planning section that collects, organizes, and presents ongoing information and intelligence about the incident for use in the IAP.

Span of control The ratio of subordinates to a single manager or supervisor. The span of control should vary from three to seven subordinates per manager. A low span of control is recommended for dynamic/high-stakes incidents.

Strike teams A group of like units managed by a strike team leader.

Supply unit A unit in the planning section responsible for ordering, supplying, and processing all incident resources.

Support branch A branch in the logistics section responsible for transport, maintenance, facilities, and supplies for the incident. This branch consists of the supply, facilities, and ground support units.

Support net A communications network for logistics support units or entities.

Tactical nets A communications network for tactical functions with the operations section.

Task forces A combination of unlike units directed by a task force leader.

Technical specialists A team of responders who serve as an information-gathering unit and referral point for both the incident commander and the assistant safety officer.

Unified planning A coordinated planning effort between multiple jurisdictions, agencies, and/or disciplines within the planning section.

Unity of command Situation in which every individual, unit, function, or entity in the ICS has only one supervisor at the incident scene.

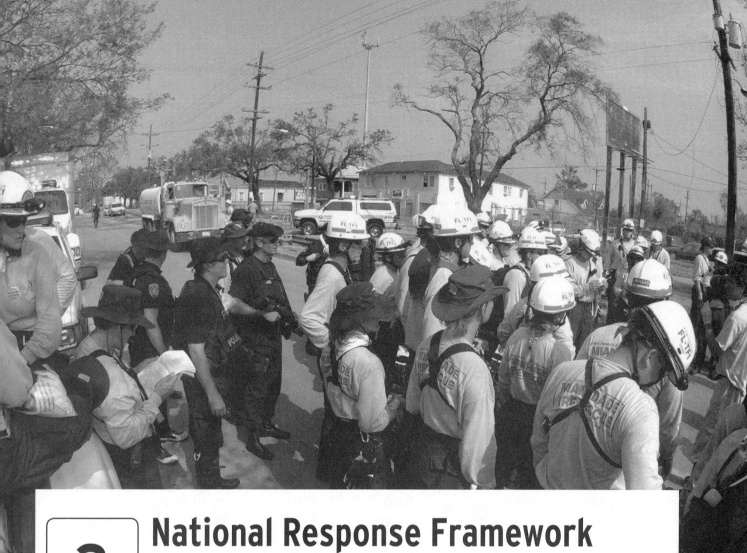

3

National Response Framework

Hank T. Christen
Paul M. Maniscalco

Objectives

- Classify the key elements in the National Response Framework (NRF).
- Summarize the philosophy of the NRF.
- Compare the NRF with the national incident management system (NIMS).
- Interpret the unified command principles within the NRF.
- Recognize and interpret the fifteen emergency support functions (ESFs) within the NRF.
- Recall and explain the eight key scenario sets that are linked with fifteen national planning scenarios.

Introduction

The former national response plan (NRP) is now superseded by the **National Response Framework (NRF)**. The NRF is a document outlining a coherent strategic framework—not a series of functional plans—for senior emergency response chiefs, emergency management practitioners, and senior executives in the private sector. The foundation of the NRF is its scalability, flexibility, and adaptable coordinating structures to align key roles and responsibilities for national emergency response and planning efforts. It articulates best practices and specific authorities for managing incidents ranging from locally controlled events to the largest of disasters.

Scalability means that the framework can be contracted or expanded according to the scope (or size) of the incident. For example, incidents as small as a pipe bomb in a rural community or as widespread as those of the anthrax attacks that concurrently impacted several states and multiple jurisdictions (federal, state, county, and local) and numerous agencies can be supported appropriately within the scalability context of the NRF (**CP FIGURE 3-1**).

The NRF adaptability, by design, establishes a responsive strategic framework to support response efforts for local responder requirements to any type of hazard or attack. This means that any responses, especially those that present large and complex issues such as a chemical leak, a terrorist attack, or a pandemic are all addressable within the adaptable NRF.

Flexible coordinating structures are incident management templates that provide a common language and organization for agencies and disciplines to integrate effectively. The integrated flexibility provides for the framework to align with all communities and disciplines. It is not a framework of rigid rules and structures. A small volunteer fire department, a suburban EMS agency, or an urban police department can apply the NRF to its mission.

Response is defined as immediate actions to save lives, protect property and the environment, and meet basic human needs. This definition is broadened in the NRF to include the execution of emergency plans and operations or actions that support short-term recovery. The emphasis of the NRF is multiagency engagement through a tiered response. This intentionally reflects the widely agreed-upon belief that all disasters are local—that the response begins at the local emergency response level and then expands through regional, state, and federal tiers (or layers) of government. The overarching philosophy of the NRF is a unified effort, a quick surge capability, and a readiness to act.

A **readiness to act posture** reflects the NRF design intention to enable a rapid and timely response capacity to an attack or disaster. This readiness philosophy commences and progressively advances from the individual citizen, household, and community level upward through county, state, tribal, and federal governments. This concept is described in the NRF as a **forward-leaning posture** because many incidents have the capability of rapidly expanding in size, severity, or complexity.

When the response mode is initiated, all activities are governed by the NIMS. The NIMS structure (review Chapter 2) ensures a unified command structure and a cohesive operational system to ensure safety for all entities engaged in the incident. The NRF and NIMS are also designed to enhance clear and concise communications between multiple agencies, disciplines, and levels. Public information management and distribution during attacks and disasters, along with pre-event citizen and community education, are other communication facets of the NRF and NIMS partnership.

The NRF is divided into five major chapters as follows:

- Chapter I—Roles and Responsibility
- Chapter II—Response Actions
- Chapter III—Response Organization
- Chapter IV—Planning: A Critical Element of Effective Response
- Chapter V—Additional Resources

The NRF organization centers on a core document with the following annexes:

- **Emergency support function annexes**— Federal resources and capabilities grouped into functional areas that are most frequently needed in a national response (e.g., transportation, firefighting, mass care).
- **Support annexes**—Essential supporting aspects that are common to all incidents (e.g., financial management, volunteer and donations management, private-sector coordination).
- **Incident annexes**—Description of the response aspects for broad incident categories (e.g., biological, nuclear/radiological, cyber, mass evacuation).

The NRF is a complex document and operational concept that cannot be addressed in a single text chapter, especially for individuals who are just becoming oriented to the framework. Our discussion of the NRF here is a review of the key points and concepts in the framework. Practitioners and other interested parties are encouraged to continue their research and inspection of the NRF, especially the varying roles agencies and personnel will be called upon to institute. The complete NRF and related annexes are available as electronic documents from the NRF resource center at http://www.fema.gov/NRF.

History

Federal planning efforts began with the 1992 federal response plan (FRP). The nascent FRP was severely tested when Hurricane Andrew devastated the Miami/Homestead, Florida, area. Many federal agencies were unfamiliar with the FRP, resulting in ineffective federal coordination in the Hurricane Andrew response effort. The FRP's foremost deficiency was the intense focus on federal roles instead of local, state, and federal coordination.

In 2004, the NRP replaced the FRP. The NRP addressed all levels of government (not just federal) into an all-encompassing response plan. After Hurricane Katrina, the NRP was modified to include the lessons learned from the 2005 hurricane season. The NRP also addressed the presidential directives such as Homeland Security Presidential Directive 5—Management of Domestic Incidents and Homeland Security Presidential Directive 8—National Preparedness, which emerged from shortfalls identified during the 2001 World Trade Center and Pentagon attacks. However, many local and state entities voiced a concern that the NRP was still based on a national-level mindset that failed to incorporate local and regional response issues.

The evolution of the NRF closely parallels the progression of the incident command system (ICS) evolving into NIMS. As a result, there is now a close relationship between the two systems. The principles of command, logistics, operations, planning, and administration/finance in NIMS provide a unified command and operational structure for agencies of all sizes and disciplines to function effectively within the overall NRF. In essence, the NRF and NIMS are closely aligned and complement each other.

The NRF attempts to address many of the concerns and shortcomings that prevailed in the FRP and NRP. The NRF is not a plan; it is a framework. This means the NRF document is a template for shared levels and responsibilities between governments, the private sector, and individual citizens. The foundation of this structure begins at the local level and progresses through regional, state, and federal levels as dictated by the needs of the incident.

NRF Strategy

The NRF is a key component in the homeland security strategy of the United States. This strategy incorporates threat analysis, lessons learned from attacks and disasters, and findings from exercises. The broad strategy of homeland security is focused on four goals:

1. Prevent and disrupt terrorist attacks.
2. Protect the American people and our critical infrastructure and key resources.
3. Respond to and recover from incidents that do occur.
4. Continue to strengthen the foundation to ensure our long-term success.

The NRF, in alignment with NIMS, centers on the third broad strategy goal of response and recovery from attacks or disaster incidents. Response must be fast, effective, and coordinated with local efforts. The community recovery process must ensure a planned and sustainable rebuilding of affected communities and infrastructures. Other strategies are supported by the NRF including the National Strategy for Combating Terrorism, the National Strategy to Combat Terrorist Travel, the National Strategy for Maritime Security, and the National Strategy for Aviation Security.

The Preparedness Cycle

The NRF addresses the three phases of emergency response: preparedness, response, and recovery. The **preparedness cycle** (**FIGURE 3-1**) includes planning,

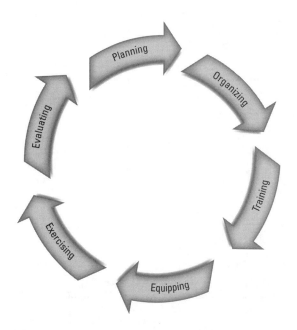

FIGURE 3-1 The preparedness cycle.

organizing, training, equipping, exercising, and evaluating for improvement. This cycle readily integrates with traditional emergency response training and exercising objectives.

Planning

Planning is the all-encompassing process of managing the entire cycle of emergency response beginning with intelligence and threat analysis, policy and procedure development, mutual aid, and strategies. These plans are written and formal. During response and recovery operations, comprehensive plans evolve into dynamic incident action plans that are developed as needs dictate to guide operational periods.

Organization, Training, and Equipment

NIMS provides a common organization structure of all agencies and entities in the emergency response continuum. NIMS is the template for a common management system with common terminology for use by all agencies and disciplines. For example, a federal law enforcement agency can effectively coordinate with a local bomb squad, a wildland fire logistics section, and a state aviation unit at a single incident.

NIMS also provides an efficient resource management system. Resources are categorized by kind and type and deployed, tracked, assigned, supported, and demobilized based on NIMS logistics organization and principles. The ESFs within the NRF align with the NIMS resource management structure to ensure effective support from federal agencies. Many states also use a hybrid of the NRF support functions as a template in their statewide emergency management plans.

Exercising and Training

Training for teams and organizations must be systematic and ongoing to ensure professionalism, qualifications, certification, and compliance with national standards. The primary purpose of exercises is to test plans and evaluate training. It is essential that exercises be realistically evaluated to identify strengths and weaknesses in planning and training. These findings should lead

to revisions in emergency planning and training programs. If lessons learned from exercises are not applied, the time and expense of exercise programs become a wasted effort.

Exercises should be interdisciplinary and interjurisdictional to ensure that plans are tested in regional and interagency venues. The Department of Homeland Security has a national exercise program with a 5-year national exercise plan that encompasses participation with local and state agencies.

Evaluation and Improvement

Response is based on key actions that deploy personnel and resources to save lives and property and protect the environment. The key response actions are:

1. Gain and maintain situational awareness.
2. Activate and deploy key resources.
3. Coordinate response actions.
4. Demobilize when appropriate.

Emergency response agencies must recognize that response actions occur within an interagency scope of operations. This is especially important when considering situational awareness. Situational awareness is an all-inclusive emergency response focus and must include emergency management, fire/rescue, law enforcement, emergency medical, public health, and public works considerations. Interagency situational awareness integrates with a common operational picture of the incident and shared information by all response agencies (**FIGURE 3-2**).

Resource activation and deployment are routinely done at the local level on a minute-by-minute basis every day. Resource management gets complicated in major incidents because resources are deployed for an extended time period over long distances from regional and/or

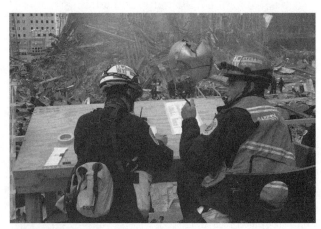

FIGURE 3-2 Situational awareness is an all-inclusive emergency response focus.

state facilities. Federal resources may be deployed from distances exceeding 1,000 miles for periods of weeks or months.

Response actions must be coordinated through a formal process. Assistance may come from communities within a region, from the state, from another state, or the federal government. The process begins with a local disaster declaration to the state government. States can initiate a disaster declaration that triggers federal assistance. At the federal level, a presidential disaster declaration allows the federal government to support states under the provisions of the Robert T. Stafford Disaster Relief and Emergency Assistance Act. It is notable that federal agencies can provide immediate assistance to local and state governments without a presidential disaster declaration when there is an immediate threat to life.

Demobilization is the safe and orderly return of resources to their original status and location. Resources must be tracked and documented to ensure effective financial reimbursement.

__Recovery__ is a shift in operational tempo from immediate lifesaving and property conservation to assistance for individuals, households, critical infrastructures, and businesses (**FIGURE 3-3**). Short-term recovery is a period that immediately follows response activities. Long-term recovery may take several years and is not within the NRF template.

NRF Roles and Responsibilities

The NRF prescribes key roles and responsibilities for all partners at the local, tribal, state, and federal levels.

It is significant that the framework also delineates roles for nongovernmental organizations and private-sector entities.

Local Roles

At the local level, elected or appointed officials are responsible for the welfare and safety of the community. These officials include mayors, city/county managers, and chief executives. These officials are not involved in tactical decisions, but they are responsible for laws, policies, and budgets that are the foundation of preparedness efforts. These officials must work with their respective community and local businesses to ensure effective decisions are made.

The emergency manager is usually the key appointed official responsible for implementing the planning and preparedness policies of senior officials. The emergency manager is responsible for developing and maintaining the local comprehensive emergency plan, maintaining a close relationship with response agencies, and conducting training and exercises that complement and support the community's emergency plan. Developing effective mutual aid and assistance agreements and conducting public education and awareness programs are additional duties (**FIGURE 3-4**). During emergency operations, the emergency manager serves as the commander of the local emergency operations center. Local agency directors are responsible for maintaining their agency capabilities at a high level of readiness and training to ensure effective response and interagency coordination within the emergency management structure.

Individuals and households have a shared responsibility for emergency preparedness that must

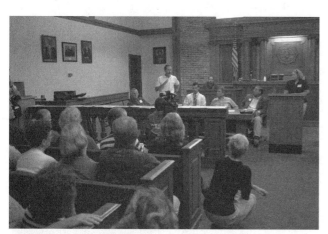

FIGURE 3-3 Arcadia, Fla., September 24, 2004. FEMA Deputy Federal Coordinating Officer Todd Davidson (standing), speaks to citizens of De Soto County at a town hall meeting to discuss recovery from Hurricane Charley.

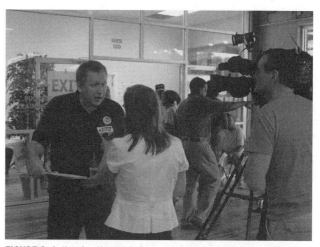

FIGURE 3-4 Keeping the public aware of the local emergency plan is one of the key components to ensuring the welfare and safety of the community.

complement emergency response efforts. Households should partner with public officials as follows:

1. Remove hazards within homes and surrounding property.
2. Maintain a home emergency kit and critical supplies.
3. Monitor communications related to public emergencies.
4. Serve in volunteer support entities.
5. Participate in citizen emergency response training.

State, Tribal, and Territorial Responsibilities

State, tribal, and territorial entities are responsible for supporting local response and recovery activities. The key state official is the governor, who is responsible for the general welfare and safety of the local governments and citizens within a state. The governor commands the National Guard and assigns missions for disaster operations. Governors have a coordination role with other states and the federal government for allocating resources and are responsible for filing a federal disaster declaration to obtain financial assistance. The director of the state emergency management agency works directly with the governor to ensure coordination among state agencies and effective allocation of response resources to local governments needing assistance.

Federal Roles

The president leads the federal response effort. The secretary of the Department of Homeland Security, appointed by the president, is responsible for federal response efforts and is the principal federal official for domestic incident management. The NRF provides specific and clear definitions for federal roles and entities as described in the following sections.

Unified Coordination Group and Staff

The **unified coordination group and staff** provide coordination in accordance with the NIMS concept of unified command (**FIGURE 3-5**).

Incident Management Teams

Incident management teams are special response teams that are interagency and regionally based to provide a rapid federal response. In addition, the Federal Emergency Management Agency (FEMA) provides initial response teams including a hurricane liaison team, urban search and rescue task forces, and mobile emergency response support.

Principal Federal Official

The **principal federal official** is representative of the secretary of DHS and is responsible for coordination of domestic incidents requiring a federal response.

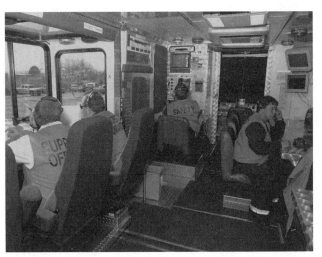

FIGURE 3-5 A unified command involves many agencies directly involved in the decision-making process for a large incident.

Federal Coordinating Officer

The **federal coordinating officer** is a focal point of coordination in the unified coordination group for Stafford Act incidents, ensuring integration of federal emergency management activities.

Senior Federal Law Enforcement Official

The **senior federal law enforcement official** is appointed by the attorney general to coordinate law enforcement operations related to the incident.

Joint Task Force Commander

The **joint task force commander** is designated by the Department of Defense to command federal military activities to support an incident.

Joint Field Office

The **joint field office (JFO)** is a temporary federal facility that provides a central location for the coordination of response and recovery activities of federal, state, tribal, and local governments. The JFO is structured and operated using NIMS and ICS as a management template. The JFO does not manage on-scene activities.

National Response Doctrine

The **national response doctrine** includes five key principles that support national response operations as follows:

1. Engaged partnerships.
2. Tiered response.
3. Scalable, flexible, and adaptable operational capabilities.
4. Unity of effort through unified command.
5. Readiness to act.

Engaged Partnerships

The term *engaged partnership* implies that local, state, tribal, and federal governments plan and respond together. This form of incident coordination includes ongoing communication and shared situational awareness. Engaged partnerships begin during the preparedness phase and progress through initial recovery efforts.

Tiered Response

In a tiered response, incidents are managed at the lowest possible level. This concept means that all incidents begin locally and expand through higher levels of government as needed. Only a small number of incidents progress to the federal level.

Scalable, Flexible, and Adaptable Operational Capabilities

Scalable, flexible, and adaptable operational capabilities are based on three important points. First, the system is scaled up or down to meet the needs of the response effort. Second, the system is flexible; it is a fluid system that changes with each specific incident. Third, the system adapts to all hazards or types of incidents.

Unity of Effort through Unified Command

Unified command is a structure in which diverse agencies and those that delineate from them share responsibilities. All major incidents and many moderate-level incidents require diverse agencies from overlapping jurisdictions. Coordination must be accomplished via a unified structure to ensure an effective effort. Unified command is especially important when military and civilian agencies share operational responsibilities.

Readiness to Act

Readiness to act is based upon the simple concept that effective day-to-day operational readiness supports the ability to always be ready. The doctrinal concept is not just for local, state, tribal, and federal partners, but most importantly about the community's role in being a prepared community.

National Response Structure

The NRF is a template for federal structures that support local response actions. The **National Operations Center (NOC)** is the primary national hub for situational awareness and operations coordination across the federal government for incident management. It provides the secretary of the DHS and other principals with information necessary to make critical national-level incident management decisions.

The NOC is a multiagency operations center that operates on a continuous 24-hour basis. Information related to hazards and threats from throughout the United States and foreign countries is monitored and analyzed by the staff and appropriate agency and private-sector representatives. These centers are discussed next.

National Response Coordination Center

The **National Response Coordination Center (NRCC)** is FEMA's primary operations management center, as well as the focal point for national resource coordination. As a 24/7 operations center, the Coordination Center monitors potential or developing incidents and supports the efforts of regional and field components.

National Infrastructure Coordinating Center

The **National Infrastructure Coordinating Center (NICC)** monitors the nation's critical infrastructure and key resources on an ongoing basis. During an incident, the NICC provides a coordinating forum to share information across infrastructure and key resources sectors through appropriate information-sharing entities such as the information sharing and analysis centers and the sector coordinating councils.

Supporting federal operations centers maintain situational awareness within their areas of responsibility and provide relevant and timely information to the NOC. Examples of these centers follow.

National Military Command Center

The **National Military Command Center** is the nation's focal point for continuous monitoring and coordination of worldwide military operations.

National Counterterrorism Center

The **National Counterterrorism Center** serves as the primary federal organization for integrating and analyzing all intelligence pertaining to terrorism and counterterrorism and for conducting strategic operational planning by integrating all instruments of national power.

Strategic Information and Operations Center

The Federal Bureau of Investigations (FBI) **Strategic Information and Operations Center** is the focal point and operational control center for all federal intelligence, law enforcement, and investigative law enforcement activities related to domestic terrorist incidents or credible threats, including leading attribution investigations.

Department of Homeland Security Operations Centers

Depending upon the type of incident (e.g., national special security events), the operations centers of other DHS operating components may serve as the primary operations management center in support of the secretary. These are the U.S. Coast Guard, Transportation Security Administration, U.S. Secret Service, and U.S. Customs and Border Protection operations centers.

Emergency Support Functions

The NRF divides federal support responsibilities into fifteen **emergency support functions (ESFs)**. Each ESF has a lead federal agency, support agencies, and a defined set of actions and responsibilities. Many state and local governments have adopted ESFs as part of their emergency operations plan (not an NRF requirement).

The federal ESFs as specified in the NRF are:

ESF No. 1—Transportation: Department of Transportation.

ESF No. 2—Communications: Department of Homeland Security (National Communications System).

ESF No. 3—Public Works and Engineering: Department of Defense (U.S. Army Corps of Engineers).

ESF No. 4—Firefighting: Department of Agriculture (U.S. Forest Service).

ESF No. 5—Emergency Management: Department of Homeland Security (FEMA).

ESF No. 6—Mass Care, Emergency Assistance, Housing and Human Services: Department of Homeland Security (FEMA).

ESF No. 7—Logistics Management and Resource Support: General Services Administration and DHS (FEMA).

ESF No. 8—Public Health and Medical Services: Department of Health and Human Services.

ESF No. 9—Search and Rescue: DHS (FEMA).

ESF No. 10—Oil and Hazardous Materials Response: Environmental Protection Agency.

ESF No. 11—Agriculture and Natural Resources: Department of Agriculture.

ESF No. 12—Energy: Department of Energy.

ESF No. 13—Public Safety and Security: Department of Justice.

ESF No. 14—Long-Term Community Recovery: DHS (FEMA).

ESF No. 15—External Affairs: Department of Homeland Security.

Emergency Management

Local, county, and state emergency management functions are guided by ESF No. 5 (Emergency Management). This function coordinates incident management and response operations, resource management, incident action planning, and financial management. Emergency management manages emergency operations centers at local, county, and state levels in coordination with federal entities.

Firefighting

Firefighting and rescue functions are guided by ESF No. 4. These functions include rural, urban, and wildland firefighting and search/rescue operations assisted and supported by federal entities. Operations are managed by incident or area commanders that are supported by local, county, and state operations centers.

Law Enforcement

Local, regional, and state law enforcement functions are guided by ESF No. 13 (Public Safety and Security). The major law enforcement functions in ESF No. 13 include facility and resource security, resource planning and technical resource assistance, public safety and security support, and support for incident access, traffic, and crowd control.

At the local level, ESF No. 13 is usually under the command of the county sheriff or municipal police chief. At the state level, ESF No. 13 is usually commanded by the state attorney general. The command and management responsibilities for ESF No. 13 are dictated by the local and state statutes, not the federal NRF.

Public Health and Medical Services

Health and medical services are guided by ESF No. 8 (Public Health and Medical Services). The primary agency assigned responsibility for ESF No. 8 is the Department of Health and Human Services. Key functions include an incredible collection of tasks including providing potable water, sanitation, food safety, veterinary services, vector control, emergency medical treatment and transport, and medical support for operations personnel, as well as managing public health, mental health, and mass fatalities. EMS agencies are the key emergency responders at the local and regional levels.

Many in the medical community and EMS response operations world have advocated for an independent ESF that is solely for addressing EMS and critical care responsibilities due to the unique and complex response requirements that these individuals face and the time-sensitive functions they perform. To date, the federal government has not acted upon this need.

Public Works

Public works and engineering functions are guided by ESF No. 3 (Public Works and Engineering). These functions include debris clearing, infrastructure restoration, emergency repairs, and engineering services. Local agencies, private contractors, military units, and state road departments are the key public works organizations.

Scenario Sets and Planning Scenarios

The NRF includes sets of key incident scenarios that are linked with national planning scenarios (**TABLE 3-1**).

Chapter Summary

The NRF replaces the national response plan and is a response template for the coordinated effort of federal,

state, tribal, and local governments, along with the private sector. The NRF complements the principles in NIMS, such as unified command and ICS. The emergency response phases of preparedness, response, and recovery are addressed in the NRF document. The key doctrine in the NRF is utilizing engaged partnerships, tiered response, scalable/flexible operational capabilities, unity of effort through unified command, and a readiness to act.

This framework defines fifteen emergency support functions and specifies a lead federal agency for each support function. The NRF includes key scenario sets and fifteen national planning scenarios.

The national response doctrine has key elements that include engaged partnerships, tiered response, scalable, flexible, and adaptable operations, unity of effort through unified command, and a readiness to act. The roles and responsibilities outlined in the framework begin at the individual and household level and progress through local, tribal, and state levels to the federal level. Roles for nongovernment agencies and the private sector are also defined in the NRF.

TABLE 3-1 National Planning and Key Scenario Sets

Key scenario sets	National planning scenarios
1. Explosives attack	Scenario 12: Explosives attack–improvised devices
2. Nuclear attack	Scenario 1: Nuclear detonation–improvised devices
3. Radiological attack	Scenario 11: Radiological attack–dispersal devices
4. Biological attack	Scenario 2: Biological attack–aerosol anthrax Scenario 4: Biological attack–plague Scenario 13: Biological attack–food contamination Scenario 14: Biological attack–foreign animal disease
5. Chemical attack	Scenario 5: Chemical attack–blister agent Scenario 6: Chemical attack–toxic industrial chemicals Scenario 7: Chemical attack–nerve agent Scenario 8: Chemical attack–chlorine tank explosion
6. Natural disaster	Scenario 9: Natural disaster–major earthquake Scenario 10: Natural disaster–major hurricane
7. Cyber attack	Scenario 15: Cyber attack
8. Pandemic influenza	Scenario 3: Biological disease outbreak–influenza

Wrap Up

Chapter Questions

1. List the four goals in the NRF strategy.
2. Describe the relationship of the NRF and NIMS.
3. List and discuss at least three elements in the preparedness cycle.
4. List three response agencies in your community or jurisdiction and describe their roles in the NRF.
5. Select a major local disaster or attack and list five or more emergency support functions and describe their functions in the event.

Chapter Project

Develop an outline of a local preparedness plan based on the NRF preparedness cycle.

Vital Vocabulary

Emergency support function annexes Areas in the NRF that explain and outline emergency support functions.

Emergency support functions (ESFs) A defined set of actions and responsibilities for fifteen federal disaster support functions including lead federal agencies and secondary support agencies for each function.

Federal coordinating officer The focal point of coordination in the unified coordination group for Stafford Act incidents, ensuring integration of federal emergency management activities.

Forward-leaning posture A preparedness and response philosophy that advances from citizens/households upward through governments to the federal level because incidents can rapidly expand and escalate.

Incident annexes The description of the response aspects for broad incident categories (e.g., biological, nuclear/radiological, cyber, mass evacuation).

Incident management teams The incident command organizations composed of the command and general staff members with appropriate functional units of an incident command system organized as regionally based interagency special response teams.

Joint field office (JFO) A temporary federal facility that provides a central location for the coordination of response and recovery activities of federal, state, tribal, and local governments. The JFO is structured and operated using NIMS and ICS as a management template. The JFO does not manage on-scene activities.

Joint task force commander Person designated by the Department of Defense to command federal military activities to support an incident.

National Counterterrorism Center The primary federal organization for integrating and analyzing all intelligence pertaining to terrorism and counterterrorism and for conducting strategic operational planning by integrating all instruments of national power.

National Infrastructure Coordinating Center (NICC) Center that monitors the nation's critical infrastructure and key resources on an ongoing basis and provides a coordinating forum to share information across infrastructure and key resources sectors through appropriate information-sharing entities such as the information sharing and analysis centers and the sector coordinating councils.

National Military Command Center The nation's focal point for continuous monitoring and coordination of worldwide military operations.

National Operations Center (NOC) The primary national hub for situational awareness and operations coordination across the federal government for incident management.

National Response Coordination Center (NRCC) A 24/7 operations center that monitors potential or developing incidents and supports the efforts of regional and field components.

National response doctrine The five key principles that support national response operations that are engaged partnerships, tiered response, scalable/flexible/adaptable capabilities, unity of effort through unified command, and readiness to act.

National Response Framework A document outlining a coherent strategic framework for senior emergency response chiefs, emergency management practitioners, and senior executives in the private sector.

Preparedness cycle The cycle of planning, organizing, training, equipping, exercising, and evaluating for improvement that integrates with traditional emergency response training and exercising objectives.

Principal federal official The representative of the secretary of Homeland Security and responsible for coordination of domestic incidents requiring a federal response.

Readiness to act posture The NRF design intention enabling a rapid and timely response capacity to an attack or disaster.

Recovery The period of short and/or long-term assistance for individuals, households, critical infrastructures, and businesses for restoration and rehabilitation from the effects of a disaster.

Response The immediate actions to save lives, protect property and the environment, and meet basic human needs, including the execution of emergency plans and operations or actions that support short-term recovery.

Senior federal law enforcement official The official appointed by the attorney general to coordinate law enforcement operations related to the incident.

Strategic information and operations center FBI focal point and operational control center for all federal intelligence, law enforcement, and investigative law enforcement activities related to domestic terrorist incidents or credible threats, including leading attribution investigations.

Support annexes Essential supporting aspects that are common to all incidents.

Unified coordination group and staff Group that provides coordination in accordance with the NIMS concept of unified command.

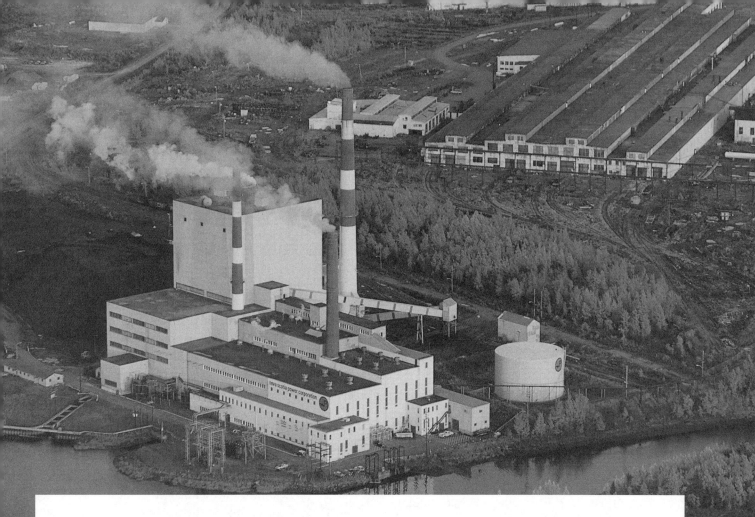

4

Critical Infrastructure Protection, Emergency Response, and Management

Dr. John B. Noftsinger, Jr.
Kenneth F. Newbold, Jr.
Benjamin T. Delp

Objectives

- Define the term *critical infrastructure*.
- List and describe the critical infrastructure sectors.
- Describe the current national policy that addresses critical infrastructure.
- List the hazards and threats in the physical and cyber components in America's infrastructure.
- List and describe the seven cardinal rules of risk communication.
- Describe the roles of the Department of Homeland Security (DHS) in critical infrastructure protection.
- Discuss the roles of the Homeland Security Operations Center (HSOC).

Introduction

<u>Critical infrastructure</u> protection is a vital component to ensuring effective and efficient emergency management practice. This chapter will explore infrastructure systems, how they are interconnected, and how these systems relate to emergency management. It is necessary to assess and identify civilian infrastructures that support communication, health, transportation, and other vital operations, which are susceptible to natural disasters, human error, and the direct target of malicious activities including terrorism and sabotage. Included in this discussion will be an examination of the cyber, physical, and human aspects of critical infrastructure systems with a specific focus on emergency management practices. Critical infrastructure systems include not just hardware and software, but the people and institutions responsible for their existence, operation, and safety.

Defining Critical Infrastructure Protection

Critical infrastructure systems have become increasingly complex and reliant on computer-based automated systems to provide the continuous operation of our critical systems. In this chapter, we will address technological and emergency management issues that affect cyber, physical, and human infrastructures.

As defined in the USA PATRIOT Act and the National Infrastructure Protection Plan (NIPP), critical infrastructures are "systems and assets, whether physical or virtual, so vital to the United States that the incapacity or destruction of such systems and assets would have a debilitating impact on security, national economic security, national public health or safety, or any combination of those matters."

The NIPP goes on to define key resources and key assets. Critical infrastructure is "systems and assets, whether physical or virtual, so vital that the incapacity or destruction of such may have a debilitating impact on the security, economy, public health or safety, environment, or any combination of these matters, across any Federal, State, regional, territorial, or local jurisdiction" (Department of Homeland Security, 2009). <u>Key resources</u> are "publically or privately controlled resources essential to minimal operations of the economy and government"(Department of Homeland Security, 2009). <u>Key assets</u> are a "person, structure, facility, information, material, or process that has value" (Department of Homeland Security, 2009).

These broadly defined infrastructure sectors all have one characteristic in common—they rely on people and technology to support and protect the systems that provide the goods and services necessary to survive as individuals and as a society. As the foundation for the function of the United States, these infrastructure sectors require attention from the policy community to ensure their continuity of operation. All levels of government have developed emergency response plans to address potential failures in critical infrastructure systems and outline best practices to ensure the safety of individuals in a disaster.

One area not specifically addressed in the list of critical infrastructure sectors is the concept of humans as a critical infrastructure. In studying the linkage between emergency management and critical infrastructure protection, it is of upmost importance that one recognizes the human element of critical systems. Without the human component, the physical systems comprising critical infrastructure will not function. Thus infrastructure assurance must include protection of the people necessary for construction, management, operation, and maintenance of critical systems.

The criticality of the human infrastructure component was dramatically illustrated by recent natural

---

Critical Infrastructure Sectors as Identified in the NIPP

- Banking and finance
- Chemical
- Commercial facilities communications
- Dams
- Defense industrial base
- Emergency services
- Energy
- Government facilities
- Health care and public health
- Information technology
- Manufacturing
- National monuments and icons
- Nuclear reactors, materials, and waste
- Postal and shipping
- Transportation systems
- Water

CRITICAL FACTOR............................

Infrastructure sectors all rely on people and technology to support and protect the systems that provide the goods and services necessary to survive as individuals and as a society.

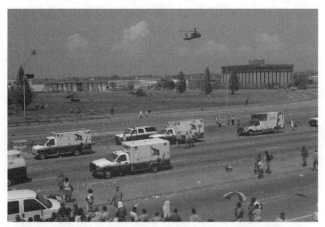

FIGURE 4-1 New Orleans, La.–August 31, 2005. Ambulances stand at the ready to transport evacuees in need of additional medical attention to outlying towns and cities with hospitals. Many victims were treated for injuries resulting from Hurricane Katrina on August 29. New Orleans was evacuated as a result of floods and damage caused by Hurricane Katrina.

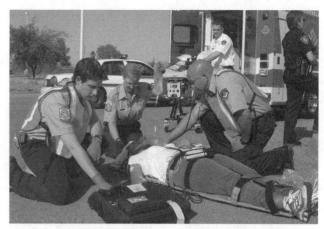

FIGURE 4-2 Emergency responders are often the first line of defense when critical infrastructure systems are threatened by natural disasters and terrorist attacks.

disasters such as Hurricane Katrina in 2005 (**FIGURE 4-1**). Evacuation planning and response hinged on the effective management of the population, including communication and leadership. Lack of planning, uncertainty of responsibilities, and poor management/coordination of the human response at all levels of government negatively affected the disaster's consequences. A complete approach to infrastructure assurance must include the human factor.

Science and technology have long been key components to defending the nation and its citizens from its enemies and in increasing the resilience of infrastructure systems from natural disasters. In the post-September 11, 2001, environment, threats to the homeland increasingly include nonmilitary, transnational organizations. Along with sound public policy and law, technological innovations will factor heavily into solutions created for the DHS. Emergency response personnel are identified as the first line of defense and response to disasters (**FIGURE 4-2**). The human element of critical infrastructure protection is best highlighted by the practices of the emergency response community.

History of Critical Infrastructure Protection Policy in the United States

Historically, the United States has been shielded geographically from physical threats to the nation's infrastructures. With friendly neighbors to the north and south and vast oceans to the east and west, the United States was somewhat isolated from attacks by external enemies. In the early 1950s, technological developments in the nuclear field allowed for the creation of improved weapons, including intercontinental ballistic missiles (ICBMs) (White House, 1997, p. 7). Both military instal-

lations and civilian infrastructures were at risk of attack from these long-range weapons. The threat posed by the former Soviet Union and its nuclear ICBM capabilities was unique in U.S. history. An enemy had never before threatened the United States from such a great distance. Technological advances in physical destruction capabilities put U.S. soil in danger of attack.

Prior to the late 1990s, federal policy addressing infrastructure protection was scarce. Not until the President's Commission on Critical Infrastructure Protection published its final report, *Critical Foundations: Protecting America's Infrastructures*, in 1997, did a national level policy initiative exist. This report was the guiding force in establishing future efforts with critical infrastructure protection.

Critical Foundations emphasized the emerging and expanding threats to infrastructure systems from cyber attacks, and increased attention was given by this report to the reliance of physical systems on cyber networks. Through the report, the president's commission called for increased sharing of information between government and industry as a means of improving the overall resiliency of critical systems. The recommendations made by this presidential commission helped to shape the future path of infrastructure protection, as many of the concepts introduced in *Critical Foundations* continue to be advocated in current policies and initiatives.

In response to the President's Commission on Critical Infrastructure Protection report, President Bill Clinton released Presidential Decision Directive 63 in 1998, which became the seminal document guiding U.S. policy in the arena of critical infrastructure protection. In Presidential Decision Directive 63, the Clinton administration stated that the "United States will take all necessary measures to swiftly eliminate any significant vulnerability to both physical and cyber attacks on our critical infrastructures, including especially our cyber systems" (White House, 1998).

Since September 11, 2001, the federal government has released four national strategy documents that outline the federal government's agenda for infrastructure assurance. These publications address homeland security, both physical and cyber security, and explicitly mention the role that the science and technology and public policy communities can play in finding solutions to combat threats to infrastructure systems. Recommended national strategy technology focus areas included the following:

- *Homeland Security* (Office of Homeland Security, 2002, pp. 68–69): Develop chemical, biological, radiological, and nuclear countermeasures; develop systems for detecting hostile intent; apply biometric technology to identification devices; improve technical capabilities of first responders; coordinate research and development of the homeland security apparatus; establish a national laboratory of homeland security; solicit independent and private analysis for science and technology research; establish a mechanism for rapidly producing prototypes; conduct demonstrations and pilot deployments; set standards for homeland security technology; and establish a system for high risk, high payoff homeland security research.
- *Securing Cyberspace* (White House, 2003b, pp. 53–60): Review and exercise information technology (IT) continuity plans; Department of Homeland Security will lead in the development and will conduct a national threat assessment, including red teaming, blue teaming, and other methods to identify the impact of possible attacks; adopt improved security protocols; development of more secure router technology; adoption of a code of good conduct; develop best practices and new technology to increase security of supervisory control and data acquisition that will determine the most critical supervisory control and data acquisition-related sites; encourage the software industry to consider more secure out-of-the-box installation and implementation of their products; research and development in areas of intrusion detection, Internet infrastructure security, application security, denial of service, communications security, high assurance systems, and secure system composition.
- *Physical Protection* (White House, 2003a): Advance modeling, simulation, and analysis capabilities including an effort to enhance data collection and standardization; enhance detection and testing capabilities with agriculture and food networks; assess transportation and security risks; improve monitoring of the water sector; enhance surveillance and communications capabilities; develop redundant communications systems for emergency response agencies; expand infrastructure diverse routing capability in the telecommunications sector; develop a national system for measures to reconstitute capabilities of individual facilities and systems within the energy sector; increase cargo screening capabilities for the transportation sector; enhance exchange of security related information in the finance sector.
- *National Infrastructure Protection Plan* (Department of Homeland Security, 2009, pp. 13–15): Protect critical infrastructure and key resources against plausible and specific threats; long-term reduction of critical infrastructure and key resources vulnerabilities in a comprehensive and integrated manner; maximize efficient use of resources for infrastructure protection; build partnerships among federal, state, local, tribal, international, and private sector stakeholders to implement critical infrastructure protection programs; continuously track and improve national protection.

Interdependencies among Critical Infrastructure Systems

Critical infrastructure systems are heavily reliant on one another to operate at maximum efficiency. The interdependent nature of these systems makes them susceptible to cascading failures and adds a level of complexity to protecting the nation's key assets. The most commonly used and farthest-reaching technology is the information technology (IT) infrastructure. Without computers and networks, our economic and infrastructure systems would not function in the manner to which we have become accustomed. Emergency managers rely on interoperable communication devices to respond to various accidents and disasters. Without a robust and resilient IT infrastructure, these communication tools would not be useful and would hinder effective response activities.

A **network of networks** now directly supports operations within all of the following sectors of the nation's economy: energy (electricity, oil, gas), transportation (rail, air), finance and banking, telecommunications, public health, emergency services, water, chemical, defense, food, agriculture, and postal (White House, 2003b, p. 6). Physical infrastructures such as electrical transformers, trains, pipeline pumps, chemical vats, and radars are also dependent on computer networks (White House, 2003b, p. 6).

These networks (**FIGURE 4-3**) are vulnerable to many types of cyber threats (including terrorist attacks, economic espionage, and random failures) and present new challenges to owners and operators of the nation's infrastructures. The high degree of automation and interconnectivity of computer networks, however, subjects them to potentially crippling and catastrophic attacks or failures.

Hazards and Threats to Critical Infrastructure Systems

The list of hazards and threats that exist to both physical and cyber components of our infrastructure is quite long. Major hazard categories include natural disasters, terrorist activities, human error, weapons of mass destruction, and mechanical failure. Solutions that combine technology with multidisciplinary research provide the most complete answers to infrastructure assurance problems. This litany of potential hazards makes it potentially challenging to those engaged in emergency response because they must be prepared to address a variety of situations, which may be caused by numerous sources. There is no single approach to addressing infrastructure protection, and emergency managers who understand the interconnected nature of critical systems and approach response from an all-hazards standpoint will be best prepared to address emergency situations and ensure the safety of individual citizens.

In the past decade, attacks against physical infrastructures have been executed successfully by exploiting technology. Emergency response personnel played key roles in mitigating further damage in each of these examples. In the 1993 attack at the World Trade Center, a truck bomb was used. In 1995, a disgruntled citizen using simple technologies and common products detonated a truck bomb at the Alfred Murrah Federal Building in Oklahoma City (**FIGURE 4-4**). Moreover, the tragic events of September 11, 2001, opened a new mode of threats to the nation's infrastructure—the use of civilian transportation systems as weapons. Based on these precedents, communities need to be on guard to anticipate and prevent terrorist use of common commercial systems and technology that are readily available within our borders.

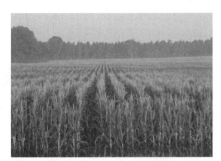

A. Agriculture needs oil and electricity to operate machinery as well as water to sustain growth. Crops, like corn, can also be used as alternative fuels.

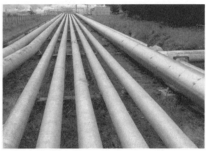

B. Electricity supplies energy and uses oil to operate and water for cooling purposes.

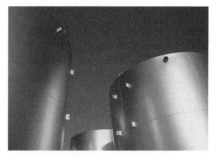

C. Oil becomes fuel for the other branches and uses water for cooling and electricity for operating machinery.

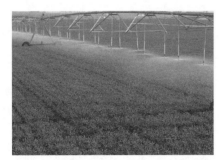

D. Water industries use power from electricity and oil, as well as for control and movement. Water is mainly used by the other branches for cooling properties as well as for power. Water is also essential for sustaining human health and life.

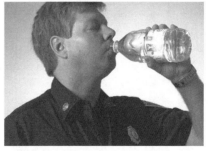

E. Humans, as the central cog of critical infrastructure, operate and manage each of the other branches as well as benefit from their use and products.

FIGURE 4-3 The interdependency of critical infrastructure.

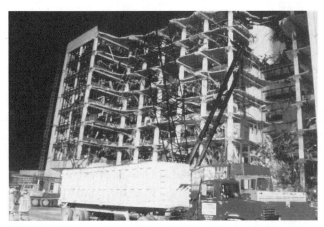

FIGURE 4-4 A scene of devastation at the Murrah Federal Building following the Oklahoma City bombing on April 26, 1995.

A primary concern is the threat of organized cyber attacks that are capable of debilitating our nation's critical infrastructures, economy, and national security (White House, 2003b). Computer networks can be attacked with little or no warning and cascade rapidly such that victims may not have time to respond. Even with warnings, victims may not have access to the proper tools and technologies to defend themselves. Efforts are under way worldwide to create models to simulate and visualize infrastructure networks.

Emergency responders must consider the interconnected nature of physical systems and cyber systems. In emergency planning, a balance must exist between physical and cyber vulnerabilities. Although attacks to physical structures often produce high numbers of victims, failures within cyber systems also create victims requiring awareness and response. Emergency response planning must now include multiple levels of consideration to how physical and cyber systems work to support each other.

While strong information security policy is of utmost importance, physical security and building design are also critical. The location of computers and servers must be well planned to prevent damage from hazards such as flooding, fire, explosion, and intrusion. Fiber-optic cable must be protected as well to prevent accidental damage from digging and malicious cutting of wires. Colocation of wires and cables introduces common, serious, single-point failure vulnerabilities to be avoided in protection design. Consequences of cable colocation were evidenced by the Baltimore train tunnel fire of 2001. This accident occurred in a tunnel with colocated fiber-optic cables whose failure interrupted telecommunications and Internet connectivity along the Washington–New York corridor.

In an increasingly complex and interconnected global community, the reliance on computers to store, transmit, and process data has grown exponentially. Wireless technology applications continue to increase society's dependence on the computer infrastructure for communication and business processes. Private-sector businesses, governments, and individuals have all become more reliant on IT to perform routine tasks. Therefore, emergency response personnel must be acutely aware of interconnected infrastructure systems and the role in which humans interact with these important elements of a modern society. Social networks are prime examples (such as Twitter and Facebook) where disaster information—some accurate and some inaccurate—can be quickly spread through an affected community.

Risk Communication Paradigms

An integral component of emergency management and critical infrastructure protection is the field of risk communication. **Risk communication** focuses on communicating disaster preparedness information and mitigation strategies to the public in order to minimize the potential effects of an event *before* said event occurs. One of the first major publications produced in the risk communication field was the 1988 guide, the *Seven Cardinal Rules of Risk Communication*, published by the Environmental Protection Agency based on the work of Vincent T. Covello and Frederick H. Allen. The guide lists seven basic rules on how to engage with the public, concerns of honesty and truthfulness, coordination efforts, dealing with the media, planning, and evaluating.

While the *Seven Cardinal Rules of Risk Communication* is still quite relevant and utilized at the local, state, and national level on a daily basis, the importance of properly communicating prior to an incident involving a critical infrastructure sector cannot be overstated.

Disastrous events involving critical infrastructure require an in-depth risk communication strategy that should be constantly evolving as technology advances and information knowledge management increases. This is due in part to the length of time a major event affecting critical infrastructure stays in the public's mind. While risk communication is a discipline with numerous concepts, strategies, and techniques, one particular aspect identified by risk communication expert Dr. Peter Sandman in his article, *Obvious or Suspected, Here or Elsewhere, Now or Then: Paradigms of Emergency Events*, focuses on three variables relevant to critical infrastructure protection. The three variables are as follows:

1. Obvious or suspected
2. Here or elsewhere
3. Now, future, or past (Sandman, 2002).

(Covello and Sandman, 2004)

Rule 1: Accept and involve the public as a legitimate partner. Disaster managers must realize in advance that the public is going to want to be involved and will find a way to be involved. It only makes sense to openly include them early on.

Rule 2: Listen to the audience. An effective dialogue will occur only after the communicators find out what is important to the public. In some cases it may be trust, caring, and courtesy, while other communities will value quantitative statistics or a combination.

Rule 3: Be honest, frank, and open. The two greatest attributes in a risk communicator's arsenal are trust and credibility. These are judgments made early on and are highly resistant to change. If answers are unknown, one should say, "We do not have the answer at this time, but are working on it." Lies and misleading will destroy any trust already gained.

Rule 4: Coordinate and collaborate with other credible sources. One of the best ways to ensure inter-organizational and intraorganizational lines of communication is to set up specific tasks early on. Agencies should know whom to contact outside of their team for information and have lines of communication already established. Once communication to the public takes place, it will look much more credible coming from many highly trained sources.

Rule 5: Meet the needs of the media. Know what the media is interested in. "The media are generally more interested in politics than in risk; more interested in simplicity than in complexity; and more interested in wrongdoing, blame and danger than in safety" (Covello & Sandman, 2004, p. 13). The overall goal with the media should be the same with the public—establish long-term relationships of trust.

Rule 6: Speak clearly and with compassion. Overly technical speech damages risk communication more than it helps. Describe technical aspects only when necessary. The public is more concerned with empathy and caring over numbers.

Rule 7: Plan carefully and evaluate performance. This essentially reiterates what risk communication is—planning. Start early on with clear objectives. Properly train staff to deal with stakeholders, the public, and other technical workers.

For example, when preparedness officials communicated with the citizens of New York City; Washington, DC; and other localities in the weeks after the events of September 11, 2001, the communication fell in the obvious/here/past paradigm. The attacks were obvious because they could be seen/heard/felt; they occurred where New Yorkers and Washingtonians resided and worked, not in a foreign city 3,000 miles away; and the attacks had already taken place. However, a California mayor's communication about those attacks would have been identified as the obvious/elsewhere/past paradigm because the incidents happened on the opposite coast from California. This distinction takes into account the physical attack on the U.S. defense industrial base (Pentagon) (**FIGURE 4-5**) and an institution of the banking and finance sector (World Trade Center). The paradigm of obvious/here/now could describe the framework for communication to the entire United States during the economic collapse following September 11, 2001, because Americans were impacted by the targeting of the banking and finance sector.

The H1N1 virus (swine flu) public health emergency highlights the distinction between obvious and suspected—the most difficult concept of the three variables as here or elsewhere and now or then are relatively easy to identify. A small number of more

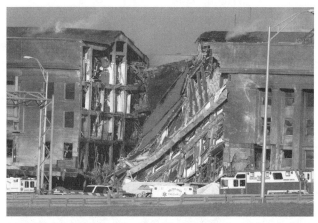

FIGURE 4-5 A 200-foot gash exposes interior sections of the Pentagon following the terrorist crash of a commercial airliner into the southwest corner of the building on September 11, 2001.

virulent cases of the flu would require the suspected distinction, without taking into account where the flu cases were occurring and the life cycle of the suspected illness. Once the H1N1 virus was identified and the number of confirmed cases reached well into the hundreds, the more virulent cases of the flu are now the swine flu pandemic, an obvious and no longer suspected event. The following list highlights six paradigms, as described by Dr. Sandman using real and hypothetical situations:

1. *Obvious/Here/Future.* Bioterrorists may someday poison the water supply. Planning now what to say if it happens is planning for an obvious/here/now emergency … but what do we say now about this future possibility?

2. *Obvious/Here/Past.* Emergencies end. When they end, the communication about them doesn't end, but it does change. What should the postemergency public dialogue look like, and how can you get ready to conduct it?

3. *Obvious/Elsewhere/Now.* September 11, 2001, and the 2002 anthrax attacks soon afterwards were obvious/here/now for a few emergency managers in a few cities. Everywhere else they were obvious/elsewhere/now—and they required a lot of communication.

4. *Suspected/Here/Now.* Someone shows up at the airport with a severe fever. The nearest doctor thinks it might be Ebola. Various health-protective steps are initiated and need to be communicated pending a more definitive diagnosis.

5. *Suspected/Here/Future.* If someone thinks he may someday face the fourth paradigm, then he faces this one now. People are likelier to cope well with the cliffhanging tension of a suspected/here/now emergency if they were aware in advance that such a dilemma might well be on its way.

6. *Suspected/Here/Past.* Some people thought there were a lot of foreign nationals taking flying lessons, but they weren't sure this was a problem and they decided not to take action. Now they have to explain why they underreacted. Others thought a weird case of chickenpox might be smallpox and did take action, and it was just a weird case of chickenpox. Now they have to explain why they overreacted (Sandman, 2002).

Understanding these characteristics of an event or future event with the potential to impact critical infrastructure will create risk communication specifically tailored to the audience; when and where the event occurred; and situations where an event has not completely unfolded. The more specific the communication is, the better chance preparedness officials will gain the trust and confidence of the public after an event occurs. While faulty communication will leave the public fearful and skeptical of the messenger (almost always government when critical infrastructure is involved), utilizing the paradigms will improve risk communication understanding, skills, and techniques, ensuring a more robust overall emergency management strategy.

The Role of the Department of Homeland Security

Critical infrastructure protection, cyber security, and emergency response initiatives are major components of the efforts of government agencies at the federal, state, and local levels. Emergency response planning varies from state to state and locality to locality, but the federal government has designated the DHS as the lead agency for policy development for critical infrastructure protection and emergency response. Within the DHS, an Assistant Secretary for Cyber Security and Telecommunications is responsible for identifying and assessing the vulnerability of critical telecommunications infrastructure and assets; providing timely, actionable, and valuable threat information; and leading the national response to cyber attacks and telecommunications attacks. The Assistant Secretary for Infrastructure Protection is charged with cataloging the nation's critical infrastructures and key resources and coordinating risk-based strategies and protective measures to secure them from terrorist attack.

As the cognizant agency for coordinating federal activities within the area of infrastructure protection and information assurance, the DHS has established programs that address policy and action necessary for the continued operation of the nation's critical systems. It's through these programs that preparedness and response activities are developed and implemented.

Critical Infrastructure Protection and Response

One major DHS initiative is the Protected Critical Infrastructure Information Program, which is designed to encourage private industry and others with knowledge about our critical infrastructure to share sensitive and proprietary business information with the government. This program is used in pursuit of a more secure homeland, focusing primarily on analyzing and securing critical infrastructure and protected systems and developing risk and vulnerability assessments assisting with recovery (DHS, 2009).

Homeland Security Operations Center

Emergency response personnel are actively engaged in protecting the nation's infrastructure through the Department of Homeland Security's **Homeland Security Operations Center (HSOC)**, which serves as the nation's center for information sharing and domestic incident management. One of the goals of this effort is to dramatically increase the coordination between federal, state, territorial, tribal, local, and private-sector partners, which provide constant watch for the safety of our nation. The center includes partners from over thirty-five agencies and receives hundreds of calls in its effort to collect and fuse information from a variety of sources on a daily basis to help deter, detect, and prevent terrorist acts and address approximately twenty incidents/cases per day. The HSOC is in constant communication with the White House, serving as a conduit of information for the White House situation room by providing the intelligence needed to make decisions and define courses of action. The information gathered and analyzed by the HSOC provides real-time situational awareness in monitoring the homeland. This program also coordinates incident and response activities and issues advisories and bulletins concerning threats, as well as coordinating specific protective measures. Information on domestic incident management is shared with emergency operations centers at all levels through the Homeland Security information network.

Information is shared and fused on a daily basis by the two halves of the HSOC that are referred to as the "intelligence side" and the "law enforcement side." Each half of the HSOC functions in conjunction with the other but requires a different level of clearance to access information. The intelligence side focuses on pieces of highly classified information and how specific details contribute to the current threat for any given area. The law enforcement side is dedicated to tracking the different enforcement activities across the country that may have a link to terrorism. These efforts highlight the relationships and coordination among all levels of government. Without the cooperation among law enforcement agencies at all levels, the HSOC would not be effective in its efforts to thwart terrorist activities.

The HSOC communicates in real time to its partners through the Homeland Security information network's Internet-based counterterrorism communications tool. This tool supplies information to all fifty states, Washington, DC, and more than fifty major urban areas. Threat information is exchanged with state and local partners to assist in planning and response activities. Participants in the Homeland Security information network include governors, mayors, state Homeland Security advisors, state National Guard offices, emergency operations centers, first responders and public safety departments, and other key homeland security partners (DHS, 2009).

The HSOC regularly disseminates domestic terrorism-related information generated by the Information Analysis and Infrastructure Protection Directorate. Information released by the HSOC comes in one of the following two forms:

1. **Homeland Security threat advisories**, which are the result of information analysis and contain actionable information about an incident involving or a threat targeting critical national networks, infrastructures, or key assets. They often relay newly developed procedures that, when implemented, significantly improve security and protection. Advisories also often suggest a change in readiness posture, protective actions, or response.

2. **Homeland Security information bulletins** are protection products that communicate information of interest to the nation's critical infrastructures that do not meet the timeliness, specificity, or significance thresholds of warning messages. Such information may include statistical reports, periodic summaries, incident response or reporting guidelines, common vulnerabilities and patches, and configuration standards or tools.

In March of 2002, President George W. Bush unveiled the **Homeland Security Advisory System** as a tool to improve coordination and communication among all levels of government, the private sector, and the American public. The advisory system not only identifies the threat condition, but it also outlines protective measures that can be taken by partner agencies. The federal government, states, and the private sector each have a set of plans and protective measures that are implemented as the threat condition is raised or lowered, thus flexibly mitigating vulnerability to attack. The HSOC is the distributor of the recommended security measures to state and local partners when the threat level is raised or lowered.

The HSOC monitors vulnerabilities and compares them to threats and pertinent intelligence, providing a centralized, real-time flow of information between homeland security partners. These data collected from across the country are then compiled into a master template that allows the HSOC to provide a visual picture of the nation's current threat status. The HSOC has the capability to do each of the following:

- Perform an initial assessment of the information to gauge the terrorist nexus.
- Track operational actions taking place across the country in response to the intelligence information.
- Disseminate notifications and alerts about the information and any decisions made.

As information is shared across agencies, HSOC staff can utilize visualization tools by cross-referencing human intelligence against geospatial data that can isolate an area of interest on the earth's surface. Satellite technology is then able to transmit pictures of the site in question directly into the HSOC. This type of geographic data can be stored to create a library of images that can be mapped against future threats and shared with our state and local partners.

The **Interagency Incident Management Group (IIMG)** is based in Washington, DC, and is comprised of senior representatives from DHS, other federal departments and agencies, and nongovernment organizations. The IIMG provides strategic situational awareness, synthesizes key intelligence and operational information, frames courses of action and policy recommendations, anticipates evolving requirements, and provides decision support to the Secretary of Homeland Security and other national authorities during periods of elevated alert and national domestic incidents.

During incidents such as Hurricanes Isabel (2003), Katrina (2005), Rita (2005), and Wilma (2005); the December 2003 orange alert; and the Northeast blackout, the IIMG was activated in less than 90 minutes and hosted assistant secretary-level members of federal agencies to provide strategic leadership (DHS, 2009).

Along with the critical infrastructure initiatives already discussed, the DHS is also focused on improving cyber security efforts. As discussed earlier in this chapter, the consequences of an attack on our cyber infrastructure can cascade across many sectors, causing widespread disruption of essential services, damaging our economy, and imperiling public safety.

The speed and maliciousness of cyber attacks have increased dramatically in recent years. Accordingly, the preparedness directorate places an especially high priority on protecting our cyber infrastructure from terrorist attack by unifying and focusing key cyber security activities. The directorate augments the capabilities of the federal government with the response functions of the National Cyber Security Division of the United States Computer Emergency Response Team. Due to the interconnected nature of information and telecommunications sectors, DHS will also assume the functions and assets of the national communications system within the Department of Defense, which coordinates emergency preparedness for the telecommunications sector.

Providing indications and warning advisories is a major function of the DHS's efforts within cyber security. In advance of real-time crisis or attack, preparedness will provide the following:

- Threat warnings and advisories against the homeland including physical and cyber events.
- Processes to develop and issue national and sector-specific threat advisories through the Homeland Security advisory system.
- Terrorist threat information for release to the public, private industry, or state and local government.

Chapter Summary

Given the distributed nature of the nation's infrastructure systems, the sharing of information between the public and private sectors and across the critical infrastructure sectors is imperative. As discussed previously, the DHS places a priority on initiatives that emphasize and facilitate the flow of information, which is crucial to preventing and responding to a disaster. While DHS has focused on the area of information sharing, greater efforts need to be taken to engage the appropriate participants. Without coordinated activities at the federal level, policy makers may be missing crucial information in a time of crisis. Data gathered by DHS must be verified and trustworthy before details are released to localities, and the communication of threats needs to be articulated clearly and early in order for appropriate measures to be taken. It is key to remember that coordination of efforts in the areas of infrastructure protection and information assurance relies on accurate and well-communicated details.

Prior to the creation of the DHS, the responsibility for the nation's efforts to secure cyber space and protect critical infrastructures was distributed within a number of federal agencies. Today, DHS is the primary organization for all cyber security and physical security initiatives. The programs highlighted in this chapter address the key areas of focus for DHS as the organization addresses an ever-evolving and growing number of threats. While all levels of government are important stakeholders in securing critical assets, only with cooperation from the private sector and individual citizens will the efforts of DHS be effective.

Wrap Up

Chapter Questions

1. Define *critical infrastructure*.
2. Describe the current national policy that addresses critical infrastructure protection.
3. List and define at least four threats in the physical and cyber components of the U.S. infrastructure.
4. List and define the seven cardinal rules of risk communication.
5. What are the roles of the HSOC?
6. Discuss the roles of the IIMG.

Chapter Project

List the critical infrastructure networks in your community, identify the key threats to each network, and define appropriate local protection and response efforts.

Vital Vocabulary

Critical infrastructure Systems and assets, whether physical or virtual, so vital that the incapacity or destruction of such may have a debilitating impact on the security, economy, public health or safety, environment, or any combination of these matters, across any federal, state, regional, territorial, or local jurisdiction.

Homeland Security Advisory System A tool to improve coordination and communication among all levels of government, the private sector, and the American public that identifies the threat condition and protective measures that can be taken by partner agencies.

Homeland Security information bulletins Protection products that communicate information of interest to the nation's critical infrastructures that do not meet the timeliness, specificity, or significance thresholds of warning messages.

Homeland Security Operations Center (HSOC) Homeland Security center that serves as the nation's center for information sharing and domestic incident management by enhancing coordination between federal, state, territorial, tribal, local, and private-sector partners.

Homeland Security threat advisories Information analysis and actionable information about an incident involving or a threat targeting critical national networks, infrastructures, or key assets.

Interagency Incident Management Group (IIMG) Senior representatives from DHS, other federal departments and agencies, and nongovernment organizations to provide strategic situational awareness, synthesize key intelligence and operational information, frame courses of action and policy recommendations, anticipate evolving requirements, and provide decision support to the secretary of Homeland Security.

Key asset Person, structure, facility, information, material, or process that has value.

Key resources Publicly or privately controlled resources essential to minimal operations of the economy and government.

Network of networks A system that directly supports the following operations within all sectors of the nation's economy: energy (electricity, oil, gas), transportation (rail, air), finance and banking, telecommunications, public health, emergency services, water, chemical, defense, food, agriculture, and postal.

Risk communication Communicating disaster preparedness information and mitigation strategies to the public in order to minimize the potential effects of an event before said event occurs.

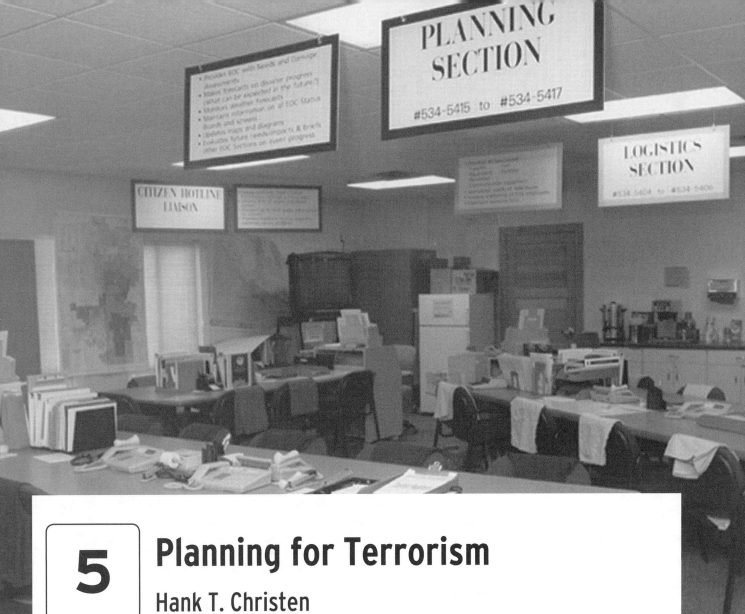

5 Planning for Terrorism

Hank T. Christen
Paul M. Maniscalco

Objectives

- Describe planning as a front-end concept.
- Recognize the importance of incorporating terrorism in an emergency operations plan (EOP).
- Outline the key National Incident Management System (NIMS) and National Response Framework (NRF) elements in an EOP.
- Distinguish between an EOP and a real-time incident action plan (IAP).
- Outline the logistics/resource management elements in an EOP.
- Describe the liaison process with support agencies in emergency planning.

Introduction

Effective response to a terrorism event is often perceived as action oriented. We picture quick and aggressive operations and tactics. This idea is hopefully accurate in a well-organized response. However, effective tactical and strategic actions cannot occur without planning.

Advanced planning is a front-end concept. This means that for positive outcomes at the back end, we must heavily load the front end. It is simply impossible to dynamically deploy in a terrorism incident and be successful without planning.

A **front-end plan** is different than a reference guide. Many disaster plans are kept in a 2-inch thick binder that includes radio frequencies, names and addresses, lists of vehicles, units, and descriptions of resources. These guides are important for reference information, but they are not documents that yield tactical guidelines in the heat of battle. There is nothing wrong with reference information—it is important, but it's not a plan that guides you through the critical steps of a disaster or terrorism incident.

An effective plan is an easy-to-read template and framework that benchmarks the critical factors of a dynamic event; the plan identifies operations and support functions that complement operations. In other words, the plan is a NIMS guide. It is important to remember that all plans suffer from a common deficiency. Namely, plans do not incorporate unexpected events. Plans address only expected or anticipated events. Unexpected events require a high-reliability organizing hallmark called **resilience**. Resilience is the ability to bounce back or recover from unexpected events. For example, the U.S. Postal Service had no plan for responding to mailed anthrax attacks. They were resilient and rewrote plans in a dynamic and unexpected environment. In summary, effective plans are a necessity but not the holy grail; expect plans to fail sometimes.

The NIMS and the NRF—Templates for Planning

Effective plans guide you through the NIMS functions and the NRF structure. The NIMS (Chapter 2) and the NRF (Chapter 3) are templates for response planning. This means all emergency response activities are managed by a command/unified staff and involve operations, logistics, planning, and administration/finance. It makes sense to use the NIMS and NRF models when developing effective operational plans.

An **emergency operations plan (EOP)** for terrorism incidents should identify key elements such as:
- Command or unified command staff
- Operations
- Logistics and **multiagency coordination systems (MACS)**
- Planning
- Administration/finance
- Liaison with state, federal, nongovernment, and private-sector agencies
- Information management
- Public information
- Safety

Who Is in Charge?

Command turf wars have no place in terrorism incidents. Emergency response agencies and policy officials have to formally determine who will manage what type of event. This may be a difficult process. Federal and state agencies have elaborate plans and statutes that identify who manages the incident, but their response may take hours or days. Local responders are always the first to arrive and the last to leave a terrorism incident.

If an event meets the federal definition of terrorism, federal agencies will have jurisdiction. In accordance with the NRF, the Department of Justice is the lead agency. The Department of Homeland Security (DHS) coordinates response activities. *Coordinate* is the key word because DHS is not a first-responder entity. This means local communities must establish scene management immediately and maintain command with a common operational picture throughout the incident. A critical step is determining who is in charge. In most local governments, the responsibility of scene management in terrorism incidents rests with the ranking law enforcement official. However, terrorism incidents are complex and require a number of agencies. This means the incident will likely involve a large EMS and fire/rescue response—possibly public health and public works—with the appropriate command responsibilities and challenges.

One solution is a single-agency incident commander, such as a sheriff or police chief, with EMS and fire/rescue operating at branch levels. The second solution is unified command. A unified command team is utilized when multiple agencies and/or disciplines have jurisdiction in a complex incident. Consider a bombing with a building collapse and mass casualties—clearly there are major EMS, fire/rescue, and law-enforcement operations that must effectively coordinate. In this case, a command post with a unified EMS/fire/law enforcement management team is the solution (**FIGURE 5-1**).

Unified command requires that all managers be located in the same area (a command post, vehicle, or an emergency operations center) to share information and maintain a common operational picture. The planning section guides this process with effective status displays, resource tracking, and comprehensive interagency action plans. Separate command posts for each major agency are not a workable solution because separated agencies and jurisdictions tend to freelance with poor interagency coordination. Unified command does not begin in the heat of battle—it starts with effective planning well before a terrorism incident. The responsibility of each agency must be specifically defined and written. Emergency management facilitates the formal development of unified command through the local comprehensive EOP.

In many ways, the informal development of unified command is more significant than the formal process. Managers must get to know each other. The corporate world uses the term **networking**. It means that various agency managers initiate mutual support by breaking bread and sharing coffee—this informal process is the first

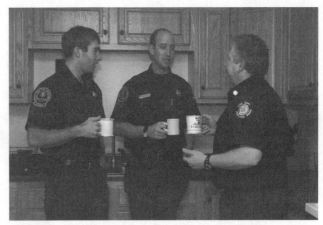

FIGURE 5-2 The informal process of building trust with colleagues or networking.

step in building trust (**FIGURE 5-2**). A community disaster committee is an excellent vehicle to schedule quarterly meetings where mutual incident command issues are discussed and agency heads develop mutual trust. Joint training exercises also facilitate interagency networking. Managers cannot meet each other for the first time in a major incident and expect to coordinate effectively.

Operations

The EOP must identify operations agencies in the local/regional area that are trained and equipped to handle specific operational problems. Obviously, EMS, fire, public health, and law enforcement have clearly defined and visible tasks. However, terrorism incidents present unique resource management and operational problems. Many of these issues require special teams that may not be available within the immediate area. Special terrorism operational requirements include the following:

1. Heavily armed tactical teams to combat terrorists with automatic weapons.
2. Hazardous materials teams equipped to detect, penetrate, and decontaminate radiological incidents.
3. EMS teams with protective equipment that triage, treat, and transport large numbers of victims.
4. A decontamination unit that decontaminates hundreds of victims in a chemical attack.
5. A public health unit that detects and tracks mass disease victims (medical surveillance/epidemiology) in a biological attack.
6. Search and rescue teams for structural collapse incidents.
7. Cyber forensics teams.

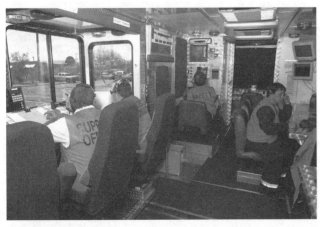

FIGURE 5-1 A command post should be coordinated by a unified EMS/fire/law enforcement management team.

These scenarios are not common incidents. At the time of this writing, few cities in the United States have the capability of managing all of these events. If special teams are not locally available, the plan must identify other sources. These resources include federal response teams, military units, state and regional agencies, and private-sector resources.

In reality, no single local government can afford all the anticipated resources. However, an effective threat assessment and planning process reveals areas of vulnerability and identifies possible operational units capable of threat response.

Resource Management

Terrorism incidents are often destructive because resources—personnel, equipment, and supplies—are consumed faster than they are replaced. A small bombing with few casualties is manageable, but a major terrorism or disaster incident rapidly depletes responders, vehicles, supplies, medications, and hospital beds. Examples of critical needs in terrorism incidents are:

- Emergency responders
- Weapons/crime scene supplies
- EMS units
- Personal protective equipment (ensembles and breathing equipment)
- Medical supplies and equipment
- Emergency Department/surgical facilities
- Detection and decontamination equipment
- Vehicles/aircraft
- Medical laboratories
- Medications/antidotes (pharmaceutical cache)
- Communications

In long-duration incidents, there is an added demand for crew rehabilitation, food/water, sleeping facilities, and sanitation measures. An effective plan addresses these resource and logistics management issues. The plan is based on the correct assumption that first response resources are immediately depleted. Resources that support the previous problem areas are outlined in the plan. There are several solutions for critical logistics needs such as:

1. Logistics caches for regional support, such as a decontamination cache of washing supplies, protective equipment, and 100 ensembles.
2. Mutual aid agreements with local, state, and federal agencies or jurisdictions.
3. A MACS to complement incident logistics activities.

4. Military support including a memorandum of understanding with local military installations and state National Guard units for critical personnel or equipment.
5. Private contracting, such as an agreement with a chemical spill response company to provide chemical spill control or radiation equipment.
6. State/federal support, such as procedures for requesting state and federal logistical support; and a nationwide pharmaceutical cache system.

Logistics caches must be packaged and stored for rapid deployment. A logistics trailer or truck is recommended. In rural systems, supplies can be stored in plastic containers for immediate loading on vehicles. Caches should not be stored in closets or back rooms where they gather dust. Supplies should be accessible, packaged, and maintained in good condition for utilization in high-impact, low-frequency incidents (**FIGURE 5-3**).

Cost and quantities are challenging issues—how much should be bought and what is affordable? The history of the local area and the political climate greatly influence the financial commitment. A selling point is that equipment caches are resources for all hazards—not just terrorism. The question of quantities is complex—there is no formula based on population or threat assessment to determine how much protective equipment or how many body bags or atropine injections a community needs. It seems obvious that high-threat urban areas need the largest caches, but what about a small college town that has a football stadium with 50,000 fans on Saturdays in autumn? Again, there is no definitive answer. In some areas of the country, communities have developed a spoke and hub system to move resources and medication as dictated by incidents and events. Routine movement of these resources is a good dress rehearsal for resource deployment in large or high-impact incidents.

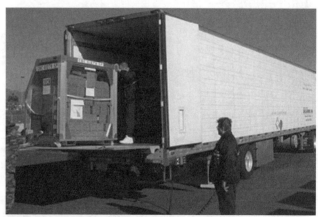

FIGURE 5-3 The Centers for Disease Control and Prevention Strategic National Stockpile can deliver one of many push packs to any location in the country within 12 hours of an emergency.

At a minimum, there should be enough medications and protective equipment for first responders and mutual aid personnel. This sounds self-serving, but the logic is irrefutable. Responders must protect themselves to ensure survivability. Key resource management points are as follows:

1. Resource management takes planning.
2. Equipment and supplies must be transferred quickly to a scene.
3. Logistics caches must be accessible and maintained.
4. Budgets and political realities will always be resource management issues.
5. Estimates of resource quantities are at best a semieducated guess.
6. Responders need certified protective equipment.

Administration

Administrative functions are omitted from most emergency plans. In normal operations, individual agencies take care of the usual administrative duties such as finance/purchasing, workman's compensation, and payroll records. During major disasters, administrative requirements escalate—normal administration is no longer suitable. For example, purchasing and contracting in the middle of the night or tracking personnel from state and national agencies are functions that local agency administrative personnel have not experienced. Many responders do not consider fiscal accountability until issues arise for expenditures that may exceed $1 million per day. To summarize, consider and plan for the administration and financial challenges of a major terrorism incident.

Comprehensive Planning

The EOP is usually developed and maintained by the local emergency management agency, an interagency disaster committee, or both. An effective emergency manager plays a coordinating role in bringing competing agencies together and implementing the EOP. Response and support agency managers should participate in the EOP development. The document should be formal and

CRITICAL FACTOR ....

An operations/logistics mindset must not interfere with the administrative needs of a major terrorism incident.

approved as indicated by appropriate signatures. When conflicts arise, the EOP serves as a template to remind participants of their responsibilities.

The EOP should establish the position of planning section chief for disasters and terrorism incidents. The planning section chief is responsible for developing the IAP, conducting planning briefings, and supervising the resource, situation, documentation, and demobilization units along with technical advisors (refer to Chapter 2).

EOP Summary

The EOP is a comprehensive plan (sometimes called a comprehensive emergency management plan) that uses the NIMS and the NRF as templates to establish an interagency plan for terrorism incidents. The key steps in the implementation phase of an EOP are:

1. Coordinate with local/regional response agencies.
2. Assign EOP responsibility to emergency management or a disaster committee.
3. Conduct a community terrorism threat assessment.
4. Identify operational and resource needs based on the threat assessment.
5. Produce a formal document signed by cooperating agency managers.
6. Perceive the EOP as an evolving document that is always a work in progress.
7. Test the EOP in exercises and revise the plan based on lessons learned.

The EOP key elements:

1. Specify who is in charge.
2. Make provisions for unified command in complex incidents.
3. Establish a command staff for public information, safety, and liaison.
4. Establish an operations section and identify operations agencies.
5. Establish a logistics section for resource management and logistics requirements.
6. Establish a planning section.
7. Establish an administration/finance section.
8. Conduct comprehensive NIMS training for all levels in the incident command system (ICS).
9. Conduct tabletop and operational exercises to test your plan.

Smaller communities are overwhelmed with the personnel demands of a full-scale EOP implementation. Remember that in any disaster, ICS positions are filled only as needed. The critical concept is that any function not assigned by the incident commander is his or her responsibility. It is important to identify critical personnel from other support agencies or mutual aid agencies and train them on their operational responsibilities per the NIMS. This is especially significant in locales that have inadequate staffing.

The Incident Action Plan

An **incident action plan (IAP)** is a plan of objectives for implementing an overall incident strategy. The IAP is a tactical plan for an operational period. Unlike the EOP, the IAP is related to a specific incident and a set of dynamic circumstances. The EOP is reference oriented, whereas the IAP is action oriented.

On routine incidents or small mass casualty events, the incident commander follows a protocol without a written plan. Planning is on the fly with the aid of a quick checklist. Major incidents need a formal IAP because escalating and dynamic variables require increased resources over an extended time period. Major incidents may geographically expand, requiring several divisions. Incidents of this nature present major planning problems, including the fact that incident or unified commanders cannot keep all of the strategies in their heads. No single individual can plan all the strategies without consultation and help. Written documents are needed to clarify and convey the strategies, objectives, and assignments to others.

The solution is a formalized IAP. When do you go formal? is a valid question. In short-duration incidents usually lasting less than one operational period, a verbal and informal plan suffices. When an incident progresses beyond an 8-hour operational period, a written plan is prepared, briefed, and distributed to operational shifts. This is especially important if 24-hour operations are continued. If night operations are scaled down, a daily briefing is adequate.

The development of an 8-hour or daily IAP is demanding for the planning section chief. Fortunately, there is a nationally accepted format developed by the National Wildfire Coordinating Group. This format has been adopted by NIMS for all-hazard incidents, including terrorism events. There are several forms associated with the IAP that serve as checklists, completed by the appropriate supervisor, and this greatly eases the IAP process. ICS forms are available via the Federal Emergency Management Agency (FEMA) ICS resource center, http://training.fema.gov/EM/Web/IS/ICSResource/ICSResCntr_Forms.htm. The forms, listed next, address critical planning areas.

1. ICS 202, Incident Objectives—includes basic strategy/objectives for the overall incident and includes critical areas such as safety concerns and forecasted weather.
2. ICS 203, Organizational Assignment List—includes operations sections with all branch directors and division/group supervisors; includes logistics section, planning section, and finance (administration) section with the respective units for each section.
3. ICS 204, Division Assignment List—a list for each branch (operations), divisions assigned to each branch, division managers, and units assigned to each division.
4. ICS 205, Incident Radio Communications Plan—lists administrative frequencies, operations frequencies, and tactical channels; lists telephone numbers for managers and key agencies; and specifies an overall communications plan, including secondary and tertiary communications networks.
5. ICS 206, Medical Plan—formalizes medical support for overhead team and on-scene responders; includes nearest hospitals, medical frequencies, and a roster of EMS units. Note: In mass casualty incidents, medical operations are delineated in ICS 204 relating to organizational assignments and division assignments.
6. ICS 220, Air Operations Summary Worksheet—lists all air units, air objectives, frequencies, and assignments.
7. Incident Map—a map, computer graphic, or aerial photo depicting the incident area.
8. Safety Plan—safety objectives and hazard warnings (prepared by the safety officer).

The formal IAP is not as overwhelming as it may appear. First, the forms serve as a checklist using fill-in-the-blank or electronic forms. Second, the IAP is a joint effort—the incident commander, operations, planning and logistics section chiefs, and specialized units such as medical, safety, weather, and communications contribute to the effort.

CRITICAL FACTOR ....

The IAP forms serve as an effective planning checklist. ICS forms facilitate the incident command process because the forms assist in maintaining span of control with checks and balances for achieving functional objectives. ICS forms are not intended to be used as checklists. However, the forms are an effective reminder of key ICS actions.

The IAP Briefing Cycle

In long-duration incidents, the IAP is presented during a formal briefing every 8, 12, or 24 hours. This is called a **planning briefing cycle**. The nature of the incident dictates the length of a shift, which is typically 12 hours in length. Some morning events use an 8-hour briefing cycle (at shift changes) or a 24-hour briefing cycle when there are diminished night operations. Effective planning section chiefs (like effective logistics section chiefs) complement and support the actions and decisions of incident commanders.

The briefing is a very important formal process. The briefing must be concise and short in duration—an average briefing of 30 minutes or less is desirable. All section-level and division-level managers, along with appropriate unit leaders, should attend the briefing—a 50-person audience or more is not unusual in a complex event. The IAP is presented by the planning section chief and includes briefings by other specialists such as weather, safety, and technical experts. The technical experts specialize in the medical, radiological, and bio-weapons fields, etc.

Copies of the IAP are distributed to each attendee. An IAP may be ten pages in length in a major disaster or terrorism incident. The IAP copies are a reference for all managers, especially the sections on communications frequencies, unit assignments, and safety procedures.

The National Wildfire Coordinating Group publishes the formal planning guidelines in the *Fireline Handbook*. The California *FIRESCOPE Field Operations Guide* contains similar material. These documents are specific to wildland firefighting, but the guidelines are adaptable to nonfire disciplines. In a 12-hour briefing cycle, IAP preparation progresses as follows:

1. Shift change—receive field observations; 1 hour.
2. Prepare for planning meeting; 1 hour.
3. Planning meeting with management staff, section chiefs, agency representatives; 1 hour.
4. Prepare IAP; 4 hours.
5. Finalize IAP; 2 hours.
6. Prepare for operations briefing; 1 hour.
7. Briefing of management staff, section chiefs, branch/division/unit supervisors; 1 hour.
8. Finalize reports; 1 hour.

The briefing cycle is a flexible guide that can be shortened or lengthened as appropriate.

To demonstrate the use of an EOP and informal and formal IAPs, consider the scenario in the accompanying case study.

CASE STUDY

It is 09:30 hours in Denney City, California. There is an explosion originating from a parked van on Center Street. One person is killed, 14 people are injured, and windows are shattered throughout the block.

A law enforcement unit arrives at 09:32; fire/rescue and EMS units arrive at 09:35. At 09:41, there is a massive explosion in a complex of government buildings immediately adjacent to the van explosion site. Many of the first responders are injured. A five-story building collapses (estimated occupancy of 500 people). The major trauma center next to the building is heavily damaged; there are multiple injuries in the hospital from flying glass.

The EOP

The Denney City EOP has several sections directly related to an explosives attack on building complexes based on the history of the Oklahoma City and World Trade Center bombings and a local emergency management threat assessment. Key response agencies immediately consult checklists based on elements of the EOP. Critical agency managers, as well as the state operations center, are immediately notified. The EOP is based on the NIMS and the NRF and identifies several critical areas, including the following:

- Command—A unified command team is specified, with unified command among law enforcement, EMS, and fire/rescue.
- Operations—The three critical operations branches are law enforcement, fire/rescue, and EMS. The EOP lists state/federal law enforcement mutual aid assets, procedures for fire mutual aid, urban search and rescue teams, regional medical response, and the activation of a disaster medical assistance team.
- Logistics—The resource management plan establishes a MACS at the EOC and lists resources for scene control, vehicles, lighting, generators, back-up communications, fuel, emergency food, construction equipment, and lumber for shoring.

- Administration/finance—Specifies that expenditures, claims, and worker's compensation issues be tracked and establishes the city purchasing director as the supervisor of expenditures.
- Planning—Establishes the activation of the EOC by emergency management and the establishment of a fully staffed planning section if the incident becomes protracted, including a resource unit and a situation unit.

The Informal IAP

Managers begin arriving and command is formally transferred from the first arriving engine company officer to a fire battalion chief. It is apparent that a major incident is in progress. A police captain and the battalion chief establish a command post four blocks from the incident. An informal IAP is developed in minutes by identifying critical factors. This plan is communicated verbally and by radio to response managers and units. The key elements are:

1. All units search their operational and staging areas for possible secondary devices.
2. The following three divisions are established: collapse division, Center Street division (including the van explosion), and trauma center division (the EOP never addressed the loss of the trauma center).
3. A reconnaissance group is established to assess damage on all sides of the original explosion.
4. Immediate control of the scene perimeter is established by law enforcement.
5. Appropriate EMS, law enforcement, and fire units are assigned to groups/divisions.
6. Triage, treatment, and transport of mass casualty incident victims throughout the incident area are addressed.

New problems include an area power failure and the loss of the downtown communications repeater. There is also disturbing information that many victims appear to have chemical injuries—a combination explosive/chemical attack is suspected. As these problems evolve, the IAP is revised accordingly.

The unified command team becomes aware in the first hour that this is a complex, long-duration incident. As a result, they request a preestablished management team for full staffing of NIMS/ICS positions. This management team is comprised of NIMS-certified personnel from a multitude of local and state response agencies.

Day Two—The Formal IAP

The planning section, in coordination with the unified command team and the logistics and operations section chiefs, develops the IAP. Emergency management maintains a MAC. The formal action plan is developed using a laptop computer and ICS forms 202-206. Copies are made for each member of the management team and all branch directors and division/group supervisors.

The second day also dawns with the arrival of federal assistance. The Federal Bureau of Investigation has a full response team assigned to law enforcement operations. A National Guard team is assigned to the hazardous materials branch for detection and decontamination. Last, state police units are assigned to law enforcement operations for perimeter security.

FIGURE 5-4 demonstrates an overview of the IAP for an incident of this level. These pages include incident objectives and safety (ICS 202) and an incident medical plan (ICS 206).

Chapter Summary

Planning for terrorism is a front-end concept. For a successful tactical outcome on the back end, effective planning must occur at the front end. The model of an effective EOP is the NIMS and the NRF. The EOP addresses the key NIMS functions of command staff, operations, logistics, planning, and administration/finance. The command component identifies who is in charge and recognizes the concept of unified management. The operations section identifies operations agencies/teams based on an emergency management threat assessment.

Terrorism incidents and disasters consume resources rapidly. The logistics section of an EOP must identify logistics needs and agencies or organizations that provide the appropriate people, supplies, and equipment. In a major event, logistical support may be regional, state,

FIGURE 5-4 Incident action plan overview example.

INCIDENT OBJECTIVES	1. INCIDENT NAME Denney City explosion	2. DATE PREPARED 3/1/2010	3. TIME PREPARED 05:37

4. OPERATIONAL PERIOD (DATE/TIME) 08:00 to 20:00

5. GENERAL CONTROL OBJECTIVES FOR THE INCIDENT (INCLUDE ALTERNATIVES)
Scene control entry/exit
Detailed secondary search
Evidence recovery and preservation
Chemical detection and decontamination
Heavy rescue
Equip and reopen trauma center

6. WEATHER FORECAST FOR OPERATIONAL PERIOD
Heavy fog restricting visibility to 10:30
Wind light from 270 deg.
50% chance rain from 17:00 to 19:00

7. GENERAL/SAFETY MESSAGE
Type of chemical(s) not confirmed in collapse area; treat entire area as hot zone.
Full PPE required in hot zones
Bio precautions for all divisions
Possible nondetonated explosives; possible secondary devices
Lightning in afternoon thunderstorms

8. ATTACHMENTS (X IF ATTACHED)

• ORGANIZATION LIST (ICS 203) **XXX**	INCIDENT MAPS (2)	Safety Message **XXX**
• DIVISION ASSIGNMENT LIST (ICS 204) **XXX**	TRAFFIC PLAN	Homestead Map
• COMMUNICATIONS PLAN (ICS 205) **XXX**	Air Operations	Structural Fire Plan
• Summary (ICS 220) **XXX**		
• MEDICAL PLAN (ICS 206) **XXX**		

202 ICS	9. PREPARED BY (PLANNING SECTION CHIEF) James	10. APPROVED BY (INCIDENT COMMANDER) Colby

MEDICAL PLAN	1. INCIDENT NAME Denney City explosion	2. DATE PREPARED 3/1/2010	3. TIME PREPARED 06:30	4. OPERATIONAL PERIOD 08:00 to 20:00

5. INCIDENT MEDICAL AID STATIONS

MEDICAL AID STATIONS	LOCATION CONTACT THROUGH DISPATCH	PARAMEDICS	
		YES	NO
Pratt treatment group	123 Pratt St.	XXX	
Center St. treatment group	704 Center St.	XXX	

(continues)

FIGURE 5-4 *(Continued)*

6. TRANSPORTATION

A. AMBULANCE SERVICES

NAME	ADDRESS	PHONE	PARAMEDICS	
			YES	NO
Denney City EMS/ mutual aid	Citywide 754 Main Ave.	555-2376	XXX	
Johnson Co. EMS	County-wide 117 Wilson St.	555-2311	XXX	

B. INCIDENT AMBULANCES

NAME	LOCATION	PARAMEDICS	
		YES	NO
Orange Co. 62, 64, 17, 28	Trauma center	XXX	
Denney City EMS 2, 4, 6, 9	Center St.	XXX	
Johnson Co. medic 4, 5, 8, 12	Hazardous materials operations–Center St.	XXX	

7. HOSPITAL NAME	ADDRESS	TRAVEL TIME (Hr)		PHONE	HELIPAD		BURN CENTER	
		AIR	GRD		YES	NO	YES	NO
Sim City Trauma Center	123 Pratt St.	N/A	1	555-2624	XXX			
Baptist Hospital	2766 Mullen Dr.	10	30	555-4555	XXX			
Mount Sinai	1749 125th Ave.	5	15	555-4002	XXX		X	

8. MEDICAL EMERGENCY PROCEDURES

All pediatric victims to Baptist; burn victims to Mount Sinai

All divisions have EMS coverage–requests for additional EMS medical branch directors

206 ICS 8/78	9. PREPARED BY (MEDICAL UNIT LEADER) Christen	10. REVIEWED BY (SAFETY OFFICER) Maniscalco

or federal and coordinated by a MACS. Critical logistics requires logistics caches (push logistics) that are quickly deployed to a scene.

An EOP also identifies an administration section and a planning section. The administration section includes a time unit, a procurement unit, and a compensation unit. The planning section consists of a resource unit, situation unit, and mobilization/demobilization unit. An EOP is a reference tool, and not a tactical guide. Terrorism incidents are extremely dynamic where critical events change in seconds or minutes. In the fog of "combat," the incident commander develops an informal and verbal IAP. The informal plan should be followed by a formal IAP if the incident is significant and/or longer in duration than a quick-response incident.

A long-duration incident (longer than a day) requires a written IAP developed by the planning section chief in coordination with the incident commander and other section chiefs. The National Wildfire Coordinating Group has developed forms for the IAP. The forms serve as a checklist for organizing the event. All section groups and divisions are given a daily briefing along with copies of the IAP.

Wrap Up

Chapter Questions

1. Define the front-end concept of planning.
2. What are the key elements in the NIMS, and how do they relate to planning?
3. What are the key elements in the NRF, and how do they relate to planning?
4. Why is administration important in a long-duration terrorism incident?
5. What are the key steps in the implementation of an EOP?
6. What are the key elements in an EOP?
7. What factors determine if an IAP is formal or informal?
8. Define an IAP briefing cycle. What are the related steps in the cycle?

Chapter Project I

Obtain an after-action report of a major incident in your community or state. Based on the incident report, develop an IAP for the incident by using ICS forms 202 and 206 (pages 8–10). Establish NIMS sections and use the branch/division concept.

Chapter Project II

You have been appointed as the emergency manager in your community. Your elation is short lived when you find out your first assignment is to develop an EOP. Develop a community EOP by observing the following principles:

- Obtain a realistic threat assessment or design a hypothetical threat assessment.
- Identify key operations agencies.
- Determine who will be the incident manager in various types of incidents.
- Identify resource entities at a local and regional level.
- Identify sources of support personnel and support agencies.

Vital Vocabulary

Emergency operations plan (EOP) A comprehensive interagency and interdisciplinary plan identifying the key elements of the terrorism response continuum using the NIMS and NRF as templates.

Front-end plan Planning for anticipated incidents rather than waiting for an incident to occur before developing a plan.

Incident action plan (IAP) A plan that contains objectives that reflect the incident strategy and specific control actions for the current or next operational period. An IAP is verbal in the early stages of an incident.

Multiagency coordination system (MACS) A system of coordinated entities and off-scene resource processes organized as a full-scale logistics system to support the resource requirements of single or multiple incidents in a local area or region. Entities in the MACS include government agencies, nongovernment agencies, volunteer organizations, and private-sector resources.

Networking A process (formal and informal) of collaboration and relationship building leading to trust and mutual support between individuals, agencies, and organizations.

Planning briefing cycle An 8-, 12-, or 24-hour cycle encompassing the development of the IAP and the conduct of an IAP briefing by the planning section chief in collaboration with the incident commander.

Resilience The organizational elasticity to bounce back or recover from unexpected events.

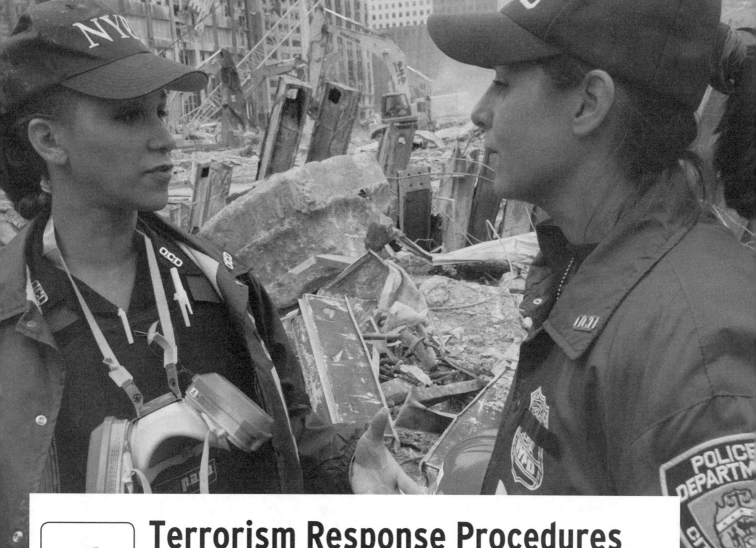

6

Terrorism Response Procedures

Hank T. Christen
Paul M. Maniscalco

Objectives

- Define convergent responders and discuss how convergent responder agencies relate to first responders.
- Discuss the critical importance of scene awareness in a dynamic terrorism incident.
- List and describe the on-scene complications present in a terrorism incident.
- List the responsibilities of the first arriving unit in a terrorism incident.
- Define the principles of 2 in 2 out and lookout, awareness, communications, escape, and safety.
- Outline the key elements in a terrorism response protocol.
- Outline critical hospital response issues.

Introduction

Response to an emergency is a routine function of public safety agencies. Thousands of times each day around the world, EMS, fire, rescue, and law enforcement agencies respond and effectively handle a myriad of incidents. However, no terrorism incident is an average or ordinary incident. Initial responders are confronted with unfamiliar, unpredictable, and unsafe scenes. There is often a combined mass casualty incident, rescue, hazardous materials incident, and crime scene scenario. No matter how global an incident becomes, it starts with convergent responders trying to assist (more on this in later paragraphs) and first responders being overwhelmed upon arrival at the scene.

While many emergency scenarios share some similar characteristics and response demands, none are routine, and all pose complex and confusing environments for the arriving emergency responders. Consider the following cases of terrorism incidents:

- **Virginia Tech University** (2007)—A single student shot and killed 31 students and teachers and wounded 17 others at multiple locations on the Virginia Tech campus.
- **Mumbai, India** (2008)—A planned and coordinated attack by at least nine Islamic extremist gunmen killed a total of 164 people and injured 308 people. The attack took place in at least ten locations and involved a combination of automatic weapons, hand grenades, and bombs. A major fire was set at the Taj Mahal hotel during the attack. The terrorists were eventually killed by Indian security forces. Similar attacks on Pakistani police stations occurred in 2009.
- **Geneva, Alabama** (2009)—A lone, heavily armed gunman attacked his family and co-workers in four separate locations in southeastern Alabama before killing himself. He began by killing his mother and setting her house on fire. There was a total of 11 dead, including a small child.
- **Oakland, California and Pittsburgh, Pennsylvania** (2009)—Within a 10-day period, four police officers were killed in Oakland and three police officers were killed in Pittsburgh. Both cases involved a single gunman.
- **Binghamton, New York** (2009)—A heavily armed gunman entered the American Civic Association where foreign immigrants were taking were taking a test for U.S. citizenship.

He killed 13 people before turning a gun on himself. Four people were wounded. No emergency responders were injured.

- **Fort Hood, Texas** (2009)—A single gunman with an automatic handgun opened fire on U.S. Army soldiers and civilians at a processing facility for personnel deploying to Iraq. Thirteen people were killed and 29 people were wounded. The alleged perpetrator, an army psychiatrist, was engaged by police officers and seriously wounded.

ABC News reported that there have been 50 mass shootings in the United States in a time period from the Virginia Tech incident to the mass killings in Binghamton. Collectively, these incidents share certain common denominators. Entire communities were terrorized. In each incident, local emergency response resources were severely stressed and initially overwhelmed. Law enforcement officers were killed or wounded in several cases. The initial response was quickly followed by intense national media exposure. The Mumbai incident was terrorism related because of the political nature of the attacks. In the other cases, individuals had differing motives, but used extreme violence to accomplish their goals. Ultimately, in each case, fire, emergency medical, and law enforcement agencies needed a robust emergency response plan and effective incident command system (ICS) to manage the incidents successfully.

First responders manage an incident for hours or possibly a day before state and federal resources arrive to support the local effort. Reliance upon state or federal assets as initial responders is unwise because regional, state, and federal resources often have extended response times. The time it takes for these resources to arrive at most emergencies creates a vast disadvantage that may result in great detriment to the responders, victims, and the community. Clearly, it is in the best interests of policy officials and emergency planners to ensure that local personnel and jurisdictions are capable of mounting an effective and sustainable response to high-impact/high-yield incidents.

Convergent Responders

Convergent responders are citizens or workers from nonemergency agencies who witness a terrorism incident and converge on the scene. In most incidents, convergent responders arrive first because attacks usually occur in a public setting where private citizens witness the incident, call 911, and take some form of action. In the cases previously discussed, convergent responders played a role in the outcomes. Fire, EMS, and law enforcement officers are known as first responders, but they almost never arrive first; convergent responders usually arrive first, and first responders usually arrive second.

Many response professionals perceive convergent responders in a negative light. Convergent responders are viewed as undisciplined and in the way. This perception is often inaccurate. In many disaster and terrorism incidents, video footage shows convergent responders digging victims out of rubble, manning hose lines, or rendering first aid to victims (**FIGURE 6-1**). Convergent responders are the people who call 911 to report a terrorism incident and provide vital incident information to the 911 operator or dispatcher. This information is often conflicting and sometimes hysterical, but multiple calls paint an initial picture that is important for determining the nature of an incident and the level of response.

Realistically, convergent responders can become victims and create a crowd, and they may hinder initial response efforts. On the surface, it appears that the good and the bad aspects of convergent responders are beyond control. This is not the case. First responder agencies are often unaware that many convergent responders are from organized and disciplined entities. At any moment, a local street may have potential convergent agencies, companies, or individuals performing work assignments. These organizations include:

1. Utility crews such as power, gas, telephone, and cable crews
2. Postal workers and express delivery services (like FedEx or UPS) workers
3. Meter readers and inspectors

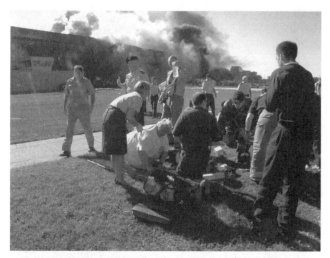

FIGURE 6-1 Arlington, Va. (September 11, 2001): Medical personnel and convergent responders work the first medical triage area set up outside the Pentagon after a hijacked commercial airliner crashed into the southwest corner of the building.

4. Transit authority, school bus and taxi drivers
5. Public works crews
6. Social workers or probation officers
7. Private security agents
8. Real estate agents
9. Crime watch and neighborhood watch volunteers

Many of these people are in radio-equipped vehicles or have cellular telephones and provide early and accurate reports of a suspicious scene or a terrorism incident in progress. Festivals, events, and public assembly buildings have security guards, ushers, ticket takers, and concession workers who are employees of formal organizations.

With training, convergent agencies are a positive initial response component. The level of training is similar to the hazardous materials awareness model. Members of convergent agencies are exposed to basic awareness material in the following subject areas:

- A brief overview of terrorism history and local threats
- Recognition of potential threats such as suspicious people, weapons, or devices
- Procedures for reporting an incident and the critical information needed by 911 communications
- Safe scene control and personal safety
- Basic first aid techniques

While it may not be practical to conduct awareness training for most of the public, adoption of the **community emergency response team (CERT)** initiative and online NIMS training is a mechanism to acquaint members of the community with an awareness of emergency actions and their roles at an incident.

It is feasible to identify agencies that are possible convergent responders, solicit their participation, and assist them with basic awareness training. This concept is similar to CERT programs or law enforcement agency training programs for developing volunteer crime/neighborhood watch organizations. Convergent responders are a viable force that the emergency service community needs to collaborate with because convergent responders usually arrive at an emergency incident first.

Scene Awareness

A terrorism incident is a dynamic and unstable scene. The area is a hot zone that may include chemical/biological/radiological hazards, individuals firing weapons (on both sides), explosive devices, secondary devices or booby traps, fires, collapsed structures, and multiple injured victims screaming for assistance. Timewise, first responders arrive when the incident is starting (stumbling into a minefield), when it is already over (sometimes responders are lucky), or somewhere in between (usually the case).

Scene awareness principles begin before the response to any incident (routine or terrorism). Familiarity with the neighborhood, the surroundings, and the violence history of the area is important. Does the area have a gang history? Are special events being held? Is the stadium full or empty? Is there recent unrest such as political protests or union/labor issues? Are special religious ceremonies being held? These questions only scratch the surface of information that response agencies must consider before the 911 call. In fact, this type of information (intelligence) should be obtained pre-event if possible and incorporated into an organization's intelligence fusion and preincident response plans.

During an emergency response, scene awareness is critical because terrorism 911 calls seldom provide accurate descriptions of incidents. An incident dispatched as a single shooting might evolve into a mass shooting with automatic weapons. A suspicious package report can become a pipe bomb explosion, and a report of respiratory distress at a stadium evolves into a chemical release with contamination and mass casualties.

While en route, responders should consider the possibility that the scene is far worse than the initial information. Key preresponse knowledge must be mentally replayed. For example, when responding to a high-profile facility for an unknown medical situation, responders should expect more than a simple medical patient. Radio traffic must be closely monitored because responders cannot afford to miss additional information about scene conditions. Local protocol must emphasize that new information be immediately forwarded to all responding units. Radio traffic from convergent responder agencies and other emergency response agencies is critical. Weather information, especially speed and direction, is also important.

When responders get close enough for the scene to appear in the distance, they need to carefully scan the landscape, especially the entire scene periphery (this is limited at night or in bad weather). This process is called a **windshield survey**. Likewise, on arrival, responders have a tendency to get tunnel vision. Tunnel vision means that responders have a tendency to concentrate on their area of responsibility. For example, EMS focuses on victims, firefighters focus on fires, and law enforcement officers focus on a crime scene. These are habits based on years of practice that are detrimental in a complex

terrorism incident. Responders need to force themselves to look around the incident. If threats are seen or suspected, responders should stop or possibly retreat. Experience and intuition should always be trusted.

Staging is another important protection posture for high-hazard incident scenes. Staging means that nonessential and support units stand by in a nearby safe zone awaiting further orders or assignments. In the ICS, the staging area is managed by a staging officer who tracks staged resources and coordinates unit assignments with the incident commander. The staging concept enhances scene safety because staging ensures minimal exposure to units that are not operating in the high-hazard zone.

Responders are especially vulnerable when exiting vehicles. For example, Fire Fighter Ryan Hummert of the Maplewood Fire Department (St. Louis County, Missouri) was shot and killed in 2008 when exiting his apparatus for a vehicle fire. A sniper also wounded two police officers before taking his own life. Step one for responders is to look for indications of an unsafe scene. This initial scene survey includes looking up, down, and around the periphery of the scene. Responders should look for any indication of people with weapons, explosive devices, or evidence of a chemical agent. Bodies or unconscious victims may unfortunately indicate a hot zone where entry requires appropriate personal protective equipment.

The Occupational Safety and Health Administration (OSHA) has established guidelines for the structural fire service that are referred to as **2 in 2 out**. These guidelines specify that two members should enter a fire hot zone, remain in personal contact, and exit together. Two others remain outside for backup purposes. This principle is similar to the buddy principle that children are taught in swimming lessons. The 2 in 2 out principle is a rule that applies to all first responders (EMS, fire, and law enforcement) in a terrorism incident when the scene is unstable. Responders must work in teams.

Another effective scene principle is one adopted from the wildland fire community and suggested for terrorism by retired Assistant Chief Phil Chovan of the Marietta, Georgia, fire and rescue department. The principle is called **lookout, awareness, communications, escape, and safety (LACES)** (**FIGURE 6-2**). These

---

CRITICAL FACTOR ....

Responders should not become blinded by tunnel vision. They should survey the entire scene, including the area above them, for threats to their safety.

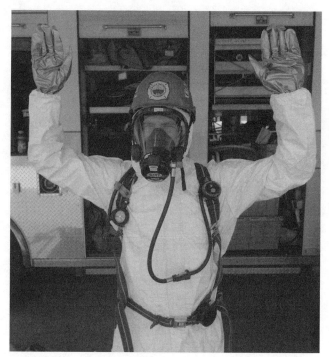

FIGURE 6-2 The LACES principle–Exposed crews must have effective communications, including direct hand signals such as holding hands in the air to signal that the responder is okay.

principles were developed from hard-learned lessons when wildland fires made sudden and unexpected changes in direction and/or intensity and trapped fire suppression crews. The same scene dynamics occur in a terrorism hot zone; especially when there is a chemical agent or automatic weapons fire.

L—**Lookout:** Someone is responsible for watching the overall scene from a safe distance and warning crews of danger.

A—**Awareness:** All members on the scene have situational awareness and are ready for dynamic changes and unpleasant surprises.

C—**Communications:** Exposed crews must have effective communications including direct voice or hand signals as well as portable radios.

E—**Escape:** Those on any unstable scene should plan an escape route and an alternate route.

S—**Safety** zones: Crews should escape to a safe area that provides distance, shielding, and/or up-wind protection.

Consider a mass-shooting example where a 911 caller describes shots fired with one possible victim in a warehouse. A first EMS unit finds a single victim by the doorway. A law enforcement unit declares the scene secured. A second EMS unit and engine company arrives and enters a large open floor space and finds six victims. The scene is quiet but does not look or feel right. Fire fighters begin searching in pairs using the 2 in 2 out principle. An EMS commander arrives and places himself as a lookout watching the street and the crime scene. Crews in the area look around the periphery and above (awareness). The lookout suddenly spots three men with weapons moving on the far side of the building. He broadcasts an evacuation message (communications) to the fire and medical crews who run along an escape route and retreat behind an industrial trash container (escape and safety). Heavy gunfire breaks out, but responders are safe because they used the LACES principle.

Active Shooter Response

On April 20, 1999, at Columbine High School near Littleton, Colorado, fourteen students were killed and twenty-one injured over a period of 22 minutes by two disturbed active shooters. It was a massacre that on-scene officers will never forget. It was also a wake-up call.

Before the Columbine shootings, law enforcement tactics dictated that responding officers protect the perimeter and wait for special weapons and tactics (SWAT) units instead of tactically engaging a shooter. This was sound wisdom in the pre-Columbine era because shooters almost always barricaded themselves with (or without) hostages and sometimes committed suicide. It made sense to wait for a SWAT unit and a negotiator to respond because they had the weapons, training, and protective equipment to ensure a successful outcome.

The Columbine situation was different. The shooters intended to die, not negotiate. They moved from one area to another, randomly shooting victims of opportunity. This pattern was repeated in other workplace shootings, a shopping center in Salt Lake City, Utah, and in university shootings including Virginia Tech and Northern Illinois University.

There were common threads in each of these cases. First, the incidents were well planned. The shooters were familiar with the layout of their crime scene. Second, they were well armed with handguns, assault rifles, shotguns, and in some cases explosives or incendiary devices. They carried extra ammunition and frequently reloaded. Last, they were shot by officers or committed suicide. Negotiations were not part of their plan. Today's **active shooter response** procedures are based on *quick action* by whatever group of law enforcement officers initially arrives. An effective active shooter policy *requires* a minimum of four officers to aggressively enter a building or structure with the intent of engaging an active shooter or shooters. In some agencies, a team of two or three officers can *choose* to engage a shooter. The primary objective is to save lives by neutralizing the shooter.

An active shooter response team uses a diamond-type formation consisting of a point officer, two utility officers, and a rear guard officer. Each officer has a designated function. The point officer is responsible for the front of the team. Utility officers offer side protection as unsecured areas are approached, and the rear officer protects the team from a rear attack.

An active shooter response team does not conduct a thorough search. The objective is to accomplish a primary sweep to locate victims and the shooter. In long-duration incidents, a coordinated search is necessary, but this is not an objective in the early response stage.

An equally significant objective is clearing the immediate area for rescue and medical treatment by fire/rescue and EMS units. Rescue and medical personnel do not have the training, weapons, or protective equipment to function in an uncleared area. It is essential that areas are cleared quickly to save lives.

The foundation of the active shooter response philosophy is *quick and coordinated engagement* instead of waiting for SWAT units. A rapidly assembled strike team must engage active shooters to save lives. Because active shooter incidents result in mass casualties, it is important to coordinate response actions with fire/rescue and EMS agencies.

The **law enforcement incident command system (LEICS)** provides a framework for managing and supporting active shooter incidents. Essential LEICS functions are organized using the ICS template and include command, a law enforcement operations section, a safety officer, and fire/EMS branches. Planning and logistics functions are established and expanded based on the needs and requirements of the incident. Further discussion of LEICS is beyond the scope of this text.

New Scenes—New Surprises

Twenty-first-century terrorism scenes offer new problems previously unseen by civilian responders. It is important to understand that first responders are not heroes to everyone. In fact, the purpose of an incident or attack may be to harm the emergency response troops.

Remember that any terrorism incident is a high-impact incident, which means there is a detrimental effect on a community's ability to deliver other 911 services. If possible, public safety managers should utilize the military principle of uncommitted reserves for 911 services and/or other terrorism incidents. In small communities, this principle requires early initiation of mutual aid resources and support. In summary, these managers must be prepared for diversions; there's no rule against having two simultaneous terrorism incidents occur on a very bad day.

Another trend is tactical ultraviolence. Terrorists, criminals, political militias, and street gangs carry the latest automatic weapons and wear body armor. Often law enforcement officers are outgunned. Responders are threatened by projectiles and fragmentation from concrete, glass, wood, and metals. There is also a danger of fire and EMS teams being caught in a crossfire between law enforcement officers and perpetrators.

The best defense is to avoid entering a ballistic hot zone by observing the scene awareness principles. The only protections for exposure to shooting are distance, concealment, and shielding. Concealment is the act of hiding to prevent detection. Shielding is the use of solid objects that cannot be penetrated by projectiles or explosive fragments. In most cases, vehicles are not effective for shielding. Although law enforcement officers might require body armor for shielding, fire and EMS responders who are in an area requiring body armor are in the wrong place.

Along with bombings and shootings, consider the brutal reality of a **chemical/biological/radiological (CBR)** hot zone. Biological mass casualties on a single scene are unlikely because biological effects take days or weeks to manifest themselves. Victims with biological ailments will be dispersed throughout a region, state, or the nation. Chemical attacks and radiological weapons are another story. First, the dispatch information is unlikely to paint a clear picture. The incident may begin with a report of a single victim having respiratory distress in a mass crowd venue such as a stadium, auditorium, or airport. Second, the usual indicators of a hazardous materials incident may not be present. The location might be benign of hazardous materials storage or transportation facilities and not have identifiable containers, placards, material safety data sheets, or shipping papers. First responders may not immediately recognize a chemical incident, and it could take hours before chemical agents are positively identified.

First responders must look for indicators and remember several important points, including:

1. Suspect a chemical agent in cases with several nontrauma victims with similar symptoms.
2. Check for multiple victims scattered throughout a crowd or facility.

3. Look for convergent responders who are symptomatic; beware of direct exposure or transfer of mechanism of injury from victims to responders.
4. If odors are noticed, responders must don breathing equipment and protective ensembles immediately.
5. In extreme cases, bodies may indicate a hot zone.
6. Radio traffic from other units is a key information source.
7. Establish a hot zone fast; remove walking victims.
8. Call for special teams quickly; control hot zone entry.
9. Set up a decontamination area for mass casualty victims.

Scene awareness in a chemical attack saves the lives of responders and victims. First responders must survey the scene, establish a hot zone, and observe safe hot zone entry principles. In all terrorism incidents, preparedness begins before arrival. Responders must use their senses and suspect anything that does not sound, look, or feel right. Use the safety principles of 2 in 2 out and LACES. Lastly, remember that the purpose of the incident may be to kill or injure first responders.

The First Arriving Unit

The first arriving unit has a drastic effect (positive or negative) on the progress of the incident because scene management and incident command builds from the bottom up. This means the first arriving unit is the incident commander and is responsible for operations, logistics, and planning. Obviously, this is an impossible task without prioritization.

CRITICAL FACTOR ....

Proper actions by the first responding units are critical for an effective outcome.

Getting help is the first priority. This process begins by making a quick scene survey and giving a radio report. The initial report involves taking command and describing the incident such as mass shooting victims or multiple nontrauma victims. A call for a number of people having food poisoning at the local food court could be a chemical incident. The first arriving unit must ensure that an initial report is acknowledged by dispatchers before taking further action.

Initial units should try to determine the scope of the hot zone, an approximate number of victims, and a mechanism of injury by questioning convergent responders or victims. It is critically important to transmit scene threats over the dispatch radio system and ensure that dispatchers relay this information to other units and agencies. Critical threat information includes:

1. Shooters on the scene or perpetrators with weapons
2. Suspicious device(s)
3. A possible CBR hot zone

As help arrives, the first arriving unit assigns operations actions. Command is relinquished by the first arriving unit when a senior officer, supervisor, or manager arrives. This process is done on a face-to-face basis and announced over the dispatch radio channel.

The following example demonstrates the responsibilities of the first arriving unit:

CASE STUDY 1

A call is dispatched for respiratory difficulty at a religious institution during worship services. Rescue 7 arrives at the front entrance. The first thing they see before even entering the building is that there are two victims on the building steps; they are experiencing respiratory difficulty with no apparent trauma. Several convergent responders are removing other victims from the building and everyone is coughing.

The unit transmits the following report: "Rescue 7 has 58th Street command; we have multiple respiratory victims; send two additional rescues and a chief officer; command post is in front of 5530 58th Street."

The Rescue 7 paramedic sends her EMT partner into the building to begin triage and obtain a victim count. The EMT stops at the doorway after discovering at least ten victims inside gasping for breath. The building interior is too hot to enter.

The paramedic orders the EMT out of the area and transmits the following report: "58th Street Command, emergency traffic; we have at least ten respiratory victims in the building. Declaring a hot zone in the interior and front entrance for unknown chemical agent; request a full first-alarm fire response and the hazardous materials team; request law enforcement for scene control; notify emergency management."

Scene Control

In any emergency incident, scene control is a difficult issue. Terrorism incidents present new and challenging scene control problems. The objective of scene control is to establish a secure perimeter around the scene/hot zone for the purpose of controlling entry and exit from the incident area (**FIGURE 6-3**). Entry control prevents civilians or media from converging on the area. Effective scene control also establishes entry/exit points where personnel and units are logged in/out for accountability purposes. Unfortunately, terrorism hot zones are very dynamic (the scene can grow in many directions). Shooters on the move or rooftop snipers expand an incident by several blocks. The discovery of an unexploded device or a secondary device requires an evacuation area of 1,000 feet or more in every direction including up and maybe down.

Preventing victims from leaving the hot zone is a new scene control issue unfamiliar to most responders. In a CBR incident, it is important to keep victims in an evacuation area to prevent contaminated victims from spreading the mechanism of injury. When victims leave in many different directions, they contaminate vehicles, people, and buildings (**FIGURE 6-4**). In urban areas, commuters board trains or return home in their cars, only to later present at suburban emergency rooms.

The solution to this problem is difficult. First, there is no corporate memory of a large civilian CBR incident. However, if large-scale industrial accidents are indicators, there will be great difficulty in control-

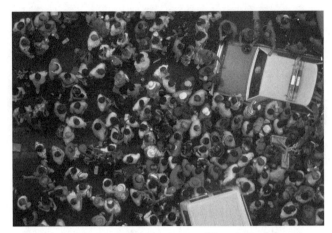

FIGURE 6-4 Victims leave incidents in many different directions and endanger effective scene control.

ling victim exits. Many victims will leave before first responders arrive, especially if untrained convergent responders are eager to transport them. Other victims will heed warnings to stay in place, but later grow impatient while waiting for decontamination. Lastly, some victims will resist the indignity of stripping down to their underwear to have themselves and their loved ones scrubbed by men or women in hazardous materials suits.

Responders should realize that many victims will initially leave the scene. This is why it is crucial for medical facilities to have an aggressive decontamination plan. Secondary victims have to be decontaminated as dictated by practicality. In most cases (not all), basic steps of clothing removal and washdown, done quickly, will suffice. Responders who lose control should at least settle for the clothing removal. Some alarmists raise the issue of using force to contain grossly contaminated victims to prevent further injury to rescuers or civilians. In reality, such force is not acceptable because the officers exerting the force must be fully suited for protection from the victims (this is an opinion based on educated guesses and a few case histories). The Tokyo sarin gas attack was an incident in which victims were not effectively confined. The victims scattered from the hot zone, unknowingly transmitted the mechanism to emergency responders, and in some cases contaminated medical facilities.

The following example demonstrates some practical scene control issues:

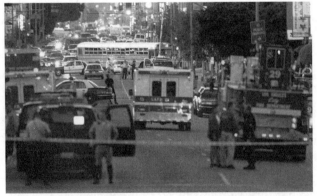

FIGURE 6-3 Isolating the hot zone is a vital step in gaining control of an incident.

CASE STUDY 2

A crime syndicate plans a multimillion-dollar armored car robbery. To create a diversion, a street gang is subcontracted to explode a chlorine tank car on a downtown railroad siding. At 12:07 p.m. on a blustery November Tuesday, the tank car has a violent pressure rupture caused by 2 pounds of strategically placed plastic explosives.

Ten people are killed almost immediately. Within minutes, 160 people are injured from acute chlorine exposure. Thirty convergent responders and three police officers approach the scene and are immediately overcome by chlorine gas.

The incident generates an immediate second-alarm fire response and the arrival of two EMS units. Units approaching from the north see a large green fog accumulating in the low-lying area around ground zero. A chlorine cloud is seen drifting south. Units approaching from the south begin driving into the chlorine cloud and have to divert their response.

Mass casualties are reported including bodies. Many victims are staggering in all directions from the scene. Some victims are leaving in taxis and private vehicles. Victims receiving minimal exposure are moving farther away or going back to their offices.

Scene Control Procedures

- There is a dynamic hot zone at ground zero that is moving south.
- Victims are diverted to three staging areas (west, north, east) for decontamination and medical treatment.
- An evacuation is conducted south of the incident.

Scene Control Issues

- Many victims exit before scene control is established. Within 10 minutes, the two nearest hospitals are inundated with contaminated victims arriving in private vehicles.
- In spite of a heavy chlorine odor, media, bystanders, and friends or relatives of the victims begin trying to enter the victim treatment areas.
- Because of a slow decontamination process, many walking wounded victims are becoming adamant about leaving to go home or get personal medical care from their private physicians.
- Within 1 hour, multiple 911 calls are being received for victims in offices, transit stations, and residences.
- For the next 48 hours, reports are continually received about patients presenting at suburban emergency rooms as far as 50 miles from the incident.
- The scene requires entry by hundreds of EMS, fire, and law enforcement responders.
- CNN breaks the story, opening the floodgates for every conceivable type of media response. Media pressure to get closer and closer to ground zero escalates.

Scene Control Solutions

- Hospitals throughout the region are alerted. The importance of decontamination before admission is stressed.
- On-site monitoring is used to determine the extent of the hot zone. The perimeter is reduced accordingly.
- A law enforcement perimeter is established in the crime area. All evidence is properly preserved, photographed, cataloged, and removed.
- Scene entry points are established for public safety personnel to control warm zone and hot zone access. A local personnel accountability system is effectively utilized.
- All receiving hospitals initiate entry control procedures. Contaminated vehicles are diverted to a remote and secured parking lot (not the emergency room [ER] driveway). Arriving victims are diverted to a decontamination area outside the building for clothing removal and initial wash-down. No victim is permitted entry into any hospital area without being decontaminated.
- Calls to 911 from outside the incident area are handled by a beefed-up response force of mutual aid units and recall personnel. Records from all chlorine exposure victims are separately maintained for inclusion into a final after-action report. All cases are also reported to law enforcement for future investigation.
- The media is instructed to establish a media pool. The media pool is given a closely supervised, escorted tour of areas cleared by the safety officer and law enforcement.

Effective control of an incident perimeter places a high drain on law enforcement resources. Consider controlling a chemical hot zone encompassing a four-square-block area. This hypothetical area requires an officer at every intersection, which is a minimum of eight units for control. To place a unit halfway down each block on the perimeter requires sixteen law enforcement units. This is a commitment of resources that severely taxes even the largest urban police or sheriff's department.

Another issue is maintaining law enforcement response times for 911 services unrelated to the major incident. A third consideration is that many units are engaged within the perimeter in a mass shooting or bombing scenario.

Major terrorism incidents requiring perimeter security are high-impact law enforcement incidents. Effective sealing of a large urban area is very difficult and resource intensive under the best of circumstances. If possible, the scene area should be reduced as soon as practical. In the previous example, if the four-square-block area was reduced to two square blocks, the number of perimeter control units are reduced from eight to six units.

Wind change is an uncontrollable factor in a chemical incident. A 90-degree wind change or a change in wind speed that optimizes a chemical plume footprint greatly changes the size and/or location of the hot zone. Sudden changes make effective perimeter control impossible in the short term because of a shifting and dynamic perimeter. Such changes require altering the evacuation zone—a step that cannot be done well on the run.

The last significant factor is public reaction—the CNN factor. A media evacuation announcement often draws people to an area. These people are not the helpful convergent responders discussed earlier. Civilians attempting to enter an evacuated area include bystanders, photographers, residents, and parents entering an area to retrieve their children. This situation is universal; onlookers and parents will always present scene control problems.

Response Training

The emergency responder survival skills required for living through a terrorism incident require development and training. The most important component is the implementation and daily use of NIMS. The ICS component within NIMS must be the gold standard for the activities of response and support agencies (see Chapter 2).

All agency members, including nonresponders, must be trained in basic NIMS as a starter. The NIMS must pervade all areas of agency operations, not just emergencies. Daily business should be conducted using NIMS forms and jargon. These actions result in NIMS and ICS becoming an organizational way of life. For example, agencies can use the ICS boilerplate for meeting agendas. Agenda items are listed under four columns entitled operations, logistics, planning, and administration. Weekly or biweekly plans are distributed using the official ICS incident action plan form. It is important to use ICS every day in all facets of an agency to ensure that when emergencies, disasters, or terrorism incidents unfold, responders will know how to effectively operate.

Convergent responder awareness is another important training objective. Trained convergent responders provide valuable crisis management information (intelligence) and early assistance in the response effort. The first step in convergent responder training is identification of relevant government agencies and utilities, with private businesses identified on a separate list. The next step is to provide training for employees of government agencies and solicit cooperation from utilities and private businesses.

Using a traditional brick and mortar classroom to train a myriad of agencies in a convergent responder program is time consuming and expensive for all parties. Virtual training is one solution. Using the Internet, e-mail, online social networks, and teleconference calling, information and basic awareness programs can be disseminated to any organization. Virtual technology is also useful to monitor certification and new employee orientation. By effectively using educational technology, response agencies become a training source with minimal expenditure of personnel. Private businesses can determine when to utilize the material and schedule employee awareness sessions. At the least, response agencies should provide a convergent responder training video supplemented by handouts or virtual files.

For major high-threat events, specialized convergent responder awareness training should be conducted for security guards, staffers, ushers, maintenance personnel, concession workers, tour guides, and others. This includes events such as major religious activities, political conventions, presidential visits, political issue rallies (pro-life, pro-choice, animal rights, etc.), and major sporting events. Before the 1996 Olympics, thousands of Atlanta workers received terrorism awareness training. Such a program is time consuming and expensive, but a single truck driver reporting a suspicious incident can prevent an attack plan from becoming a tragic incident.

Special response teams have national standards and training certification levels that must be maintained. This sounds like a given, but in some locales, special team activity is infrequent and the specialists lose their edge. These teams, including SWAT units, SWAT medics, search and rescue teams, and hazardous materials teams, also need terrorism awareness programs.

All emergency responders must be trained in scene awareness. The principles of 2 in 2 out and LACES should be in a written protocol and part of a scene awareness program. All terrorism incidents, especially the small ones, should be reviewed for scene awareness issues. An effective postincident analysis is also a good training aid.

Medical Facility Response

A terrorism incident requires medical facilities to alter their general mode of operation and support the medical demands of the incident. Granted, hospitals do not respond by driving to a scene, but they do respond by preparing for unusual patients in mass numbers.

The initial element in hospital preparation that drives the rest of the hospital response system is communications. Medical receiving facilities must be alerted early in the incident chain via the same process used in standard mass casualty procedures. Early warning gives facilities time to prepare for a patient onslaught. Information about the type of incident and numbers of victims is critical. For example, ten mass shooting victims, thirteen bombing victims, or twenty chemical attack victims all trigger different preparedness actions.

Communications are assured (or have a high potential for success) through the use of correct protocol and technology. Local protocol must specify that terrorism incidents initiate immediate notification of appropriate receiving facilities. Medical facilities must be in the receiving loop when EMS crews transmit scene information (**FIGURE 6-5**).

A protocol for hospital communications must require feedback from critical medical facilities. In many systems, EMS and/or fire communications are monitored in the ER. There are many reasons why initial information about a terrorism incident may not be heard on a busy night. One-way monitoring is not reliable. Protocols should require that medical receiving facilities acknowledge receiving notification of an unusual incident.

Medical facilities should have several layers of technology to ensure receipt of communications. There must be auxiliary power and backup systems to compensate

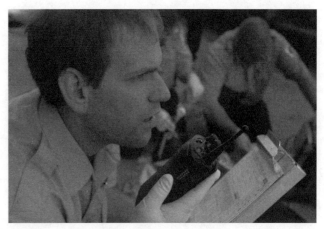

FIGURE 6-5 First responders should provide hospital facilities with initial information about a terrorism incident.

for the failure of private systems and electrical power. At the least, a secondary system must back up the telephone system.

Hospital security is a key nonmedical element in hospital response procedures. Workplace violence and gang-related mass shootings sometimes migrate from the scene to the ER. The number one cause of workplace death for physicians and nurses is gun violence. Assailants in several case histories have gone to the ER attempting to finish off their victims.

Hospital security should be immediately alerted when mass shooting victims are being transported to the facility. Armed officers should secure entry to the ER and related treatment areas.

Contaminated victims en route to an ER require a different type of security plan. Security officers should initiate a complete medical facility lockdown. Every effort must be made to protect the facility from contaminated victims bypassing decontamination procedures. Erik Auf der Heide, in his book, *Disaster Response*, noted that in mass casualty incidents, over 50 percent of the victims arrived at the hospital in private vehicles or by other means. Hospital personnel cannot expect all chemically exposed victims to arrive via EMS in a clean condition.

If the decontamination area is separate from the ER entrance, security officers must direct arriving vehicles (EMS and private cars) to the decontamination corridor. In any terrorism incident, the CNN factor goes into hyperdrive. Victims' friends and relatives follow the

CRITICAL FACTOR ....

Victims may also present at physician offices or emergency care centers hours or days later.

media swarm. Both situations require security control. All private vehicles are assumed to be contaminated and must be diverted from driveways to a vehicle staging area. The vehicles are decontaminated later after victim removal.

Unfortunately, some hospitals use contract security officers who are not permanently assigned to the facility. An officer assigned to a hospital one day may have been at a park on the previous day. This is especially true on weekends. For this reason, security checklists and protocols for officers should be written in a pocket guide format and issued to each security officer, especially officers on rotation. The pocket guide procedures should be brief and consist of critical factors only—the usual 2-inch-thick notebook is too much. Remember that if a facility has contracted security that frequently rotates, traditional methods of orientation and training will not suffice.

Reliance upon local emergency response agencies to augment hospital capacity to manage victim load or decontamination is unwise. This dependency is discouraged because most, if not all, emergency assets will be either committed to incident operations (on the scene) or responding to 911 calls unrelated to the terrorism incident.

Chapter Summary

Local agencies are the cornerstone of an effective terrorism response. Managers at these agencies should plan to be self-sustaining for 12 to 72 hours before federal help arrives. As convergent responders arrive before first responders, it is important to identify convergent responder agencies and develop an awareness training program for them.

A terrorism scene is a hostile workplace environment, and focusing on victims instead of overall scene awareness is an unsafe practice. Responders must use their senses and look around before charging in. First responders must be aware of chemical threats, shooters in the area, and primary or secondary explosive devices. Responders must use the buddy system when entering an unsecured scene by applying the 2 in 2 out principle and the wildland firefighting principle of LACES. Likewise, the trend of mass shootings and tactical ultraviolence means more exposure to ballistic hot zones. Responders must survey the peripheral areas of a scene, including roofs or other high places, and use the principles of distance and cover for self-protection.

The NIMS and ICS are the boilerplate for management of terrorism incidents. Response agencies must learn, implement, train, exercise, and operate using NIMS. Scene control is a critical factor in a terrorism event and has high impact on law enforcement. Victims, witnesses, and possible assailants must be kept on the scene. Other groups, such as media, onlookers, and friends and families of the victims, will attempt to enter the scene.

Essentially, all emergency responders must be specially trained for terrorism incidents. This training includes NIMS proficiency, scene awareness, and special team training. Medical facilities must initiate response protocols for processing and treating mass casualty terrorism victims. Facility response begins with effective communications to provide early scene information, and hospital security is a critical factor in medical facility preparedness. In a mass shooting, the ER must be physically protected from possible perpetrators. In a chemical attack, contaminated victims must be diverted to the decontamination area and the facility should be locked down.

Wrap Up

Chapter Questions

1. What are convergent responders? What are their strengths and weaknesses?
2. List the public and private convergent responder agencies in your community.
3. What are the unsafe conditions that may be present at a terrorism incident?
4. What is the 2 in 2 out principle? Discuss the LACES principle.
5. What is the importance of NIMS in terrorism incidents?
6. List and discuss the major scene control issues in a terrorism incident.
7. What procedures should be initiated by a medical facility when contaminated victims are en route?

Chapter Project

Research the response procedures of your local fire, EMS, and law enforcement agencies. Determine how effectively these procedures address tactical violence scenes. Develop a comprehensive terrorism operational procedure based on the concepts and key issues discussed in this chapter.

Vital Vocabulary

2 in 2 out A firefighting safety principle dictating that when two members enter a structure or high-hazard area, two additional members are standing by outside the hazard area for the purpose of immediate rescue and/or support.

Active shooter response The quick action by whatever group of law enforcement officers initially arrive on scene by aggressively entering a building or structure with the intent of engaging an active shooter or shooters. The primary objective is to save lives by neutralizing the shooter.

Chemical/biological/radiological (CBR) An incident or threat involving chemical, biological, or radiological devices or weapons.

Community emergency response team (CERT) An organized team of community citizens trained to respond to local disasters and perform actions that mitigate death, injury, property loss, and quality of life.

Convergent responders Citizens or workers who witness a terrorism incident and converge on the scene, call 911, and take action before first responders arrive.

Law enforcement incident command system (LEICS) Law enforcement incident management functions organized by the ICS template.

Lookout, awareness, communications, escape, and safety (LACES) Scene safety procedures based on having a lookout, situational awareness, functioning communications among units, and an escape route leading to a safe zone.

Staging A safe area near the incident scene where nonessential and support units, managed by a staging officer, stand by awaiting further orders or assignments.

Windshield survey Careful scan of the incident scene from a vehicle, especially the entire scene periphery, to determine hazards or threats.

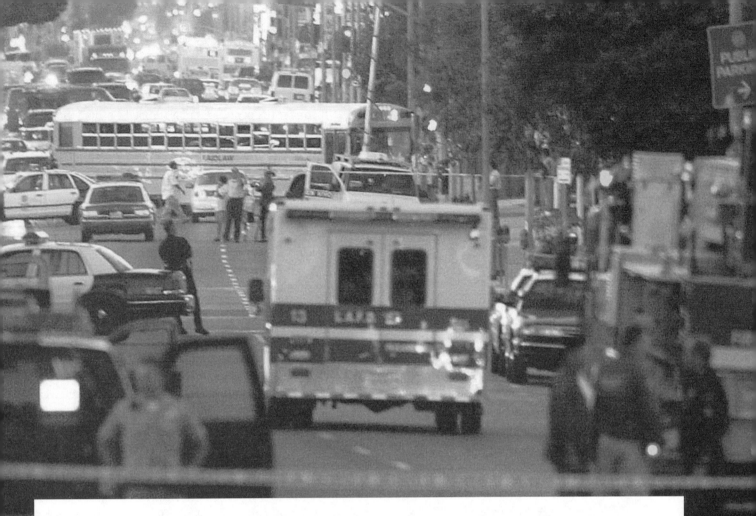

7

Operations Security, Site Security, and Terrorism Incident Response

Paul M. Maniscalco
Hank T. Christen

Objectives

- Discuss the definitions of operations security (OPSEC) and site security.
- Describe the difference between OPSEC and site security.
- List the five critical component steps of OPSEC.
- Discuss and describe the intelligence cycle.
- Recognize how OPSEC integrates with the incident command system.
- Discuss the challenges of implementing and sustaining site security.
- Describe the integration of OPSEC and site security for terrorism incident response.
- Recognize the importance of evidence preservation and the role of responders in protecting evidence for law enforcement agencies.

Introduction

When preparing organizations and individuals for response to a high-impact/high-yield emergency incident, some of the most often overlooked requirements are OPSEC and site security.

Bound inextricably with coordination and integration strategies for response, OPSEC and site security are often compromised in the heat of the battle. Responders, with nothing but the best of intentions, converge on the scene of an incident implementing strategies that, pre-event, have failed to address these most important aspects of the incident response and management strategy. The discipline to apply the principles of OPSEC and site security following a preestablished, organized, and well-practiced plan is crucial given the nature of the threat and the variety of conditions that may present themselves. Failing to address these critical security tenets prior to an event amounts to failing to protect the protectors.

OPSEC

Terrorist attacks present the contemporary emergency response manager or chief officer with more complex challenges and greater probable risks. Site security and OPSEC are multifaceted concepts, bringing together elements ranging from pre-event protection of information concerning an organization's activities, intentions, or capabilities to operational issues such as scene access, traffic control, and evidence protection. Due to the fact that this involves so many different aspects of disaster response, and because it cannot be completely achieved without full integration of each of those aspects, site security is best understood broadly. Robust control of the incident and proximal areas should be the desired goal. This includes maintaining command and control over the human and material flow into, out of, and around the site, providing for the security and safety of responding personnel, providing these responders with the ability to perform their jobs, ensuring personal accountability and the fulfillment of performance requirements.

For an OPSEC program to be effective, personnel must be aware of OPSEC concerns, implement OPSEC countermeasures when appropriate, and be observant of potential collection activities directed at their organization. This is possible only if the members of the organization understand the range of threats affecting their organization and actively support the OPSEC program.

OPSEC Purpose

OPSEC as a formalized strategic concept was developed in 1988 under the provisions of National Security Decision Directive 298, The National Operations Security Program. **OPSEC** is a tool designed to promote operational effectiveness by denying adversaries publicly available indicators of sensitive activities, capabilities, or intentions. The goal of OPSEC is to control information and observable actions about an organization's capabilities, limitations, and intentions to prevent or control the exploitation of available information by an adversary. The OPSEC process involves five steps, which are discussed in greater depth later in this section. These steps are:

1. Identification of critical information
2. Analysis of threats
3. Analysis of vulnerabilities
4. Assessment of risks
5. Application of appropriate countermeasures

The overarching OPSEC framework comences with an assessment of the entire organization/activity in order to determine and identify what exploiable but unclassified evidence or classified or sensitive activities could be acquired by an adversary through known collection capabilities—human or technological.

Indication of sensitive activities is often the consequence of publicly available information that can be found via a variety of sources including agency Web sites, press briefings, open house events, scheduled exercises, and deliberate probing of the 911 system by false alarm responses or monitoring daily response actions. This information can then be pieced together to develop critical information and understanding of agency response tactics, techniques, and procedures. Sensitive activities indicators can originate routine administrative, logistics, or operational activities, and if identified, these observations are analyzed via known collection capabilities of an adversary to be employed to exploit vulnerabilities and place responders at risk. An agency chief officer, manager, or safety officer uses this disciplined threat and vulnerability assessment process to determine the current OPSEC state of affairs and guide the agency through the selection and adoption of countermeasures to diminish or eliminate the threat.

OPSEC Process

OPSEC considerations must be integral to the process of planning for and integrated with all response doctrine and standard operating procedures (SOP) irrespective of whether they are sensitive operations or not. Similar to the adaptation and adoption of safety principles and engineering controls to keep responders safe, OPSEC tenets should be an integral component of that strategic process.

Early implementation of OPSEC in the agency response planning process encourages and sustains a heightened awareness by all personnel for maintaining a protective posture for agency-critical information and capabilities. In order to be effective in this arena, the OPSEC planning process requires an unambiguous comprehension of the specific activity's mission and agency organizational and operational plans and doctrine. An effective OPSEC program should be seamlessly integrated into an agency's culture and reinforced by policy, SOPs, and utility in all operational aspects.

The OPSEC planning process must identify and incorporate strategic/tactical countermeasures, where appropriate and feasible, that are necessary to complement physical, information, personnel, signals, computer, and communications security measures. The synergy of the OPSEC system provides an agency with total integration of security countermeasures to blunt vulnerabilities and enhance safety of the responders. An agency might implement OPSEC countermeasures including but not limited to amendment of existing standard operating administrative procedures; application of cover, concealment, and deception techniques; and other OPSEC measures that can degrade an adversary's capability to exploit vulnerabilities. Developing a sustainable and cost-effective security countermeasures program that is tailored to meet the identified threat is one of the central benefits of an agency OPSEC program.

Even though the OPSEC system paradigm is often described as a five-step process, the delineated steps were never intended to be interpreted/implemented as an incremental or sequential execution. The program strengths of the OPSEC process are that it is structured to be dynamic and flexible to facilitate an adaptive progression that meets the specific and unique needs of an organization and the operational environment of its jurisdiction. The global strength of the OPSEC process is acknowledged in the final report of the Joint Security Commission where the commission identifies the tenets of OPSEC as the U.S. government's fundamental basis for risk management.

The five steps of the OPSEC process involve the following:

1. **Identification of critical information**—Critical information is factual data about an organization's intentions, capabilities, and activities that the adversary needs to plan and act effectively to degrade operational effectiveness or place the potential for organizational success at risk. The OPSEC process identifies critical information and determines when that information may cease to be critical in the life cycle of an operation, program, or activity.

2. **Analysis of threats**—Threat analysis consists of determining the adversary's ability to collect, process, analyze, and use information. The objective of threat analysis is to know as much as possible about each adversary and its ability to target the organization. It is especially important to tailor the adversary threat to the actual activity and, to the extent possible, determine what the adversary's capabilities are with regard to the specific operations of the activity or program.

3. **Analysis of vulnerabilities**—Vulnerability analysis requires that the OPSEC analyst adopt an adversarial view of the activity requiring protection. The analyst attempts to identify weaknesses or susceptibilities that are exploited by the adversary's collection capabilities. The vulnerability analysis process must identify the range of activities that can be observed by the adversary, the type of information that can be collected, and the specific organizational weaknesses that the adversary can exploit. Based on this knowledge, the OPSEC analyst determines what critical information the adversary can derive based on the known threat and assessed vulnerabilities.

4. **Assessment of risks**—Risk assessment is the heart of the OPSEC process. In a risk assessment, threats and vulnerabilities are compared to determine the potential risk posed by adversary intelligence collection activities targeting an activity, program, or organization. When the level of vulnerability is assessed to be high and the adversary threat is evident, then adversary exploitation is expected, and risks are assessed to be high. When the vulnerability is slight, and the adversary's collection ability is rated to be moderate or low, the risk may be determined to be low, and no protective measures are required. Based on the assessed level of risk, cost/benefit measures can be used to compare potential countermeasures in terms of their effectiveness and cost.

5. **Application of appropriate countermeasures**—In the final step, countermeasures are developed to protect the activity. Ideally, the chosen countermeasures eliminate the adversary threat, the vulnerabilities that can be exploited by the adversary, or the utility of the information. In assessing countermeasures, the impact of the loss of critical information on organizational effectiveness must be balanced against the cost of implementing corrective measures. Possible countermeasures should include alternatives that may vary in terms of feasibility, cost, and effectiveness. Based on the

probability of collection, the cost effectiveness of various alternatives and the criticality of the activity countermeasures are selected by the program manager. In some cases, there may be no effective means to protect information because of cost or other factors that make countermeasure implementation impossible. In such cases, the manager must decide to accept the degradation of effectiveness or cancel the activity.

As described, threat analysis is the critical foundation of the OPSEC process. Fundamentally, the assessed threat level determines the extent of the agency's vulnerability and risk. These findings provide agency leadership with the requisite information to make informed decisions relative to mitigating vulnerabilities as well as how to select the most effective countermeasure strategies to achieve the same. Subsequently, it is critical that threat assessment findings truthfully reflect the entirety of the intelligence collection effort that targets the agency.

The Intelligence Cycle

Intelligence is the product resulting from the collection, collation, evaluation, analysis, integration, and interpretation of collected information. The intelligence cycle represents an investigation protocol by which information is acquired, produced, analyzed, and then made available to parties who have a direct need to know or have access based upon specific and definitive agency responsibility (such as the OPSEC officer or fusion center liaison) or operational involvement in a specific matter directly related to this intelligence product. This cycle **(FIGURE 7-1)** is based upon five distinct functions that govern a critical component of this disciplined process. The five functions are:

1. Planning and direction
2. Collection

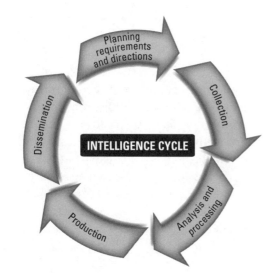

FIGURE 7-1 Intelligence cycle.

3. Processing
4. Production
5. Dissemination

Each segment of the intelligence cycle has a specifically crafted function that provides valuable contributions to the end product of the entire process. The functions are described as follows:

1. **Planning and direction**—This step involves the management of the entire intelligence effort, from the identification of a need for data to the final delivery of the intelligence product to the consumer. The process consists of identifying, prioritizing, and validating intelligence requirements; translating requirements into observables; preparing collection plans; issuing requests for information collection, production, and dissemination; and continuously monitoring the availability of collected data. In this step, specific collection capabilities are tasked based on the type of information required, the susceptibility of the targeted activity to various types of collection activity, and the availability of collection assets.

2. **Collection**—This step includes both acquiring information and provisioning that information to processing and production elements. The collection process encompasses the management of various activities, including developing collection guidelines that ensure optimal use of available intelligence resources. Intelligence collection requirements are developed to meet the needs of potential consumers. Based upon identified intelligence, requirements collection activities are given specific tasks to collect information. These tasks are generally redundant and may use a number of different intelligence disciplines for collection activities. Task redundancy compensates for the potential loss or failure of a collection asset. It ensures that the failure of a collection asset is compensated for by duplicate or different assets capable of answering the collection need. The use of different types of collection systems contributes to redundancy. It also allows the collection of different types of information that can be used to confirm or disprove potential assessments. Collection operations depend on secure, rapid, redundant, and reliable communications to allow for data exchange and to provide opportunities for cross-cueing of assets and tip-off exchanges between assets. Once collected, information is correlated and forwarded for processing and production.

3. **Processing**—This step involves the conversion of collected information into a form suitable for

the production of intelligence. In this process, incoming information is converted into formats that can be readily used by intelligence analysts in producing intelligence. Processing includes such activities as translation and reduction of intercepted messages into written format to permit detailed analysis and comparison with other information. Other types of processing include video production, photographic processing, and correlation of information collected by technical intelligence platforms.

4. **Production**—This step is the process of analyzing, evaluating, interpreting, and integrating raw data and information into finished intelligence products for known or anticipated purposes and applications. The product may be developed from a single source or from collection and databases. To be effective, intelligence production must focus on the consumer's needs. It should be objective, timely, and most importantly accurate. As part of the production process, the analyst must eliminate information that is redundant, erroneous, or inapplicable to the intelligence requirement. As a result of the analytical effort, the analyst may determine that additional collection operations are required to fill in gaps left by previous collection or existing intelligence databases. The final intelligence product must provide the consumer with an understanding of the subject area and draw analytical conclusions supported by available data.

5. **Dissemination**—This step is the conveyance of intelligence to the consumer in a usable form. Intelligence can be provided to the consumer in a wide range of formats including verbal reports, written reports, imagery products, and intelligence databases. Dissemination can be accomplished through physical exchanges of data and through interconnected data and communications networks.

An agency OPSEC manager must be familiar with the intelligence cycle for three essential reasons. First, awareness allows the OPSEC manager to assume a role in the required intelligence production to effectively support the agency OPSEC initiative. OPSEC managers must be acutely aware of the range of threats confronting the agency to ensure they implement effective countermeasures that deny adversaries access to data that provide critical information.

Next, comprehension of the intelligence cycle and associated functions provides the agency OPSEC manager with the critical insight and threat perspec-

tive to develop protective measures in order to thwart adversary collection activities that could undermine response effectiveness and responder safety. The OPSEC manager's knowledge of an adversary's collection methods and patterns allows the program manager to develop effective countermeasures that hide or distort indicators that could be used against the agency and its personnel.

Lastly, knowledge of the adversary's analytical biases is used to develop deception programs that deceive the adversary by confirming erroneous perceptions. For example, expectations that agency credentials are exploitable to the point of personnel counterfeiting IDs, believing that official vehicles can be stolen from vendors, or that uniform articles can be acquired without proper credentials allow the adversary to exploit the public's trust and confidence in an agency by masquerading as responders to launch an attack.

The importance of a coherent and seamlessly integrated OPSEC program in the contemporary public safety and emergency response agencies' SOPs cannot be overstated. In the changing world, where emergency responders are no longer viewed as noncombatants and are being targeted as part of the larger terrorist plot, adoption and implementation of a robust, integrated OPSEC program is an obligation, not a luxury. Organizations such as the International Association of Emergency Medical Services Chiefs (IAEMSC), International Association of Fire Chiefs, and the International Association of Chiefs of Police all have OPSEC and operations site security best practice reference documents that one can access and use when crafting one's own agency protocols. An example of the reference sheet from the IAEMSC is listed herein for review **(FIGURE 7-2)**.

CRITICAL FACTOR ....

This chapter segment does not presume to present an exhaustive, comprehensive representation of intelligence processes and OPSEC processes; however, it does provide the learner with the opportunity to develop a fundamental, analytical, historical, and theoretical understanding for further research on the general subject of intelligence and OPSEC. Learners are encouraged to discuss these issues in greater detail with their intelligence officer liaisons and local/regional fusion center representatives. Additionally, information and training on OPSEC can be obtained through a variety of sources, including the Federal Law Enforcement Training Center and the Interagency OPSEC Support Staff at www.ioss.gov, or IOSS, 6411 Ivy Lane, Suite 400, Greenbelt, MD 20770; (443) 479-4677.

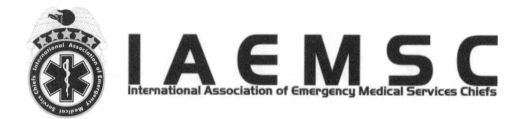

Position Statement 2009-001

Recommended EMS Agency Operational Security Measures:

With the heightened state of threat for terrorist incidents, greater operational security and situational awareness needs to be adopted by EMS members and organizations. Consistent with our assessment of this threat, the IAEMSC has adopted the following position with respect to EMS organizations sharing threat information with their members and the protection of the physical assets that identify EMS members and the vehicles required to deliver EMS services.

EMS organizations should seriously contemplate adopting the following initial steps for their operational security assessment:

EMT's and Paramedics:

- Members should be provided with a security briefing regarding present or emerging threats to their safety or the integrity of the EMS mission. The briefings can take many forms such as meetings, information sheets or supervisory briefings conducted at the commencement of a tour of duty. This provides a common operating picture of the present environment.

- Members should be provided the opportunity by their respective EMS organizations to develop a greater sense of operational security and situational awareness. While the threats EMS faces are not new, they continually change requiring greater acuity and understanding. Training opportunities exist via a number of resources that can be employed to accomplish this goal. Many programs are offered at no cost to the agency through the US Department of Homeland Security. IAEMSC members are encouraged to review the references in the "members only" section of the website for additional information or to contact the IAEMSC for additional information & assistance with identifying and securing the proper resource/program to satisfy and remedy your agency's requirements.

Vehicles:

- Accountability of all vehicles—marked and unmarked—this includes tracking vehicles that are in-service, off service – reserve status, off-service–repair status and those that are going for salvage.

FIGURE 7-2 IAEMSC-recommended EMS agency operational security measures.

- EMS vehicles when unattended should NOT be left running or the keys left in the ignition.

- Tracking of vehicle access must include:
  - ✓ Insure that off service vehicles at EMS stations are secured in such a manner that significantly increases the difficulty of unauthorized access and use. Routine and random vehicle audits are encouraged.

  - ✓ Routine and random audits of vehicle and station key access logs. Inventory of keys should be conducted to account for all keys. Take requisite security corrective measures should keys be discovered unaccounted for.

  - ✓ Insure that EMS vehicles that are off premise for service are accounted for especially when not in direct possession of the EMS organizations. This includes, in addition to government based repair facilities, contracted vendor services that require the vehicle to be shipped off site such as radio repair firms, mechanical and bio-medical repair and warranty service. EMS organizations are strongly encouraged to discuss security measures with repair facilities and vendors to confirm that they understand the requirements to secure the vehicle and your compliance expectations. Such requirements might be:

    - Securing the vehicle overnight inside when facility is closed.

    - Not leaving the keys in the vehicle.

    - Not allowing the vehicle to be taken off vendor premise for any reason other than directly related to the repair and return of the unit to the owning organization.

    - Reporting to the EMS organization and Law Enforcement officials any unusual interest in the vehicle while in their possession.

- Decommissioned vehicles slated for resale, but not to another bona fide emergency response organization, or vehicles scheduled for salvage, should be stripped of agency identifying markings by complete removal or destruction by grinding. Uninstalling of emergency warning devices and other EMS markings is strongly encouraged.

Uniforms and Identification Articles:

- Safeguard agency patches and ID cards to insure defense against unauthorized access.

- Adoption of counterfeit resistant identification credentials that incorporate a photo of the authorized member.

FIGURE 7-2 *(Continued)*

- Alert uniform store vendors of the need to establish and verify the identity of an individual seeking to purchase your uniform articles. This should be accomplished by verifying agency Identification Credentials. More comprehensive processes such as a contact number with your agency to verify identity against the database of authorized active members should be considered.

###

Reviewed and Approved:

International Association of EMS Chiefs
Quarterly Meeting – August 18, 2007
Denver, Colorado

Updated and Approved:
Quarterly Meeting – February 8, 2008
Raleigh, North Carolina

Annual Review – Approved: January 29, 2009

For More Information: IAEMSC
                           PO BOX 27911
                           WASHINGTON, DC 20038-7911

                           www.IAEMSC.org

                           1-877-442-3672

FIGURE 7-2 *(Continued)*

Incident Management/Unified Command as the Foundation for Safety and Security

The framework that makes for effective and successful deployment of OPSEC and site security strategies is the incident management/unified command (IM/UC) structure as articulated in the *National Response Framework* (NRF) and the National Incident Management System (NIMS). Many OPSEC and site security issues are addressed by properly applying these disciplined and standard structures, practices, and protocols. For example, interagency integration problems involving the establishment of a chain of command, which produced many of the issues that plagued security at the World Trade Center site in the aftermath of the September 11, 2001, terrorist attacks, could have been significantly ameliorated by the implementation of an effective IM/UC early in the incident and the immediate establishment of a workable security perimeter.

Simply restating the requirement for implementing the IM/UC system, which has already been established with the release of the NRF and the resulting NIMS, is not the purpose here. Moreover, this chapter section seeks to address the issue of the role OPSEC and site security plays in the response to a terrorist incident within the framework of the IM/UC process.

Although it is in the blood of every individual who chooses to devote his or her life's work to responding when others are fleeing, we must resist the urge to run in without fully understanding what we face beyond a door, on the other side of a cloud of smoke, or around a corner. Although this is easier said than accomplished, in a terrorist event, our survival to fight another day depends on projecting or knowing what threats lie ahead.

The organizational protocol that is established by IM/UC is simply the framework by which OPSEC/site security is efficiently, effectively, and successfully established; in other words, it is required but not self-sufficient. While not a panacea, IM/UC implementation is crucial for us to remediate the hard lessons learned in the recent past, fixing the strategic and operational problems inherent in past responses and implementing standards for OPSEC and site security.

The adoption and implementation of the NIMS–IM/UC framework addresses and corrects a large portion of site security issues by the talents and service provided via the law enforcement community at the command post. It is important to note, however, that not all of these issues are terrorism specific, and the UC concept should be allied at most emergency scenes.

Many of the difficulties inherent in the massive response of multiple agencies are as prevalent in an earthquake as in a dirty bomb attack. What makes the issue of OPSEC/site security so important and unique in the context of terrorism is the particular nature of the threat. The unpredictability of terrorism creates conditions that are fluid, requiring speed and flexibility of thought and action as well as thorough planning and preparation. Furthermore, the targeting of responders and "soft targets" such as healthcare facilities and schools makes this an even more complex matter to address and manage to ensure one's safety and the safety of those responders who are being coordinated at the scene.

In analyzing many major recent terrorist attacks, numerous areas of concern consistently emerge. By identifying each of these and focusing on the pitfalls of the response at the time, as well as stating how the response could have been improved, responders can learn lessons and establish best practices for future incidents. These concerns fall into two general categories. The first category involves those concerns that are potentially present in any sort of disaster and that are remedied by the proper implementation of IM/UC. These include:

- Victim rescue in the immediate aftermath of an incident
- Personnel needs including work shifts to ensure proper rest, adequate personal protective equipment, and continuation of normal EMS/law enforcement/fire services over the course of the event
- Organizational integration/interoperability communication issues
- Public relations, including providing information to dignitaries, media, charities, and families of victims/missing
- OPSEC/site security
- Staffing support for other elements

The second category of concern addresses those concerns unique to terrorism that cannot be addressed simply by the implementation of IM/UC, thereby requiring further attention and creativity. These include:

- Search for secondary devices and hostile threats to the scene and responders
- Perimeter establishment and access control
- Traffic and crowd control
- Evidence recovery and protection

OPSEC/Site Security–Challenges of a General Nature

The importance IM/UC plays in enabling successful OPSEC/site security cannot be overstated. Perhaps the key component in OPSEC/site security is communication and coordination among responders, and the primary focus of IM/UC is just that. The following section addresses each aspect of OPSEC/site security that is helped by the implementation of IM/UC, including multiple examples from recent terrorist attacks where such implementation resulted in saved lives or property, and suggestions on implementing site security at future incidents or events.

Victim Rescue

The first challenge to OPSEC/site security is victim rescue in the immediate aftermath of an incident **(FIGURE 7-3)**. This is the initial and most dramatic problem faced by all responders during and immediately following a terrorist attack. As mentioned briefly before, a driving characteristic that defines all responders is the natural instinct to rush forward, nobly doing whatever one can to quickly save as many lives as possible. For the safety of the responders and the victims, some restraint and organization must be exercised, or the overall incident outcome may become negative, and people may die needlessly. The lasting images from the events of September 11, 2001, are of the hundreds of first responder personnel rushing to the scene to help all who were victimized by these horrible attacks. One striking example in a day full of actions hampering, hindering, and preventing all good intentions was the Shanksville, Pennsylvania, plane crash site, which on September 11, 2001, was overwhelmed and severely congested due to the phenomenon of response units, both on and off duty,

making their way to the scene either by self-dispatch or by convincing dispatchers to send more help. The resulting chaos clogged the scene, severely complicating command and control, and confusing perimeter maintenance. Additionally, similar conditions emerged in New York City after the mayor announced on television that all available resources should be brought to bear at the World Trade Center site. This resulted in numerous well-meaning individuals self-dispatching to the scene, creating an incredible problem with respect to validation of personnel claiming to possess certain capabilities, skills, certifications, and licenses, as well as personal accountability for those operating on the scene during the initial days postevent.

This area of OPSEC/site security primarily deals with ensuring an effective response rather than an unorganized, potentially dangerous, and surely less effective response. Implementation of IM/UC could have diminished the reported congestion and ensuing confusion at both events because it states that off-duty response personnel should not respond to an incident unless directed to do so. Although operational doctrine dictates that you man your post until otherwise directed, the reality is that such a situation rarely exists. The instinct to respond is powerful and is complicated by the "touch the plane" phenomenon, in which people feel they have to be at the disaster scene so they can tell others that they were there when it happened. Therefore, it is incumbent on the agency and organization leaders to stress and practice operational discipline that demands coordination and adherence to strict deployment protocol.

Another relevant example is the Bali bombing of October, 2002. As with all responders, the Bali responders rushed in to help victims and save as many lives as possible. However, OPSEC/site security was nonexistent, and many more lives were in danger in the event of coordinated secondary attack. Though it is difficult to find fault with the selfless actions of such responders, it is crucial that this emotional response be tempered by reason and the knowledge that restraint and discipline are not only necessary, but required to keep responders safe and ensure that the investigation is not fouled by responder crime scene contamination thwarting attempts to bring the perpetrators to justice.

Finally, there is the example of the brave responders to the World Trade Center attacks. In their zeal to charge into the scene and save as many people as possible, the tunnel vision they experienced most likely contributed to an ineffective assessment of the prevailing danger and catastrophic structural failure of the towers. This is a tremendously unique incident in our history with no historical reference point, and the multiple planes em-

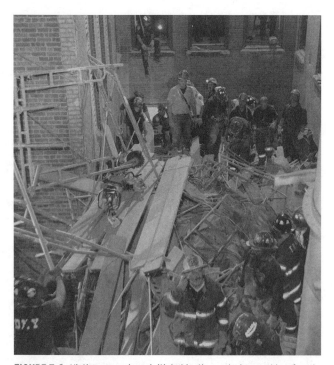

FIGURE 7-3 Victim rescue is an initial objective and a key problem faced by all responders during and after a terrorist attack.

ployed in the attack were effective secondary devices of significant proportion.

OPSEC/site security involves understanding the situation to the greatest degree of accuracy possible, including the possibility that attempting to rescue victims immediately may not be the wisest, safest, or most appropriate course of action. Though it may seem that delaying rescue efforts is tantamount to abandonment of our duty to act and is contrary to the oath many of us swear to, in the end, lives may be saved by taking the time to fully assess the situation in a coherent fashion prior to operational response execution.

Personnel Needs

The security needs of response personnel are a major issue to be addressed in planning for response to a high-impact/high-yield emergency incident. The needs are varied and complex, complicated, and resource demanding during and after a terrorist event. These demands are further amplified given the dual threat of the likelihood of hazardous materials being present and the active intent of the terrorist(s) to hurt or kill as many people as possible, including responders.

One good example of personnel needs was the 1997 sarin attacks in the Tokyo subway. Japanese medical personnel lacked proper personal protective equipment; more than 20% of the staff of St. Luke's International Hospital exhibited some sort of detrimental physical effects after treating victims of the attack. Had the hospital planned properly and equipped the facility/personnel, in addition to regularly training all employees, the instances of secondary contamination would have been greatly reduced.

The most recent and well-known example of responders lacking proper personal protective equipment was the September 11, 2001, attacks. Early on in the response, heavy particulate asbestos and other hazardous materials contaminants, including Freon and cadmium, were found at the site, yet there were responders without proper protective equipment. This was attributed to both poor planning and logistics acquisition problems, because there was simply not enough equipment to go around—indicating that planners failed to grasp the scope or even believe that an attack of that magnitude could occur—and on poor logistics management, because some of the needed equipment was present (on-scene) but was not distributed properly.

There is another critical aspect to protecting responders in a traditional sense; personnel rest and rehabilitation are critical to the success and sustainability of an operation. Although responders are often willing to work to the point of exhaustion, doing so is danger-ous to the responders, the victims, and the effectiveness of the operation. Fatigue creates more victims through poor decision making, increased stress, frustration, and impaired judgment. The medical profession continues to address the effects of sleep deprivation and fatigue due to errors directly traced back to exhausted healthcare providers. Several well-publicized studies that chronicle the effects of long work hours in life-and-death, stressful environments reveal that errors have produced increased morbidity and mortality in the patients being cared for by these well-meaning professionals. Studies conducted over the last several years reveal that moderate sleep deprivation produces impairments in cognitive and motor performance equivalent to illegal levels of alcohol intoxication.

The last thing any coordinated response should have to deal with is victims among the responding rescue workers. To help prevent and ensure the equitable and safe distribution of personnel, IM/UC has instituted a system by which the incident commander assigns shifts to the workers, thereby forcing rest on the weary, whether they realize they need it at the time or not. The final personnel issue to be addressed is the continuation of public services, including EMS, medical, law enforcement, and fire service, through the end of the incident and into the recovery and mitigation stages.

Sustaining 911 response capacities for the entire community must be a significant goal that all agencies strive to achieve. Just because the agency is confronted with a large disaster in the community does not alleviate it from the obligation to ensure the best possible planning efforts to at least attempt to provide appropriate management of all emergencies in the community. Clearly the fiscal implications of having a sustainable and robust response system that can handle any and all 911 calls at all times are strictly cost prohibitive. The burden sharing that has become widely accepted is the use of mutual aid compacts between communities, regions, and now states under the Emergency Management Assistance Compact. The key to sustained successful operation is embracing this concept and employing it on a regular basis. Further, a review of response protocols for uniformity, ensuring interoperability, and having a shared vision of application of OPSEC and site security tactics are integral on "game day."

Hospitals share the same concerns for their facilities and staff. During the planning phase for responding to disasters, hospital planners must take the time to consider a number of issues that previously did not require their attention. Such matters include increased security, physical management of patient flow, personal protective equipment, decontamination strategies, staff training, and personnel support. One such hospital failure that resulted in much national media attention occurred in Florida during the hurricane season of 2004. In this case, Florida Hospital-Ormond Memorial fired or suspended about 25 nurses for not working during Hurricane Frances. Some nurses were fired for not calling in, not showing up, or refusing to work, while others were suspended for not completing a shift. The hospital stated that under hospital policy, critical care employees are required to work during a disaster. Some nurses responded in media accounts alleging that they were not trained to deal with these extreme scenarios and also questioned who would protect their families. No matter the reason, staffing rosters that were expected to be populated based upon the internal disaster plan were not, leaving the facility in a lurch to cover staff vacancies and sustain operations.

Another unfortunate occurrence in the aftermath of disasters is civil unrest and criminal activity. Police presence is often distracted and concentrated at the site of the disaster, coverage is weakened in the areas where law enforcement officers would normally patrol or deploy, and if the presence is weakened enough, citizens might loot nearby houses, commercial districts, and in some cases emergency response equipment. Examples of this were found during and after countless disasters, including Hurricane Charley's landfall in Florida, and there were unsubstantiated accusations of looting by the responders themselves in the September 11, 2001, attacks on New York City. In 2005, after Hurricane Katrina hit New Orleans, there was considerable media attention on allegations of emergency responder and law enforcement involvement in looting. In 2009, there were still grand jury investigations regarding numerous allegations that were leveled at responders ranging from thefts to abuse of authority and civil rights violations.

Community planners, responders, and emergency services personnel must also consider the likelihood of a situation where events have created a large scale area that is too dangerous for anyone to enter or in which to respond. Responders must ask themselves two questions—and answer honestly. (1) In such a given situation, what are the primary responsibilities of responders in getting people out, keeping people from entering, and making sure that the area remains contained? (2) Are we currently prepared to evacuate, relocate, secure, and effectively close a significant portion of or an entire city as was necessary during the 1986 Chernobyl nuclear power plant disaster or Hurricane Katrina?

Proper and effective deployment of law enforcement officers is a key aspect of incident management, NIMS, and the NRF. With proper law enforcement tactical implementation, the lion's share of criminal activity or any form of civil disorder can be mitigated. The implementation strategy also provides for more effective coordination of responders at the scene, affording a higher level of coherence to ensure that security of all personnel, integrated operations, investigatory processes, and sustained evidentiary recovery can be achieved.

A similar concern exists for fire services in the wake of a disaster, specifically in fire-heavy disasters. The typical response for the fire service is to rush to the scene of a major blaze, such as the World Trade Center, and engage as quickly as possible to control the threat and resolve the problem. One can only imagine the collateral dangers if coincidental fires emerge in other parts of a city, particularly in the event of a secondary terrorist attack. The successes of mutual aid are clearly evident in the various responses to a number of large-scale disasters, but especially on September 11, 2001.

Emergency management professionals often speak of the secondary attack. How many communities, agencies, and/or organizations responsible for response and recovery actually have plans in place for a controlled, coordinated, organized deployment in the face of a growing disaster? Can the existing response plans and operational doctrine withstand a campaign event challenge?

Despite what most would believe, and as horrible as the September 11, 2001, attacks were, the United States has yet to experience a true mass casualty, mass fatality event that overwhelms the capabilities of the affected community and the country. As emergency responders and leaders, we must revisit the pain and shock we all felt on September 11, 2001, when almost 3,000 people were murdered. Three thousand sounds like an unimaginable number, but to our enemies, based upon their stated intent to inflict harm, 3,000 is a training exercise.

Integration

Integration issues are a central consideration in any emergency response, but they are critical for a large-scale incident. The most obvious example of this is in the immediate aftermath of the September 11, 2001, attacks on the World Trade Center in New York City. Lack of interoperability between fire and police radios was found to be a major problem during the response to the 1993 bombing of the World Trade Center, and unfortunately, the same problem reared its ugly head on September 11, 2001. Due to this failure and overloaded radio equipment, fire fighters in World Trade Center tower 1 were unaware of reports of the imminent collapse of the tower from a New York Police Department (NYPD) helicopter and therefore did not initiate their own evacuation. This lack of communication resulted in an increased number of casualties that might have been avoided. The proper implementation of IM/UC, which stresses both horizontal and vertical information sharing, would have required interoperable radios, and the NYPD helicopter in the air above the World Trade Center would have been able to relay the information regarding the collapse directly to the fire department, allowing fire fighters to have a fuller depth of understanding for the events and begin evacuating.

The Moscow theater siege of October 2002 is another tragic example of the cost of lives lost when agencies are not integrated. Chechen terrorists took over the theater, claimed the patrons as hostages, and were killed when Russian commandos pumped a toxic gas into the theater, which rendered both terrorists and hostages unconscious, in some cases killing them. The refusal and delay by Russian authorities to release information regarding the type of gas used to subdue and incapacitate the Chechen terrorists rendered medical personnel unable to properly diagnose and treat the nearly 650 hostage victims of the gas, 117 of whom perished in the rescue. The unfortunate reality is that authorities in the Spetsnaz (Russian Special Forces, who carried out the raid) did not involve the medical community or on-site medical responders. If the Spetsnaz had coordinated the assault and included a medical component in tactical operations, the critical medical communication and coordination would have positioned the rescue attempt for greater success, saving additional lives because the medical knowledge, treatment, and response capabilities would have been on scene and poised to effectively intervene when called upon.

The Press and Dignitaries

Public relations is an important aspect of OPSEC/site security because outside factors such as the media and the victims' families can seriously complicate a response or errantly alter public understanding and perception of the response actions and effectiveness. An example of the lack of OPSEC/site security with respect to the media causing major problems was evident during the Beltway sniper shootings of October 2002. The sniper pair left notes for the police with specific instructions not to be relayed to the press, and allegedly made numerous requests for the media not to be involved in the interaction between the sniper and police. The press obtained this information through the notorious unnamed source and

went public with information that not only jeopardized the investigation, but also put many lives in danger. The resulting lack of trust between the snipers and the police impeded communication between investigators and the perpetrators, slowing the investigation as authorities shifted focus toward damage control.

The media is a valuable asset when responding to an incident, provided relations take place in a controlled, efficient manner. An example of the positive and negative role the media can play in responding to an event was during the sarin attacks in Tokyo. The most common and frustrating problem during any response is a lack of information and communication. In the Tokyo incident, personnel at local hospitals had no idea what type of hazardous material or contaminant was creating their medical problems. The hospital personnel dealing with the unknown became aware of the substance from watching the local television broadcasts. Coincidently, physicians who had experience with sarin and the effects on humans were also watching. The resultant communication between the physicians viewing the news coverage and the hospitals correctly identified the culprit substance. Concurrently, the media was criticized for filming while people suffered and died instead of helping them to the hospital.

Media coverage of terrorist events can be a double-edged sword, and it is up to planners to ensure that the benefits of having the media present are not outweighed by the disadvantages. This entails having a **public information officer (PIO)** who is trained prior to an incident on the successful discharge of the PIO duties that are integrated into the command structure to assist with response information dissemination and management of the media **(FIGURE 7-4)**. The PIO must work closely

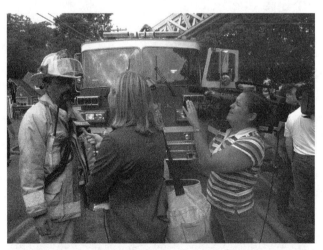

FIGURE 7-4 The public information officer is trained prior to an incident on the successful discharge of the PIO duties integrated into the command structure and can therefore assist with response information dissemination and management of the media.

with the OPSEC officer to determine what information is shared with the media so that the released information does not compromise the integrity of the investigation or the safety of responders operating at the scene.

In the event of a major disaster, it is common practice for government officials of all levels to visit the site to offer reassurance, including governors visiting the areas devastated by disaster in their states and the president coming to the scene of a disaster to lend support and witness the operations in person, such as after September 11, 2001. It is necessary to have strict OPSEC/site security to maintain the safety of these dignitaries. Concurrently, OPSEC/site security is also structured to ensure the dignitaries or their entourages do not disrupt operations, disturb the scene, or hinder investigations. While the visit of these dignitaries is important to reassure the public, it must not come at the cost of successfully executing the local or state recovery efforts or the strategies in the NRF. As has been stated, planning cannot take place in a vacuum; plans to deal with the onslaught of media and dignitaries must be a part of the ongoing community response to any event that may overwhelm a community's ability to operate under normal daily conditions. Therefore, meet, greet, and planning meetings must be conducted with all involved parties to include the local media representatives with the primary goal that all participants have a job to do and planning prior to the worst case scenario will allow for the completion of the mission in a safe and cooperative manner. All egos, preconceived assumptions, and negative relationships must be checked at the door.

OPSEC/Site Security Demands for Off-Site Operations

OPSEC personnel must also take into account the issue of security and staffing support for elements of the response not located directly at the event site, such as joint or regional operation centers, joint or regional information centers, multiagency coordination centers, morgues, food distribution, and donation reception sites. While these sites may not be physically located inside the incident perimeter, they are likely targets. These critical areas are vulnerable to being compromised or attacked by a variety of means including, but not limited to physical attacks with arms, explosives, criminal acts, and hazardous material dispersal.

Law enforcement officials, such as federal marshals or local police or security forces, must be present to ensure protection and sustained operation of these vital services. It is vital to the success and continuation of

the response that community planners, local, city, and county emergency managers and responders (career and volunteer) meet on a regular basis prior to a catastrophic emergency to promulgate prudent operational response doctrine, to ensure OPSEC and site security, and lastly to test planning strategies through comprehensive robust exercising activities.

OPSEC/Site Security for a Terrorist Incident

It isn't enough simply to adopt and fully implement the NIMS–IM/UC framework in order to control and overcome the majority of OPSEC/site security issues, although it is important to note that the majority of concerns, challenges, and problems faced by EMS, medical personnel, law enforcement, security personnel, and fire service are not unique to terrorism/weapons of mass destruction events. The implementation of a plan and/or a system to alleviate identified problems and to avoid new problems is only as good as the training that is provided to familiarize all those who will utilize the plan and/or system. It is impossible and may border on negligence to expect that people, agencies, departments, and communities will be able to utilize plans designed to place everyone on the same sheet of paper without coherent and comprehensive ongoing training and exercising.

In the case of a natural disaster, for example, the difficulties inherent in the massive response of multiple agencies remain. The logistics involved in mobilizing personnel, equipment, and resources coupled with emotions, hungry, tired victims, and those nefarious few who are bent on taking advantage of victims in need creates circumstances that will derail the best laid plans. Now, add to that a situation where these very same people are asked to respond, faced with all the normal obstacles, but have had little or no time to be acquainted with the new plan and even less time being trained on the plan's usefulness, purpose, and operational guidance. You now have the current scenario in place; add to this already chaotic, stressful, and incredibly frustrating event the current severity and the particular nature of the threats we face in the post–September 11, 2001, era.

The unpredictability of terrorism presents conditions that are highly fluid and subject not only to the whims of nature or the physics of a damaged building but to the advanced plans and suicidal determination of well-trained terrorists. Additionally, a garden variety terrorist does not abide by Occupational Safety and Health Administration requirements, does not apply for permits, does not worry about the adequacy of financial support, does not follow labor laws and/or legal restraints preventing action, and the list goes on and on. The terrorist groups that have been identified, and most likely those we have yet to uncover, commit, plan, train, and act in an organized, efficient, and effective manner.

An organizational structure adequate to deal with such an elusive threat, represented by NIMS–IM/UC, only provides the means by which proper measures can be successfully implemented. This is not a question of whether a strategy will be properly followed, but what the strategy entails. The plan in no way provides implementation funding, training and educational funding, staffing backfill, or overtime funding, allowing comprehensive training and education, equipment acquisition, and maintenance. Any plan is only as good as the assumptions it is based on, and a plan certainly is useless when those utilizing the plan have yet to see the plan, be familiar with it, and receive training in plan implementation.

The critical issue is the priority that must be given to OPSEC/site security at all incidents, not just those eventually identified as terrorism related. Adoption of this position creates a familiarity with OPSEC and site security for all responders and becomes institutionalized into the way we do business 24 hours a day, 7 days a week.

The after action reports from numerous major terrorism incidents clearly reveal shortcomings in OPSEC/site security that warrant significant emphasis and close attention by agencies developing their terrorism/WMD response plans in concurrence with NIMS–IM/UC.

There is a striking convergence of properties that characterizes this second group of OPSEC/site security concerns: that they cannot be solved by organizational reform alone, and that they are all particularly pertinent in a terrorist attack. This highly interconnected list for scene management includes perimeter establishment, access and egress control, personal accountability, evidence protection and chain of custody, and the search for secondary devices and threats. Solving the inadequacies in these areas requires not just that the organizational structure exists, but that it be imbedded in a prominent position within the incident command structure.

Establishing a Perimeter

The effective establishment of a perimeter is often a crucial aspect of gaining control over the scene of an attack. Establishing a perimeter has ramifications in all aspects of maintaining OPSEC/site security. Force protection cannot be assured, evidence cannot be protected, chain of custody cannot be guaranteed, and access to the scene cannot be controlled with a porous or haphazard creation of a perimeter.

The overall response to the 1995 terrorist bombing of the Alfred P. Murrah Federal Building in Oklahoma City, Oklahoma, is an excellent model of what was right and what was wrong. There were three layers of perimeters quickly established by morning on the day after the bombing; the inner perimeter was designed to provide limited access to only those personnel authorized to participate in the rescue/recovery work and the criminal investigation, a staging area that also served as a buffer for workers, and a limited traffic access cordon. Unfortunately, an effective perimeter was not established immediately and the site quickly became overwhelmed with hundreds of well-meaning people who wanted to help in any way they could. The problem was that no control existed over any area of the dangerous site and one convergent responder—a nurse—was killed early on due to falling debris.

The eventual establishment of an effective perimeter was accomplished by close coordination of disparate agencies and proper utilization of their abilities along with the securing and construction of fencing. At the World Trade Center site on September 11, 2001, in admittedly more trying circumstances, "Perimeter security was not adequately established, allowing large numbers of unnecessary personnel to enter" (McKinsey & Company) due in large part to a 5-day delay in the creation of an adequate credentialing system and the construction of a fence. It took an extra 4 days at the World Trade Center to establish security even approaching the perimeter set up at the Murrah Federal Building. The potential repercussions for this sort of inattention are massive.

Another example of the need for perimeter security is the case of a 1997 bombing of a women's clinic in suburban Atlanta, where Eric Rudolph is alleged to have planted a secondary explosive device timed to detonate upon the arrival of personnel responding to the initial explosive event. A CNN camera crew filming an interview with a witness of the initial blast caught the nearby second explosion on film; both media and civilians were endangered because they were allowed access to an area surrounding the scene, which should have been secured.

The uncontrolled scene increases the potential and likelihood that individuals not involved in the initial catastrophic event will become victims as a result of a secondary attack, the hazardous material (if present) will be spread to a wider area, and the criminal investigation will be hampered or evidence destroyed. Ground zero at a terrorist attack, therefore, demands special attention to the formation of perimeters as a necessary prerequisite to full OPSEC/site security implementation.

The cooperation and discipline required to ensure security and safety does not and will not happen overnight or because it is the right thing to do. All aspects of scene control must be carefully planned, practiced, and exercised on an ongoing basis. It is impossible to expect two completely divergent disciplines to come together and cooperate without the right training and education. A vital perspective to understand in this matter is the doctrinal conflict that this creates—attribution versus intervention. One large group of responders is running in to tear the scene apart to look for victims and survivors and to treat the injured (intervention). The other large response group requires the meticulous preservation of evidence and maintaining the site just as it was found (attribution).

There is no question that each group has a vital and important role and responsibility—none more important than the other. It is naïve and irresponsible for any responding person, agency, group, or department to expect these two parallel forces to eventually meet in the middle without long-term focused efforts aimed at settling the differences and ensuring that both jobs are completed efficiently and timely. A mutual respect must be achieved through policy and reinforced through exercising if the contemporary emergency response and public safety professions realistically expect to bridge the intervention–attribution gap. This can only be accomplished well before the incident response through regular meetings, educational sessions, training, and effective exercising opportunities. Failure to address this coordination factor pre-event will result in a response that resembles a cacophony—not the desired symphony.

Scene Evidence Preservation

As previously stated, ensuring the preservation of evidence is another fundamental aspect of OPSEC/site security in the event of a terrorist attack. Consider the Oklahoma Department of Civil Emergency Management after action report, which outlines the problems that presented themselves because of the large number of volunteers who were incorporated into rescue operations without being registered or identified. "Since the site was a crime scene, all our volunteers were required to be critically screened before they could work at the bomb site" (Oklahoma Department of Civil Emergency).

Fortunately, authorities implemented this system to rectify the unimpeded access people were afforded; about 30 unauthorized convergent responder volunteers were evicted from one floor alone. This was not handled as well at the site of the 2002 Bali bombings.

There, "the crime scene was seemingly ruined and unprotected" (Pastika) due, in addition to unavoidable circumstances involved in the response, to "the public's curiosity," (Pastika) which was apparently allowed to hinder the investigation despite the fact that a police line had been set up.

The removal, addition, destruction, or alteration of material, whether intentional, unintentional, or simply the product of an inexperienced volunteer seeking a souvenir, could be a major hindrance to the proper conduct of the criminal investigation and identification of those responsible. Even the most minute and seemingly unimportant pieces of evidence often prove to be irreplaceable in these situations, and they cannot afford to be compromised. To the untrained eye, the aftermath of a terrorist attack is a pile of debris or a chaotic mass of humanity. To the trained criminal investigator, the scene is a roadmap that tells the complete story of the circumstances leading up to the event and the event itself. As noted previously, the control of access to the site of a terrorist incident through well-guarded and protected perimeters and a secure credentialing system that does not allow for forgeries is the only way to guarantee the integrity of the crime scene.

The Influence of Traffic and Crowd Control upon an Incident Scene

Traffic and crowd control make up an extremely important aspect of scene OPSEC/site security, especially in the wake of a terrorist attack. With this aspect, OPSEC/site security takes on a much broader impact subsequent to the flow of people and materials in and out of the site itself, and the city or general area in which the attack has occurred is impacted by activity elsewhere. The frightening nature of terrorism, especially for cases in which chemical, biological, radiological, or nuclear (CBRN) substances are implicated either by fact or by speculation, could result in mass hysteria and chaos. In the absence of accurate, timely information from authorities, rumor mongering can take root, leading to potentially disastrous public panic. Something in the vein of an uncontrolled, large-scale attempt to flee a city in the midst of reports of a CBRN incident could freeze attempts to contain the attack or worse, prompt more people into the affected area, and risk exposure to a greater slice of the population.

Consider the description of the evacuation of coastal Florida at the approach of Hurricane Floyd in 1999: "Even many of those not in evacuation zones fled at the sight of satellite images on the news, which depicted a monstrous Floyd larger than the entire state of Florida … the result was a transportation nightmare" (Kriner).

The Florida public, frightened by memories of 1992's Hurricane Andrew, is akin to today's nationwide memory of September 11, 2001; combined with sensationalizing factors such as talk of a hurricane engulfing a state or the imminent citywide release of a chemical agent, they can easily produce wholesale disorder. Full control of the site of a terrorist incident area requires that the information being disseminated from a scene be released in multiple media and methods of communication to dispel rumors, with an eye to directing the public to the proper course of action. Emergency response managers and chief officers cannot lose sight of the fact that our communities are made up of cultures that interpret the same information in different ways. Keeping in mind the cultural, language, and educational barriers that make up each community requires extensive preparations to ensure a complete information sharing plan of action. Concurrently, traffic and crowd control of the entire surrounding area must be fused with information control to ensure that on-site efforts receive proper support and aid.

Control of human traffic also has great importance in its localized form. In the rush to leave a scene to avoid injury or seek medical attention, it is very possible that citizens will unintentionally carry hazardous substances, particularly CBRN material, with them. Depending on the nature of the agent that has been introduced, the failure to contain contaminated people or other material could lead to secondary contamination of individuals or property.

The 1995 sarin nerve agent attack on the Tokyo subway system is an example of the difficulties and effects associated with the uncontrolled vector of contaminated victims. In that incident, over 4,000 affected victims, some contaminated and off-gassing, sought medical treatment without official transport. This means that a very large number of people who either came into contact or had a good chance of coming into contact with sarin were moving freely throughout the city. It is fortunate that the toxicity of the sarin used in the attacks was not potent enough to kill many more and the associated off-gassing that occurred resulted in illness and not death.

Citizens seeking medical assistance were not treated by responders prepared with on-scene decontamination assets, causing a high rate of secondary exposure among the medical staff at unspecialized facilities. Containment of the incident area includes, therefore, the ability to bring specialized treatment to the site, because "agent absorbed by cloth may be released as a vapor by the cloth for 30 minutes or more after exposure" (CBWinfo.com). Again, because the sarin was put together quickly and was only 30% pure, the agent did not lead to any serious injuries to people not in direct contact with the dispersal device. However, it is startling that such an impure chemical mixture was able to affect over 20% of the hospital workers treating victims who hadn't been in direct contact with the sarin dispersal device and had been transported from the scene over an extended period of time. The lesson is clear—in responding to an attack in which biological, chemical, or radiological weapons are suspected, establishing control of the traffic of people both in and out of the area is crucial for the protection of the scene victims and those would-be victims in the surrounding communities.

Secondary Devices or Threats

Perhaps the most pressing and worrying element of concern is that of secondary devices and threats targeting responders and evacuating civilians. Terrorism poses a distinct, highly dangerous hazard and challenge in itself, but the potential for secondary attacks and fallout aimed at even more casualties to responders further complicates the big picture and attempts to control the aftermath. Terrorism aims to cause as much damage or harm to as many people as possible, so a follow-up attack should be a primary consideration, not merely considered a marginal possibility.

The previously mentioned example of Eric Rudolph and his involvement in abortion clinic bombings is relevant here as well. The detonation of a bomb outside of an Atlanta night club 1 week after the women's clinic blast where a secondary attack was successful provided responders with enough warning to suspect a similar tactic in the Atlanta night club bombing. Fortunately, the responders remained diligent, and the secondary device that Rudolph allegedly planted was located and rendered safe before it killed or injured responders. Similar terror tactics were used extensively by several international terrorist organizations, most notably the Real Irish Republican Army and the Colombian paramilitary guerilla group known as the Revolutionary Armed Forces of Colombia. Real Irish Republican Army guerilla forces "have operated a two-bomb strategy, hoping secondary devices 'catch' security forces rushing to the scene of the first" (CNN). The adoption of such tactics by the enemies of the United States, given their resourcefulness and excellent access to information, should certainly not be discounted.

Regardless of the recent elevated concerns and attention given to this phenomenon, preparation for such a scenario was lacking. In the aftermath of the collapse of the World Trade Center towers, the initial rescue phase was followed by a massive recovery effort. Within a day or so after the two towers collapsed, there were already thousands of workers on the scene. Following the attacks, estimates placed the number of volunteers and workers from all disciplines at ground zero at 30,000 to 40,000. At the same time, however, "risk of secondary attack was not made a priority as the rescue effort was vigorously pursued" (Senay). The buildings in the immediate vicinity were not searched for 4 days; it took months to clear all structures properly. There was no standard procedure for obtaining resources such as military aid to augment this task and expeditiously proceed with the search and clearance process.

Failure to secure a perimeter immediately and control site access, as just mentioned, left avenues open through which to strike. In addition, the majority of the nation's federal response and leadership to the disaster was housed in two Manhattan hotels surrounded by response vehicles brightly decorated with a wide variety of responding agencies' logos, decals, and identifying placards. The worst kept secret in the city of New York was where all the federal responders were resting, recuperating, and spending their down time. There is no question that a well-planned or even a last-minute secondary attack would have produced a very high number of casualties due to the large number of vulnerable personnel in the area. Such an attack would have crippled the New York response, but more importantly, the secondary attack at that particular time would have crippled the nation due to the message it sent to those not directly affected by the events in New York and Washington, DC, elevating the appearance of capacity and potency of the terrorist attackers.

Numerous tactics could be applied in a secondary attack. The potential for snipers to receive training and apply it with startling effect was demonstrated by the killing spree undertaken by the Beltway snipers, John Allen Muhammad and Lee Boyd Malvo. Powerful and accurate weapons such as shoulder-fired rocket-propelled grenades and American-made Stinger missiles, in addition to heavily proliferated small arms, are obtainable through the international black market and have been proven to be deadly in small-scale guerilla conflicts in Africa, the Middle East, and across the globe. Suicide attacks come in many forms, including vehicle-borne improvised explosive devices and explosives strapped on or secreted in the body of an individual; both tactics have proven to render devastating effects. It is clear, therefore, that there is both a real threat and a worrisome example in which this threat was not prepared for sufficiently. The NYPD report makes this apparent: "NYPD lacked systematic intelligence and threat assessment function and had difficulty assessing risk of further terrorist attack in weeks after 9/11" (McKinsey & Company). But given this historical perspective and embracing a desire to enhance response safety, readiness, and capacity, the contemporary emergency response leader can use these events and context as a platform for moving ahead with refinement of existing plans to address gaps that might exist to afford their communities and responders a better degree of safety.

Chapter Summary

Operational security and site security are the most important concepts that are engaged through a conscientious, comprehensive effort to protect and secure vital infrastructure before, during, and after a catastrophic event. To ensure that OPSEC and site security is a concept that is embraced and promoted, dialogue with all traditional and nontraditional response agencies should occur on an ongoing basis prior to "game day." These meet-and-greet-and-break-bread gatherings require the checking of egos at the door and the establishment of a real goal-oriented working session. Where possible, agencies should assign, support, and fund the position of OPSEC officer to address and coordinate these responsibilities. This requirement also includes the creation of memoranda of understanding detailing the roles, duties, and responsibilities of all agencies and responders assisting in the development of long-term working relationships all aimed at security, safety, and preservation of life.

Wrap Up

Chapter Questions

1. List and discuss the definitions of OPSEC and site security.
2. Discuss the differences between OPSEC and site security.
3. List and discuss the five steps of the OPSEC process.
4. Diagram and subsequently discuss the components of the intelligence cycle.
5. Identify what agency is charged with fostering widespread adoption of OPSEC at the national, state, tribal, territorial, and local agency levels. What support does it provide to these constituent agencies?
6. Discuss why site security is an important strategic and tactical consideration at emergency response scenes.
7. Outline the critical components of establishing and sustaining site security operations and how they integrate into the incident command system process.
8. Discuss the importance of evidence protection and the value emergency responders afford law enforcement when responders take protective measures to recognize and preserve suspected evidence at the scene of an incident.
9. Identify and discuss the importance of personal accountability at the scene of an incident and how OPSEC and site security can augment this process. Additionally, describe what measures for personnel authentication can be employed by integrating OPSEC and site security into local response policy and operational doctrine.

Chapter Project I

Develop a sample OPSEC policy for your agency that addresses each of the five steps in the OPSEC process. Remember to allow for integration of mutual aid response assets into the protocol.

Chapter Project II

Review a past large-scale incident, examining the response for site security compliance. Discuss the pros and cons of the response and how you would improve/enhance the site security operation.

Vital Vocabulary

Intelligence The product resulting from the collection, collation, evaluation, analysis, integration, and interpretation of collected information.

OPSEC A tool designed to promote operational effectiveness by denying adversaries publicly available indicators of sensitive activities, capabilities, or intentions.

Public information officer (PIO) The position within the incident command system responsible for providing information about the incident. The PIO functions as a point of contact for the media.

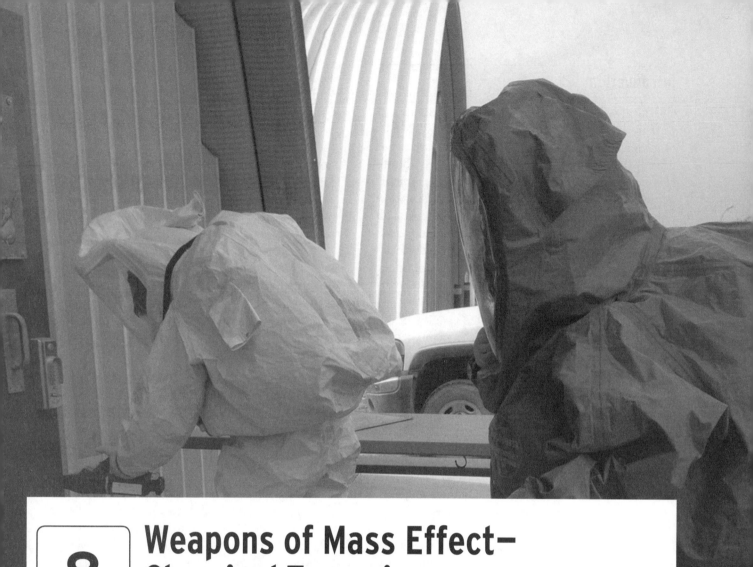

8

Weapons of Mass Effect– Chemical Terrorism and Warfare Agents

Paul M. Maniscalco
Dr. Christopher P. Holstege
Dr. Frederick R. Sidell

Objectives

- Understand the importance of preparedness for a chemical attack.
- Recognize the characteristics of nerve agents.
- Outline victim treatment procedures for nerve agent exposure.
- Outline treatment procedures for cyanide exposure.
- Define vesicants and list the symptoms for exposure to specific vesicants.
- Recognize the symptoms of exposure to pulmonary agents.
- Define the common riot control agents.
- Recognize the importance of triage in mass victim incidents.

Introduction

Chemical warfare agents are chemical substances that were developed for use on the battlefield to kill, injure, or incapacitate. For 79 years, from their first use in 1915 in World War I until 1993, the intentional use of these chemicals to kill, injure, or incapacitate was limited to battlefield use. The requisite tactics and necessary technology for chemical terrorism events are unmistakably notable from using chemical weapons designed to meet military needs. Chemical terrorism can be defined as an asymmetric warfare tactic employed by nonmilitary actors against noncombatant (civilian) targets.

At the first World Trade Center attack in New York City in 1993, the attackers integrated cyanide into the construct of the explosive device they manufactured. Fortunately, the expected dissemination did not efficiently occur with the violent explosion; the explosion rapidly consumed the integrated product, rendering the tactic ineffective. In June 1994, the religious cult Aum Shinrikyo disseminated one of these agents, sarin, throughout an apartment complex in Matsumoto, Japan, with the intent of causing widespread harm or death to people. In March 1995, the same group released sarin on the Tokyo subways, causing injuries in over 1,000 people and death in 12. Terrorists had a new weapon—a chemical weapon.

Rogue individuals and organizations continue to possess or have access to these weapons. There are probably several dozen countries with the capacity to manufacture these chemicals, and some of these countries are known to be sponsors of terrorist groups and acts of terrorism. In addition, instructions for the synthesis of these agents are widely available to terrorist groups and rogue individuals in books, on the Internet, and in other places such as militia newsletters.

Some very toxic chemicals are regularly manufactured in large amounts in this country and are transported daily on our highways and railways. Chemicals such as cyanide, phosgene, and chlorine, all of which were once military agents, are widely used in large amounts (**CP FIGURE 8-1**). Many commonly used pesticides have very similar properties to nerve agents.

With the ever-increasing number of toxic chemicals in the world and the existence of rogue organizations that are willing to use them to further their causes, it is essential that communities and emergency response organizations prepare to confront the challenges presented by a chemical terrorist event.

Terrorist incidents involving military chemical agents are, from an individual victim treatment foundation level, not much different from a regular hazardous materials incident; victim care is the same. The critical differences are: (1) it is a deliberate release and (2) most likely it is a high-impact/high-yield incident with numerous victims.

Overall, there are differences between an accidental spill of a toxic chemical and a deliberate release of the same chemical. Probably the most important difference is the fear and anxiety generated in the community and among the emergency responders who must deal with unknown factors. This fear and anxiety may be present in possible victims, who do not know and who cannot be immediately reassured that they have not been harmed, or it might be present in responders who fear a secondary hostile device at the scene designed to injure them. Many more agencies become involved in a deliberate release incident, including emergency medical services (EMS), fire/rescue, emergency management, law enforcement, and all levels of government that will converge on the scene in an effort to assist. The site of a deliberate incident is a crime scene, a chemical hot zone, a biological hot zone, and in most cases a high-impact/high-yield multiple casualty incident. These events result in EMS and the medical community playing a significant lead role in consequence management. Between delayed onset of symptoms, decontamination practices, victim tracking, and other relevant activities, EMS and hospitals must remain attentive to victim signs and symptoms that may indicate a sentinel event of an attack.

Delivery/Dissemination

Chemical agents are disseminated in many ways. Bombs, rockets, mines, and other explosive devices are used by the military. When these explode, some of the agent remains as liquid, some immediately evaporates to form vapor, and some will exist as small droplets of the agent suspended in air, or an aerosol. These small droplets eventually evaporate and become a vapor. The result is a hazard from the liquid agent, both as the original liquid and as the aerosol droplets (which neither remain long nor travel far) and a hazard from agent vapor. Agents can also be sprayed from airplanes during battlefield use, as some agents were during the Vietnam War.

Liquid chemical agents might be employed with an explosive device by nonmilitary users. The user would have to make the device, which is not without hazard, and then detonate it in the right place at the right time.

CRITICAL FACTOR ....

The emergency response community must be prepared for a consequence response to a chemical attack.

Other means of disseminating the agent are more likely. Insecticides are sprayed from airplanes and helicopters in both crop dusting (**FIGURE 8-1**) and mosquito eradication. This is an obvious and expensive way to disseminate an agent, but it is effective for spreading it over a large area providing the weather and winds are favorable. Vehicle-mounted spray tanks can be driven through the streets of a target area to disseminate an agent. For example, in Matsumoto, the agent was spread from the back of a vehicle in which a container of agent was heated (to help it to evaporate), and the vapor was blown through the street by a fan. Indoor areas might be attacked by putting an agent in the air system, and rooms could be thoroughly and quickly contaminated by the use of a common aerosol spray can. There are other methods of disseminating liquids.

Nerve Agents

<u>Nerve agents</u> are toxic materials that produce injury and death within seconds to minutes. The signs and symptoms caused by nerve agent vapor are characteristic of the agents and are not difficult to recognize with a high index of suspicion. Very good antidotes that will save lives and reduce injury if administered in time are available.

Nerve agents are a group of chemicals similar to, but more toxic than, commonly used organophosphate insecticides such as Malathion. Nerve agents were developed in Germany during the 1930s for wartime use, but they were not used in World War II. They were used in the Iran–Iraq war. They were also used by the religious cult Aum Shinrikyo in Japan on two occasions; the first use injured about 300 people and killed seven in Matsumoto in June 1994; the second killed

12 and injured over 1,000 in the Tokyo subways in March 1995.

The common nerve agents are tabun (GA), sarin (GB), soman (GD), GF, and VX (GF and VX have no common names) (**CP FIGURE 8-2**).

The nerve agents are liquids (not nerve gases) that freeze at temperatures below 0°F and boil at temperatures above 200°F (**CP FIGURE 8-3**). Sarin (GB), the most volatile, evaporates at about the rate of water, and VX, the least volatile, is similar to light motor oil in its rate of evaporation. The rates of evaporation of the others lie in between. In the Tokyo subway attack, sarin leaked out of plastic bags and evaporated. Serious injury was minimized because the rate of evaporation of sarin is not rapid, so the amount of vapor formed was not large. If the sarin had evaporated more rapidly (e.g., like gasoline or ether), much more vapor would have been present, and more serious injury in more people would have occurred.

Nerve agents produce physiological effects by interfering with the transmission between a nerve and the organ it innervates or stimulates, with the end result being excess stimulation of the organ. Nerve agents do not actually act on nerves. Instead, they act on the chemical connection of the nerve to the muscle or organ. Normally, an electrical impulse travels down a nerve, but the impulse does not cross the small synaptic gap between the nerve and the organ. At the end of the nerve, the electrical impulse causes the release of a chemical messenger, a neurotransmitter, which travels across the gap to stimulate the organ. The organ may be an exocrine gland, a smooth muscle, a skeletal muscle, or another nerve. The organ responds to the stimulus by secreting, by contracting, or by transmitting another message down a nerve. After the neurotransmitter stimulates the organ, it is immediately destroyed by an enzyme so that it cannot stimulate the organ again. Nerve agents inhibit or block the activity of this enzyme so that it cannot destroy the neurotransmitter or chemical messenger. As a result, the neurotransmitter accumulates and continues to stimulate the organ. If the organ is a gland, it continues to secrete; if it is a muscle, it continues to contract; or if it is a nerve, it continues to transmit impulses. There is hyperactivity throughout the body.

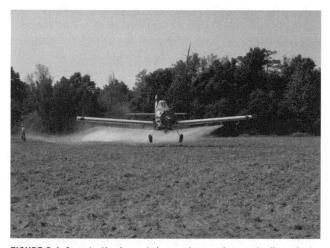

FIGURE 8-1 Crop dusting is an obvious and expensive way to disseminate an agent, but it is effective for spreading it over a large area providing the weather and winds are favorable.

Nerve agents perform the following actions within the human body:

- Block the activity of an enzyme (called acetyl-cholinesterase)
- Cause too much neurotransmitter to accumulate (acetylcholine)
- Cause too much activity in many organs, glands, muscles, skeletal muscles, smooth muscles (in internal organs), and other nerves

In the presence of nerve agent poisoning, exocrine glands secrete excessively. These glands include the tear glands (tearing), the nasal glands (rhinorrhea or runny nose), the salivary glands (hypersalivation), and the sweat glands (sweating). In addition, the glands in the airways (bronchorrhea) and in the gastrointestinal tract secrete excessively in the presence of nerve agents.

The clinically important smooth muscles that respond are those in the eye (to produce small pupils, or miosis), in the airways (to cause constriction), and in the gastrointestinal tract (to cause vomiting, diarrhea, and abdominal cramping).

Skeletal muscles respond initially with movement of muscle fibers (fasciculations, which look like rippling under the skin), then twitching of large muscles, and finally weakness and a flaccid paralysis as the muscles tire.

Nerve agents affect the following:

- Lacrimal glands (tearing)
- Nose (rhinorrhea)
- Mouth (salivation)
- Sweat glands (diaphoresis)
- Bronchial tract (in airways causing wheezing)
- Gastrointestinal tract (cramps, vomiting, diarrhea)
- Skeletal muscles
  - Fasciculations, twitching, weakness, paralysis
- Smooth muscles
  - Airways (constriction)
- Central nervous system
  - Loss of consciousness
  - Convulsions
  - Cessation of breathing

Among the nerve-to-nerve effects are stimulation of autonomic ganglia to produce adrenergic effects such as hypertension (high blood pressure) and tachycardia (rapid heart rate). The exact mechanisms in the central nervous system are less well defined, but the result is loss of consciousness, seizures, cessation of breathing (apnea) because of depression of the respiratory center, and finally death. Early effects also include stimulation of the vagus nerve, which causes slowing of the heart (bradycardia), or stimulation of the sympathetic system to cause tachycardia.

The effects that occur depend on the route of exposure and the amount of exposure. The initial effects from a small amount of vapor are not the same as those from a small droplet on the skin, and the initial effects from a small amount of vapor are not the same as those from a large amount of vapor. Exposure to nerve agent vapor produces effects within seconds of contact. These effects will continue to worsen as long as the victim is in the vapor atmosphere but will not worsen significantly after the victim is removed from the atmosphere.

Exposure to a small concentration of vapor will cause effects in the sensitive organs of the face that come into direct contact with the vapor—the eyes, the nose, and the mouth and lower airways. Miosis (small pupils) is the most common sign of exposure to nerve agent vapor. Reddened, watery eyes may accompany the small pupils, and the victim may complain of blurred and/or dim vision, a headache, and nausea and vomiting (from reflex mechanisms). Rhinorrhea (runny nose) is also common, and after a severe exposure the secretions might be quite copious. Increased salivation may be present. Agent contact with the airways will cause constriction of the airways and secretions from the glands in the airways. The victim will complain of shortness of breath (dyspnea), which, depending on the amount of agent inhaled, may be mild and tolerable or may be very severe. These effects will begin within seconds after contact with the agent. They will increase in severity while the victim is in the vapor, but will maximize within minutes after the victim leaves the vapor.

Sudden exposure to a large concentration of vapor, or continuing exposure to a small amount, will cause loss of consciousness, seizures, cessation of seizures with cessation of breathing and flaccid paralysis, and death. After exposure to a large concentration, loss of consciousness occurs within seconds, and effects progress rapidly to cessation of breathing within 10 minutes.

Vapor Exposure

Small Concentration

- Miosis (red eyes, pain, blurring, nausea)
- Runny nose
- Shortness of breath
- Effects start within seconds of contact.

Large Concentration

- Loss of consciousness
- Convulsions
- Cessation of breathing
- Flaccid paralysis
- Effects start within seconds of contact.

A very small, sublethal droplet of agent on the skin causes sweating and muscular fasciculations in the area of the droplet. These may begin as long as 18 hours after agent contact with the skin and generally will not be noticed by either the victim or medical personnel. A slightly larger, but still sublethal droplet will cause those effects and later cause gastrointestinal effects, such as nausea, vomiting, diarrhea, and cramps. The onset of these are also delayed and may start as late as 18 hours after exposure. A lethal-sized droplet causes effects much sooner, usually within 30 minutes of contact. Without any preliminary signs, there will be a sudden loss of consciousness and seizures followed within minutes by cessation of breathing, flaccid paralysis, and death.

Effects from skin contact with a liquid droplet will occur even though the droplet was removed or decontaminated within minutes after contact. Rapid decontamination will decrease the illness but will not prevent it. Nerve agent liquid on skin will cause effects that begin many minutes to many hours after initial contact. After the effects begin they may worsen because of continued absorption of agent through the skin.

Liquid on Skin

Very Small Droplet
- Sweating, fasciculations
- Can start as late as 18 hours after contact

Small Droplet
- Vomiting, diarrhea
- Can start as late as 18 hours after contact

Lethal-Sized Droplet or Larger
- Loss of consciousness
- Convulsions
- Cessation of breathing
- Flaccid paralysis
- Usually starts without warning within 30 minutes

Management of a nerve agent casualty consists of removing the agent from the victim (decontamination) or the victim from the agent, administration of antidotes, and ventilation if needed. EMS providers must have proper personal protective equipment during these operations.

For the antidotes to be effective, the victim must be removed from the contaminated area and/or the agent must be removed from the victim's skin. Although the antidotes are quite effective, they cannot overcome the effects of the agent while the victim is continuing to breathe the agent or while the agent is still being absorbed through the skin. Skin decontamination will not remove an agent that has been absorbed into the skin. Even if the agent is not yet through the skin, effects may start as long as several hours after skin decontamination.

Removing the victim from the area of contamination or the vapor area should be rather simple in a normal hazardous materials incident, but the complexities of a mass casualty terrorism event present some unique challenges. If the agent was released inside a building or other enclosed space, moving the victims outside should suffice. If the agent was released outside, victims should be removed and triaged far upwind.

Removal of the agent from the skin must be done as early as possible. It is unlikely that you will see a living victim with visible amounts of nerve agent on his skin. However, if this occurs, remove it (the substance) as quickly as possible. Flushing with large amounts of water or wiping it off with dirt or any other convenient substance will help. If clothing is wet, suggesting agent exposure, remove the clothing as quickly as possible. This should be done in the hot zone before the victim reaches the decontamination site in the warm zone. Although the agent is removed from the surface of the skin, the agent that has already penetrated into the skin cannot be removed, and absorption will continue; the victim may worsen despite antidotes.

The antidotes for nerve agent poisoning are atropine and an oxime, 2-pyridoxime chloride or 2-PAMCl (Protopam). They act by different mechanisms. Atropine blocks the excess neurotransmitter and protects the site on the organ that the neurotransmitter stimulates. As a result, the glands dry and the smooth muscles stop contracting (such as those in the airways and gastrointestinal tract). However, atropine has little effect on the skeletal muscles, and these muscles may continue to twitch despite an adequate dose of atropine.

The initial dose of atropine is 2 mg to 6 mg. This dose might seem high to those accustomed to administering it for cardiac or other purposes, but it is the amount necessary to overcome a total-body excess of the neurotransmitter. After the initial dose, a dose of 2 mg should be administered every 5 to 10 minutes until (1) the secretions have diminished considerably, and (2) breathing has improved or airway resistance has decreased (if the victim is being ventilated). Tachycardia (rapid heart rate) is not a contraindication to atropine

CRITICAL FACTOR ....

Treatment for nerve agent exposure involves decontamination, administration of antidotes, and ventilation.

use in these victims. Atropine can be administered by an intramuscular (IM) route, an intravenous (IV) route, or by an endotracheal route. Atropine administered by IV to animals hypoxic from nerve agent poisoning has caused ventricular fibrillation, so good advice is not to administer it by this route until ventilation has begun.

The oxime, 2-PAMCl, attacks the complex of the agent bound to the enzyme and removes the agent from the enzyme. As a result, the enzyme can resume its normal function of destroying the neurotransmitter. Despite the fact that this drug sounds like a very effective antidote, it does not reverse the effects seen clinically in the glands and smooth muscle. It does reduce the skeletal muscle twitching and weakness. It is almost totally ineffective when used against poisoning from one nerve agent, soman (GD), but it is unlikely that identification of the agent will be made before the initial therapy, and use of the oxime in the usual doses will do no harm.

The initial dose of 2-PAMCl is 1 gram given slowly (over 20 minutes or longer) in an IV drip. More rapid administration will cause hypertension (which can transiently be reversed by phentolamine). The 2-PAMCl should not be titrated with the victim's condition as atropine is, but it should be administered at hourly intervals for a total of three doses.

A third drug, diazepam (Valium) or a similar benzodiazepine anticonvulsant, should be used for any convulsions and as rapidly as possible.

The military originally had an autoinjector device called the MARK I with two spring-powered injectors, one containing atropine (2 mg) and the other 2-PAMCl (600 mg) (CP FIGURE 8-4). The latest iteration of this countermeasure is a single unit autoinjector with two chambers called the "antidote treatment—nerve agent, autoinjector" (ATNAA). The ATNAA provides atropine injection and pralidoxime chloride injection in separate chambers as sterile, pyrogen-free solutions for intramuscular injection. The ATNAA is a specially designed unit for automatic self-administration or buddy administration by military personnel. When activated, the ATNAA sequentially administers atropine and pralidoxime chloride through a single needle. There is a civilian version of the ATNAA that is called the DuoDote, manufactured by Meridian Medical Technologies, which is intended as an initial treatment of the symptoms of organophosphorus insecticide or nerve agent poisonings (CP FIGURE 8-5).

The autoinjector is a very effective and fast way to administer the antidotes, and use of this causes the drugs to be absorbed faster. Instructional material for both the ATNAA and DuoDote can be found in the reference section of this text.

When treating an unconscious victim severely affected by nerve agent poisoning, gasping for air or not breathing, seizing or postictal, the responder should take care of the airway, breathing, and circulation first. When an airway is inserted and ventilation is attempted in a severe nerve agent victim, the airway resistance will be so great that most devices used for ventilation will not be effective, making ventilation impossible. It might be best to IM administer the antidotes first. This ensures that some air will be moved when ventilation is attempted.

A victim might be exposed to vapor only and be out of the vapor environment and be walking and talking when first seen. This victim might be relatively asymptomatic or may be very uncomfortable from shortness of breath but generally is in no danger of loss of life. There may be miosis with red, watery eyes, rhinorrhea, a headache or eye pain, nausea and vomiting, and shortness of breath with auscultatory sounds of airway constriction and secretions. Atropine (2 mg, IM or IV) will reduce or eliminate the shortness of breath and most of the rhinorrhea, but not the eye effects (miosis, pain) or the nausea and vomiting. The responder should start 2-PAMCl (1 gram, slow IV drip).

Initial Antidote Use

Vapor Exposure

- Miosis and/or runny nose—no antidotes unless eye pain is severe (eye drops)
- Shortness of breath—2 or 4 mg of atropine depending on severity; 2-PAMCl by slow drip
- Unconscious, convulsions, severe breathing difficulty; moderate to severe effects in two or more systems—6 mg of atropine IM; 2-PAMCl by slow drip; ventilation

Liquid on Skin

- Local sweating, fasciculations—2 mg of atropine; 2-PAMCl by slow drip
- Vomiting, diarrhea—2 mg of atropine; 2-PAMCl by slow drip
- Unconscious, convulsing, severe breathing difficulty; moderate to severe effects in two or more systems—6 mg of atropine IM; 2-PAMCl by slow drip; ventilation

In all cases, follow with 2 mg of atropine every 5 to 10 minutes until improvement occurs using the amount of wheezing (bronchospasm) as an indicator of when to administer subsequent doses.

Systemic atropine (IM, IV, and endotracheally) has almost no effect on the eyes unless large amounts are administered. If eye pain/headache or nausea and vomiting are severe, these are relieved by topical application of atropine or homatropine eye ointment. These medications will cause severe blurring of vision for about 24 hours, and it is best not to administer them unless the pain or vomiting is severe. The slight reduction in vision (dimness, slight blurring) caused by the agent is less than that caused by the medications. Miosis by itself (without pain or nausea) should not be treated.

If dyspnea is more than moderate and if the victim is still capable of walking and talking, the initial dose of atropine should be 4 mg. Whether the initial amount is 2 mg or 4 mg, an additional 2 mg should be administered in 5 to 10 minutes if there is no improvement in the victim's condition. More should be given at similar intervals if necessary, but in most instances the initial 2 mg will reduce the symptoms.

A more severely affected victim will be unable to walk or talk. He will be unconsciousness with severe breathing difficulties or not breathing, perhaps convulsing or postictal with copious secretions and muscular twitching. A severely affected victim may also be one who has moderate or severe signs in two or more organ systems (respiratory, gastrointestinal, muscular, and central nervous systems). The eyes and nose are not considered in this evaluation. This victim should initially be given 6 mg of atropine (IM, not IV), and an IV drip containing 1 gram of the oxime should be started. Ventilation begins after the antidotes are administered. Diazepam or a similar anticonvulsant should be administered. Atropine should be continued at 5- to 10-minute intervals until there is improvement.

A small liquid droplet on the skin will cause sweating and fasciculation at the site, and if this is noted, the victim should receive atropine (2 mg, IM) and 2-PAMCl (1 gram in a slow IV drip). A slightly larger droplet initially will cause gastrointestinal effects (nausea, vomiting, diarrhea, cramps), and a victim with these symptoms should receive the same drugs in the same amounts. A victim with either the small droplet or the larger droplet might worsen, and atropine should be continued at intervals. The onset of these effects may be as long as 18 hours after contact with the agent. Any victim suspected of contacting a liquid agent should be kept under observation for 18 hours.

A large, lethal-sized droplet of agent will cause sudden loss of consciousness followed by seizures, cessation of breathing, flaccid paralysis, and death. These effects begin within 30 minutes of contact with the agent, and there are usually no preliminary effects before the loss of consciousness. Management is the same as for severe vapor exposure, with early decontamination if therapy is to be successful.

You can save a victim with a heartbeat by timely and adequate therapy. Occasionally an arrested victim can also be saved. One victim from the Tokyo subway incident had no heartbeat when he was taken into the hospital, but he was adequately treated. He walked out of the hospital several days later.

Cyanide

Cyanide, like the nerve agents, can cause serious illness and death within minutes. Cyanide was not successful as a warfare agent in World War I for several reasons, including: (1) it is volatile and tended to evaporate and be blown away by a breeze; (2) it is lighter than air and will not stay close to the ground where it can do damage; and (3) the dose to cause effects is relatively large, and, unlike other agents, it causes few effects at lower doses.

Some forms of cyanide are gases under temperate conditions (hydrogen cyanide, cyanogen chloride), and other forms are solids (sodium, potassium, or calcium cyanide). Hundreds of thousands of tons of cyanide are manufactured, shipped, and used worldwide annually. It is used in the manufacture of certain synthetic products, paper, and textiles; in tanning; in ore extraction; in cleaning jewelry; in printing; and in photography. It is in the seeds of some foods and is in the cassava plant—a staple in certain parts of the world. It is produced when synthetic materials (e.g., plastics) burn. Cyanide has been associated with killing. For centuries it has been used for assassinations and is used in the gas chamber for executions. People sometimes ingest cyanide with suicidal intent. It was taken by the followers of the Reverend Jim Jones for suicide and was illicitly placed in Tylenol bottles in the Chicago area years ago.

The human body has a means of detoxifying or neutralizing small amounts of cyanide, and this is very effective until the system is overwhelmed. The body combines cyanide with a form of sulfur, and the nontoxic product is excreted. When the body runs out of sulfur, effects appear.

Cyanide causes biological effects by combining with an enzyme that is in cells, and stopping or inhibiting its activity. This enzyme normally metabolizes oxygen in the cell so that the cell can function. When cyanide stops the activity of this enzyme, the cell cannot function and dies. There is plenty of oxygen available in the blood, but the cell cannot use it so it does not take it from the blood.

The effects of exposure to a small concentration of vapor or the initial effects from drinking cyanide are relatively nonspecific. They include a brief period of rapid onset, gasping respiration, tachycardia, anxiety, altered mental status, seizures, hypotension, dysrhythmias, chest palpations/tightness, tachypnea, diaphoresis, low pulse oximetry even with presence of oxygen, skin pale to slightly reddish color, deep breathing, feelings of anxiety or apprehension, agitation, dizziness, a feeling of weakness, nausea with or without vomiting, and muscular trembling. As more cyanide is absorbed, consciousness is lost, respiration decreases in rate and frequency, and seizures, cessation of breathing, and disturbances in heart rate and rhythm follow. After inhalation of a high concentration of vapor, seizures can occur within 30 seconds, and cessation of breathing and disturbances of cardiac rhythm follow. Death occurs in 6 to 10 minutes after exposure.

Large Amount by Inhalation

Hyperventilation: 15 seconds
Convulsions: 30 seconds
Cessation of breathing: 3–5 minutes
Cessation of heartbeat: 6–10 minutes

Management

Hydroxocobalamin 5g IV
> or

Amyl nitrite pearl
Sodium nitrite IV (10 mL; 300 mg)
Sodium thiosulfate IV (50 mL; 12.5 g)
> and

Ventilation with oxygen
Correction of acidosis

Cyanogen chloride causes the effects of cyanide as listed previously. However, it is very irritating (similar to the riot control agents) and will produce burning of the eyes, the nose, and airways. It has a pungent odor.

There are few findings on physical examination. The skin is said to be cherry red (because of the red, oxygenated venous blood), but this is not always present. The pupils are normal in size or slightly large, secretions are relatively normal, and there are no muscular fasciculations, all of which serve to distinguish cyanide poisoning from nerve agent poisoning.

In the laboratory, cyanide can be measured in blood. Also, there will be more than the normal amount of oxygen in venous blood, and there may be a metabolic acidosis. Management consists of removing the victim from the contaminated atmosphere (or by removing the poison from the victim), and administering antidotes and oxygen.

Hydroxocobalamin

Hydroxocobalamin, a vitamin B_{12} precursor, is now available in multiple countries as an antidote for cyanide poisoning. In 2006, it was approved by the U.S. Food and Drug Administration. Hydroxocobalamin complexes cyanide, forming cyanocobalamin (vitamin B_{12}). One molecule of hydroxocobalamin binds one molecule of cyanide. The U.S.-approved adult starting dose is 5 g administered by IV infusion over 15 minutes. Depending upon the severity of the poisoning and the clinical response, a second dose of 5 g may be administered by IV infusion for a total dose of 10 g. Hydroxocobalamin has few adverse effects, which include allergic reaction and a transient reddish discoloration of the skin, mucous membranes, and urine. No hemodynamic adverse effects other than a potential mild transient rise of blood pressure are observed.

The Cyanide Antidote Kit

The cyanide antidote kit (**CP FIGURE 8-6**) contains the following three components: (1) amyl nitrite; (2) sodium nitrite; and (3) sodium thiosulfate. Amyl nitrite is available in a pearl. This should be broken and placed in a breathing bag for the victim to inhale. Instructions state that this should be held under the victim's nose for him or her to breathe. Sodium nitrite is packaged in an ampule containing 300 mg in 10 mL for IV administration. Amyl nitrite should be used only until the sodium nitrite can be administered by IV. The third component is a sulfur compound, sodium thiosulfate. When this is administered, the body can resume the normal process of tying up cyanide with sulfur to form a nontoxic substance. An ampule contains 12.5 g in 50 mL for IV administration. These three antidotes should be given sequentially to a victim who is unconscious and/or not breathing. Oxygen should be administered, even though the oxygen content of blood is normal. The acidosis should be corrected.

Vesicants

Vesicants are agents that cause vesicles or blisters. They may be of animal, vegetable, or mineral origin, such as some types of sea creatures, poison ivy, and certain chemicals. Other things, such as sunlight, can produce blisters. Vesicants have been used as chemical warfare agents. Several have been developed for this purpose, but only one—sulfur mustard (**CP FIGURE 8-7**)—has been used. The other major chemical warfare vesicant is lewisite.

CRITICAL FACTOR ....

Cyanide antidotes are: hydroxocobalamin or amyl nitrites, sodium nitrite, and thiosulfate.

Sulfur mustard was first synthesized in the early 1800s and was first used on the battlefield in World War I. During that war it caused more chemical casualties than any other agent; however, only about 3 percent of these casualties died. Iraq used it extensively during its war with Iran, and pictures of some casualties were in the media during that period. Its use has been alleged in some other conflicts over the past 80 years.

In the early 1940s, nitrogen mustard (developed for military use), a close relative of sulfur mustard, was used in the treatment of cancer, the first chemical to be used for that purpose.

Sulfur mustard (mustard) is a light yellowish to brown oily liquid that smells like garlic, onions, or mustard (the reason for its name). Its boiling point is over 200°F, and it freezes at 58°F. The low freezing point hinders its battlefield use in cool weather, and it is often mixed with another chemical to lower the freezing point. It does not evaporate very quickly, but large amounts of mustard, particularly in warm weather, produce a vapor hazard.

Mustard causes cellular damage and death with subsequent tissue damage. The mechanism by which it does this has not been entirely clear, but the best evidence suggests that it damages DNA, which then prevents further cellular functioning and leads to cellular death. Although its best-known effects are those on the tissues, the agent directly contacts the skin, the eyes, and the airways. When it is absorbed into the body in adequate amounts, mustard damages many tissues such as bone marrow, lymphoid tissue, and the gastrointestinal tract. Its effects are similar to those caused by radiation, and it is a radiomimetic agent.

Once liquid or vapor mustard is in contact with an epithelial surface, the skin, the eye, or the mucosa of the airways, it penetrates that surface quite rapidly, and enough is absorbed within a minute to cause cellular damage. Decontamination after a minute will not prevent tissue damage, but it will reduce the amount of ensuing damage. Once into tissue, the chemical reactions within the cell that eventually result in clinical effects begin. Once mustard touches a body surface, irreversible damage is done in cells within minutes.

Upon contact with the skin, the eyes, or the airways, mustard causes no immediate clinical effects. There is no immediate pain, redness, or blister formation. The victim usually does not know he or she has been exposed. The itching and pain of erythema, the irritation of the conjunctiva, or the irritation and discomfort in the upper airways do not appear until many hours later. The period without signs or symptoms is called the latent period, and it can range from 2 to 24 hours after contact. Commonly these effects begin in 4 to 8 hours after contact.

At the site of an incident or spill involving mustard, there will be no victims with signs and symptoms of mustard exposure. Hours later, the pain, irritation, and discomfort will start, and the victims will seek medical care.

The initial effects in the eyes after exposure to mustard vapor are irritation or burning, and the victim will complain of grittiness in his eyes. The eyes will be red, similar to the appearance of eyes with sand or dust in them. This may progress to a severe conjunctivitis, swelling of the lids, and even corneal edema (seen as an irregular light pattern on the cornea). The victim will complain of pain, irritation, and sensitivity to light. He may also complain of inability to see. This is usually because the lids are shut, either because of swelling or because of involuntary contracture of the muscles around the eye. Rarely, a droplet of mustard will get into the eyes, and this may cause more severe damage to the cornea, including ulceration and perforation.

Mustard contact with skin will initially cause redness, or erythema, which is similar to sunburn with burning and itching. If the contact was to a low concentration of vapor, this may be the extent of the injury, but more commonly small blisters develop around the edges of the redness. These gradually coalesce to form larger blisters, which are generally no worse than second degree burns. Third degree burns are very uncommon and require exposure to a large amount of liquid agent.

Mustard vapor, when inhaled, damages the mucosa or inner layer of the airways. The damage begins at the upper part of the airways (the nose) and descends to the lowermost portion, the terminal bronchioles. The amount of damage depends on the amount of mustard inhaled, which, in turn, depends on the concentration of the vapor and exposure time. The initial effects are in the nose and sinuses with burning, irritation, and perhaps some nasal bleeding. Pharyngitis, with a sore throat and a nonproductive cough, may appear, followed by laryngitis with hoarseness or complete lack of voice. Mustard damage in the lower airways causes shortness of breath and a cough productive of inflammatory and necrotic material as the agent destroys the inner lining of these small airways. Severe damage provides an ideal setting for infection 4 or 5 days later.

CRITICAL FACTOR ....

Vesicants cause vesicles or blisters.

Initial Effects

There are no immediate effects of contact with sulfur mustard; effects start potentially hours after contact.

Skin
- Redness (erythema) with burning and itching
- Blisters

Eye
- Redness with burning and itching

Airways
- Nasal and sinus pain
- Sore throat, nonproductive cough

Large amounts of absorbed mustard severely damage the precursor cells in the bone marrow, with a decrease in the white cells, red cells, and platelets in the blood. This usually happens four or more days after exposure in a severely exposed victim. The lining of the gastrointestinal tract is also severely damaged after absorption of a large amount of mustard with subsequent loss of fluid and electrolytes starting days after exposure. This effect is similar to that seen after radiation exposure.

Immediate decontamination—within a minute—should be performed to minimize the damage, but responders will not be on the scene that quickly. Skin damage will be reduced by decontamination of the contact site on the skin if done within 30 minutes, but not beyond that time.

A victim returning hours after the incident with red skin (erythema) needs no immediate care, although soothing lotions (e.g., calamine) can be applied to reduce the burning and itching. Later, areas of blistering or denuded skin must be irrigated frequently, with the application of topical antibiotics three or four times a day to these areas. Fluids do not need to be replaced in large amounts as they do after thermal burns, because mustard burns do not cause the amount of fluid loss seen in thermal burns. Care must be taken not to overhydrate victims. They will not need significant fluid replacement unless they are dehydrated from other causes.

A victim with red eyes (conjunctivitis) who is complaining of burning or irritation in the eyes should have his or her eyes washed out and a soothing ophthalmic ointment or drops applied. Because the lesion appears hours after contact with the agent, the agent is no longer in the eye because of absorption and evaporation, and the purpose of eye irrigation is to wash out inflammatory

CRITICAL FACTOR..........................

Immediate decontamination is very important with mustard exposure.

debris. Later eye care consists of regular application of a topical antibiotic and a mydriatic (to prevent future adhesions between lens and iris). Petroleum jelly should be applied regularly to the edges of the lids (to prevent adhesions). Some believe that topical steroids used within the first 24 hours only will reduce inflammation, but application should be done by an ophthalmologist.

A suggestion of airway involvement by the agent, such as nasal or sinus irritation or a sore throat with a dry hacking cough, may occur. Laryngeal damage with voice changes or hoarseness accompanied by signs of beginning lower airway damage is an indication for the immediate insertion of an endotracheal tube. Later, more severe damage will necessitate assisted ventilation including positive end-expiratory pressure and frequent sputum examinations for infecting organisms.

Bone marrow depression and severe gastrointestinal damage occur days after the initial exposure in an already severely ill victim.

All victims must be decontaminated before they enter a medical facility. When signs and symptoms appear hours after the initial agent contact, the agent will be gone from exposed surfaces by evaporation or by absorption. Later decontamination will not prevent further injury to the victim. However, liquid may be in clothing or the agent (liquid or condensed vapor) may be in hair.

Lewisite

Lewisite was developed late in World War I but was not used in that war. Japan possibly used it against China in the late 1930s; otherwise it has not been used on the battlefield. Some countries are known to have military stockpiles of lewisite.

Lewisite is an oily liquid with the odor of geraniums. Its freezing point is below 0°F, it boils at 190°F, it contains arsenic, a heavy metal, and it is more volatile than mustard.

Lewisite participates in many biological reactions, but the mechanism of cellular injury is unknown. It damages cells causing cellular death, and its biological effects are similar to those of mustard with topical damage to eyes, skin, and airways (**CP FIGURE 8-8**). It does not damage marrow, the gastrointestinal tract, or lymphoid tissue, but it does damage systemic capillaries allowing leakage of intravascular volume. This can culminate in hypovolemic shock in severe cases.

An important initial clinical distinction between lewisite and mustard is that lewisite vapor causes immediate irritation of eyes, skin, and upper airways. Lewisite

CRITICAL FACTOR..............................

Lewisite causes eye and upper airway irritation and pain on contact.

liquid causes pain or burning on whatever surface it contacts within seconds. The victim is alerted to its presence and will leave the area or remove the liquid. Mustard causes no clinical effects until the lesions develop, hours after contact.

Lewisite causes topical damage to eyes (conjunctivitis and more severe damage), skin (erythema and blisters), and airways (damage to the lining or mucosa) similar to that of mustard. Severe lewisite exposure may cause pulmonary edema, which is very uncommon after mustard exposure. Generally, the lesions from lewisite are deeper with more tissue damage than those from mustard.

Management of a victim with lewisite exposure is similar to the management of a victim with mustard exposure. The victim will usually self-decontaminate quickly because of the pain or irritation. In addition to the measures recommended for mustard lesions, there is a specific antidote for the systematic (nontopical) effects of lewisite. This is British antilewisite, a drug used for several other types of heavy metal poisoning, and is for hospital use only.

Pulmonary Agents

Pulmonary agents are chemicals that produce pulmonary edema (fluid in the lung), with little damage to the airways or other tissues. The best known and most studied of these is phosgene (carbonyl chloride), although other chemicals (e.g., chlorine) behave in this manner.

Phosgene and chlorine were major agents in World War I until the use of mustard. Their usefulness as warfare agents has diminished since then, and now they are not considered important militarily. However, both are important in industry, and large amounts of both are manufactured and shipped annually.

After inhalation of phosgene, the carbonyl part of the molecule causes damage in the thin wall between the blood vessels (capillaries) and the air sac (alveolus). As a result of this damage, the watery part of the blood leaks into the alveoli. When these become filled with fluid, air cannot enter to deliver oxygen to the blood, oxygen cannot be delivered to other tissues, and the victim suffocates in a sense. This fluid in the lungs is similar to that seen in drowning. Damage by these agents is sometimes called "dry-land drowning." Another name for this is *noncardiac pulmonary edema*, which is pulmonary edema (fluid in the lung tissue) caused by something other than heart failure.

A high concentration of phosgene causes an immediate irritation in the eyes, nose, and upper airways. This is usually transient and is followed later by pulmonary edema. An extremely high concentration will cause laryngeal edema and death within a short period of time, but this is very uncommon. The usual circumstance is that the victim inhales phosgene without immediate effects. Anywhere from 2 to 24 hours later, the victim begins to become short of breath. Initially, he or she notices the shortness of breath only with walking or other exertion, but as time passes, it is present at rest. A cough brings up clear, frothy sputum—the fluid that leaked into the lungs. If the symptoms begin late, after 6 or 8 hours, the damage is usually not severe enough to cause death, but if the effects begin early, from an hour to 6 hours after exposure, the lung damage is often severe enough to cause death despite medical care.

Initial Effects

Initial effects of pulmonary agents include the following:

- Shortness of breath with exertion, later at rest
- Cough, later with production of frothy sputum

A responder at the site may see few symptomatic victims, except possibly some with irritation of the eyes and upper airways or some exposed to extremely high concentrations who will soon have laryngeal edema. Most casualties will be minimally symptomatic, and the tendency might be to discharge them from care. This could well be a mistake. Symptoms can start suddenly, and if they begin within the first several hours, death may occur within the next several hours. Anyone who has been exposed to one of these agents must be kept under medical observation for at least 6 hours.

A victim exposed to a pulmonary agent will have two major problems for hospital management. The first is the fluid in the lungs (pulmonary edema) with resulting lack of oxygen (hypoxemia). The second is loss of fluid from the intravascular space (hypovolemia), which may lead to hypotension, shock, and organ damage.

Initial management of victims is twofold. The first and hardest thing to remember is that anyone possibly exposed to one of these agents should be kept at absolute rest with absolutely no exertion. The victim must be carried, not walked, to the ambulance. It is hard to tell a healthy person at the site of a spill or incident who has no symptoms that he or she cannot walk, but it must be done. World War I experience with these casualties shows that a victim breathing comfortably in bed might collapse and die if allowed to walk down the hall to the bathroom.

The second and more obvious part of managing a pulmonary agent victim is to provide oxygen to anyone who is short of breath. This usually will not happen while the responder is on the scene initially, but may happen when the responder provides transport later.

Riot Control Agents

Most people are familiar with **riot control agents**, otherwise known as tear gas or irritants. Three are in common use in this country. CS (or 2-chlorobenzal-malononitrile—also called o-chlorobenzylidene malononitrile) is used by law enforcement agencies and the military; phenacyl chloride—also called Mace—was used in World War I and is now in small spray devices carried for self-protection; and pepper spray, which is replacing the others for both law enforcement and military use and for self-protection.

Unlike other agents that are liquids, these are solids. The powdery particles are suspended in liquids when they are in spray devices. These agents have much in common. Their effects begin within seconds of contact, the effects last only a few minutes after the person is in fresh air, they are effective in small concentrations, and the lethal concentration is thousands of times higher than the effective concentration, which means that accidentally producing an overdose is very unlikely.

These agents cause irritation, pain, or burning on surfaces they contact, including the eyes, the nose, the mouth and airways, and the skin. Eye effects include burning, tearing, redness, and an initial involuntary temporary closing of the eyes (blepharospasm). While the eyes are closed, the victim cannot see and might be considered incapacitated. The interior of the nose burns, and there are secretions from the nose. There are secretions from the mouth, and the interior of the mouth burns. If the agent is inhaled, there will be coughing and perhaps a feeling of shortness of breath. There is an initial burning or tingling on the skin accompanied by a mild redness. Sometimes a high concentration will cause retching or gagging. The effects will gradually recede in 15 to 30 minutes after exposure has ceased.

There are potential complications that seem to be rare. If the face is close to the agent when it is dispersed with force (e.g., a spray device), the force may drive the particles into the eye. This necessitates flushing with copious amounts of water or manual removal of the particle by an ophthalmologist. The agent might precipitate a severe reaction in a person with chronic lung disease (chronic obstructive pulmonary disease, asthma, etc.) including hyperactive airways. The use of oxygen, assisted ventilation, and bronchodilators might be indicated. A person exposed to a high concentration in a hot and humid environment might develop a delayed dermatitis beginning about 6 hours after contact, with erythema developing into blisters.

People can develop tolerance to these agents. With continued exposure, the effects lessen and the exposed people can open their eyes and function relatively normally.

Triage

Triage is an ongoing process that begins with the first person to see the victim and continues through hospital management. The responder will triage at several places, including in the hot zone, in the cold zone after the victim has been decontaminated, and possibly in between. In the hot zone, the responder is encumbered with protective clothing and victim examination is not ideal. The following triage categories are generally used: immediate, delayed, and minimal.

An immediate victim is one who is in danger of loss of life unless there is intervention within a short period of time. Intervention generally has to do with airway, breathing, and circulation (the ABCs), and to this the administration of antidotes should be added. A delayed victim is one who can wait for intervention, and this wait will not affect the outcome of care. The victim is stable but will require further care. A minimal victim is one who requires care for a relatively minor injury. The care can be done quickly, the injury is not life threatening, and the victim is unlikely to require long-term care (i.e., hospitalization). An expectant victim is one who cannot be saved with the resources available or resources cannot be made available within the time the victim needs them.

Nerve Agents

An immediate victim is one who (1) is unconscious, is apneic or struggling to breathe, is convulsing or has convulsed, and has muscular twitching or is flaccid; or (2) has moderate or severe signs in two or more organ systems (respiratory, gastrointestinal, muscular, and central nervous system). This victim should be given 6 mg of atropine—IM, not IV—and a 20- to 30-minute drip of 1 g of 2-PAMCl.

A delayed victim is one who is recovering from moderate or severe effects or from the effects of several doses of antidote.

A minimal victim is one who is walking and talking. That person may be severely short of breath or vomiting, but still has muscle strength and control and can understand the spoken word enough to respond. Generally, this victim should be given 2 mg of atropine with a drip of 2-PAMCl. If the victim is extremely short of breath, 4 mg of atropine should be administered. Despite the shortness of breath, this victim is not immediate.

An expectant victim is one who is not breathing and is without a heartbeat. However, if he or she has been without cardiac activity for a very brief period of time, every attempt should be made to resuscitate the victim.

Cyanide

Cyanide victims can die within minutes after inhaling a large concentration of the agent. Those who are unconscious and not breathing but who still have a heartbeat should be classified as immediate, and the antidotes should be given as soon as possible. If a victim is conscious, he or she will be minimal and will not need antidotes. An expectant victim is one who has been without a heartbeat for many minutes.

Vesicants

Almost all vesicant victims will be delayed. They will need no immediate care, but they will need further care for their eye, skin, or airway injuries. An exception is a victim with moderate to severe airway effects including shortness of breath. He or she is immediate and needs intensive pulmonary care.

Pulmonary Agents

Although shortness of breath, the major symptom from these agents, can be faked, anyone complaining of shortness of breath within 6 hours of exposure should be classified as immediate for intensive pulmonary care. A victim with shortness of breath beginning later than 6 hours postexposure will also need care and monitoring. A victim with severe shortness of breath and copious frothy sputum within an hour after exposure is expectant, although an attempt should be made to provide maximum care.

Riot Control Agents

Victims of riot control agents will be usually classified as minimal with the exception of a victim who has a severe airway reaction to these agents or a polypharmacy scenario where underlying conditions are exacerbated and possibly require immediate care.

Early Recognition

When first responders in protective gear first enter the hot zone, they usually will not know what the toxic agent is and usually will not have a detector to tell them. They must quickly evaluate the victims based on what is seen and heard and take appropriate action. Early therapeutic intervention is needed for only two types of agents—nerve agents and cyanide. A victim exposed to a large concentration of a pulmonary agent may be in severe respiratory distress, but there is nothing that can be done in the hot zone; if the effects started before the responder arrived, probably nothing can be done elsewhere.

In most chemical mass casualty situations, the victims will exhibit a spectrum of effects. Some victims' conditions will be quite severe, and others will have minor effects, and the responder must quickly evaluate this spectrum. For example, if some victims are convulsing or are unconscious and appear to be postictal, the responder should look at other victims. The presence of miosis, runny noses, and shortness of breath or any one or two of these strongly suggests that nerve agents were the offending substance. If the conscious victims are relatively normal with a few nonspecific complaints, cyanide should be considered. If all victims are conscious with no complaints, the responder should consider that (1) no chemical agent was present, or it was present in concentrations too low to produce effects, or (2) the agent was one that produces delayed effects only, such as mustard or the pulmonary agents.

If many victims are complaining of irritation or burning in the eyes and nose, on the mucous membranes of the mouth, and on the skin, one might consider the following:

1. Riot control agents (in which case the victims will improve with fresh air)
2. Phosgene (the effects will improve, but there will be later, more severe ones)
3. Cyanogen chloride (the irritation will gradually decrease, and if the victim is conscious when help arrives it is unlikely that a lethal concentration was present)
4. Lewisite (the effects will worsen)

Refer to **TABLE 8-1** for a summary of signs, symptoms, and decontamination procedures for chemical agents.

Chapter Summary

Chemical agents are not new, and terrorist organizations have access to these substances as demonstrated by the use of sarin in a Tokyo subway attack in 1995. Many industrial chemicals such as chlorine, cyanide, phosgene, and pesticides are readily available in large quantities.

It is essential that response agencies be prepared for a chemical attack. Effective planning must include protective equipment, decontamination procedures, and antidotes. A deliberate incident is a crime scene, usually with mass numbers of victims.

Nerve agents are toxic materials that produce injury or death in seconds to minutes. Nerve agents are similar to insecticides but are more toxic.

Very good antidotes are available for nerve agents, but they must be administered quickly. Common nerve agents include tabun (GA), sarin (GB), soman (GD), and GF and VX. Effects from nerve agents show very quickly. Management of nerve agent exposure consists of decontamination, administration of antidotes, and ventilation.

The antidotes for nerve agent poisoning are atropine and an oxime, PAMCl (Protopam). Atropine blocks the excess neurotransmitters. PAMC1 removes the nerve agent from enzymes, allowing the enzymes to block the neurotransmitters. Benzodiazepines (i.e., diazepam) can be used as anticonvulsants.

Cyanide can cause serious illness and death within minutes. Cyanide affects the ability of the cells to metabolize oxygen. Treatment of cyanide poisoning can include hydroxocobalamin or using the cynanide antidote kit (amyl nitrite pearl or sodium nitrite IV and sodium thiosulfate IV). Victims should be ventilated with oxygen and acidosis should be corrected.

Vesicants are agents that cause vesicles or blisters. The most common vesicant agents are sulfur mustard and lewisite. Mustard does not cause an immediate effect; the common latent period is 4 to 8 hours after contact. Inhaled vapor causes damage to the airway and bronchioles. Victims must be decontaminated immediately and the eyes irrigated.

Lewisite produces instant effect on contact. The symptoms include immediate pain, eye damage, and airway injury.

Pulmonary agents produce pulmonary edema. The best-known agents are phosgene and chlorine. The effects of these agents are not immediate, but shortness of breath followed by pulmonary edema follows hours after exposure. Exposed victims with no symptoms must be kept under medical observation for at least 6 hours. Initial victim treatment includes keeping the victim at rest and administering oxygen.

Riot control agents are known as tear gas and irritants. They include tear gas, Mace, and pepper spray. Effects begin in seconds but last only a few minutes after the victim is removed to fresh air. These agents cause pain, burning, and irritation to the contact body surfaces. The use of oxygen is indicated.

Triage is an ongoing process in a chemical exposure incident. The triage categories are immediate (critical), delayed, and minimal (walking wounded). A critical victim is one who is unconscious, apneic, or convulsing. Almost all vesicant victims will be delayed. Most riot control victims will be in the minimal or walking wounded category.

Early responders must quickly evaluate the scene. Rapid therapeutic intervention is needed only for nerve agents and cyanide. If a victim shows severe pulmonary distress from a pulmonary agent, nothing can be done in the prehospital setting.

The use of positive pressure ventilation and albuterol nebulizers has been shown to improve the noncardiac pulmonary edema condition. The extent of treatment offered by a responder is dependent upon the type of incident, number of victims and your local treatment and MCI protocols. The learner is encouraged to review the guidance documents provided by local authorities.

In mass casualty incidents, victims will exhibit a spectrum of effects. Responders must quickly don protective equipment and triage all victims to determine treatment categories.

TABLE 8-1 Chemical Agents: Symptoms and Treatment

Agent	Signs and symptoms	Decontamination	Immediate treatment/ management
Nerve agents (GA, GB, GD, GF, VX)	**Vapor:** *Small exposure–* Miosis, rhinorrhea, and mild dyspnea. *Large exposures–* Sudden loss of consciousness, convulsions, apnea, flaccid paralysis, copious secretions, and miosis. **Liquid on skin:** *Small to moderate exposure–* Localized sweating, nausea, vomiting, and feeling of weakness. *Large exposure–*Sudden loss of consciousness, convulsions, apnea, flaccid paralysis, and copious secretions.	Large amounts of water with a hypochlorite solution.	Administration of atropine and pralidoxime chloride (2-PAMC1); diazepam in addition if casualty is severe; ventilation and suction of airway for respiratory distress.
Mustard (HD, H)	Asymptomatic latent period (hours). Erythema and blisters on the skin, irritation, conjunctivitis, corneal opacity, and damage in the eyes; mild upper respiratory signs, marked airway damage; also gastrointestinal effects and bone marrow stem cell suppression.	Large amounts of water with a hypochlorite solution.	Decontamination immediately after exposure is the only way to prevent/limit injury/ damage. Symptomatic management of lesions.
Lewisite (L)	Lewisite causes immediate pain or irritation of skin and mucous membranes. Erythema and blisters on the skin and eyes and airway damage similar to those seen after mustard exposure develop later.	Large amounts of water with a hypochlorite solution.	Immediate decontamination; symptomatic management of lesions the same as for mustard lesions; a specific antidote British antilewisite (BAL) will decrease systemic effects.
Phosgene oxime (CX)	Immediate burning and irritation followed by wheal-like skin lesions and eye and airway damage.	Large amounts of water.	Immediate decontamination; symptomatic management of lesions.
Cyanide (AC, CK)	Initially may have dyspnea, weakness, and dizziness.	Skin decontamination is usually not necessary because agents are highly volatile. Wet, contaminated clothing should be removed and the underlying skin decontaminated with water or other standard decontaminates.	Antidote: intravenous sodium nitrite and sodium thiosulfate. Supportive care: oxygen and correct acidosis.
Pulmonary agents (CG)	Eye and airway irritation, dyspnea, chest tightness, and delayed pulmonary edema.	Vapor: fresh air. Liquid: copious water irrigation.	Termination of exposure, ABCs of resuscitation, enforced rest and observation, oxygen with or without positive airway pressure for signs of respiratory distress, other supportive therapy as needed.

(continues)

TABLE 8-1 Chemical Agents: Symptoms and Treatment (continued)

Agent	Signs and symptoms	Decontamination	Immediate treatment/ management
Riot control agents (CS, CN)	Burning and pain on exposed mucous membranes and skin, eye pain and tearing, burning nostrils, respiratory discomfort, and tingling of the exposed skin.	*Eyes:* thoroughly flush with water, saline, or similar substance. *Skin:* flush with copious amounts of water, alkaline soap and water, or a mildly alkaline solution (sodium bicarbonate or sodium carbonate). Generally, decontamination is not required if wind is brisk.	Usually none is necessary; effects are self-limiting.

Source: Medical management of chemical casualties handbook, 2nd ed. (1995). Aberdeen Proving Ground, MD: Chemical Casualty Care Office, United States Army Medical Research Institute of Chemical Defense.

Wrap Up

Chapter Questions

1. Discuss several reasons why your community should be prepared for a terrorist chemical attack.
2. What are the methods of disseminating a chemical agent?
3. Define nerve agents. How do they act on the body?
4. List five common nerve agents.
5. What are the symptoms of nerve agent exposure?
6. What is the treatment for nerve agent exposure? Name three antidotes.
7. Discuss the symptoms of cyanide poisoning. What are the antidotes for cyanide exposure?
8. What are vesicants? What are the signs of vesicant exposure? What is the treatment?
9. Define lewisite. How does lewisite exposure differ from mustard exposure?
10. What are pulmonary agents? What is the treatment for severe exposure?
11. List three riot control agents. What are the symptoms and treatment for exposure?
12. What are the triage categories in a chemical attack with mass victims? Describe typical symptoms of a victim in each category.

Chapter Project

You are an EMS training officer in an organization that has no chemical attack training program. Your goal is to develop guidelines for first response fire units and EMS units. Develop a written chemical response guideline that includes the following key elements:

- Categories of chemical agents
- Symptoms at onset and long-term symptoms
- Advanced life support care for each type of agent including antidotes
- Basic life support treatment procedures
- Safety guidelines
- Triage categories and related symptoms

Vital Vocabulary

Cyanide A toxic material, like the nerve agents, can cause serious illness and death within minutes, but is also volatile and lighter than air.

Hydroxocobalamin A vitamin B_{12} precursor that is now available in multiple countries as an antidote for cyanide poisoning.

Lewisite An oily liquid with the odor of geraniums that contains arsenic and a heavy metal and is more volatile than sulfur mustard.

Nerve agents Toxic materials that produce injury and death within seconds to minutes.

Pulmonary agents Chemicals that produce pulmonary edema (fluid in the lung), with little damage to the airways or other tissues.

Riot control agents Solids suspended in liquids as powdery particles; often used in spray devices and used commonly in the United States.

Sulfur mustard (mustard) A light yellowish to brown oily liquid that smells like garlic, onions, or mustard and causes cellular damage and death with subsequent tissue damage.

Vesicants Agents that cause vesicles or blisters.

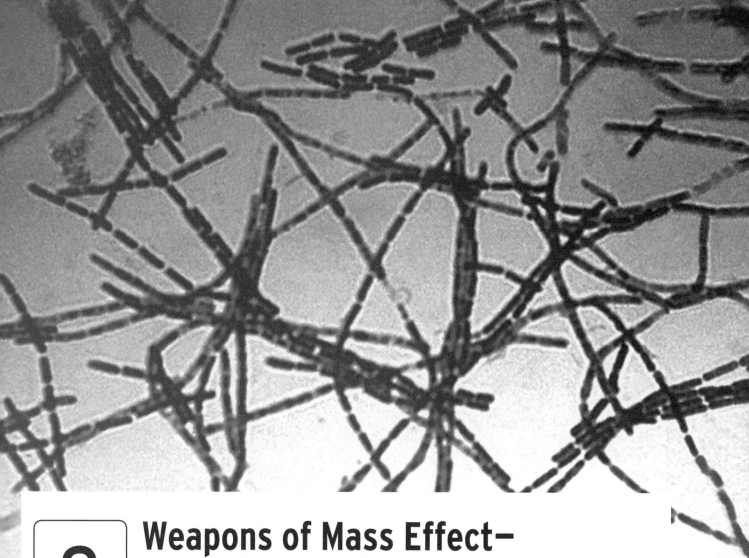

9 Weapons of Mass Effect–Biological Terrorism

Dr. Charles Stewart
Paul M. Maniscalco
Hank T. Christen

Objectives

- Define the concept of biological warfare.
- Know the history of biological warfare.
- Understand and be able to apply the concepts of biological threat assessment.
- Define the importance of biological protective equipment.
- Outline the types of biological agents including the chemical effects, detection, and prophylaxis/treatment of *botulinum* toxins, *Clostridium* toxins, ricin, saxitoxin, staphylococcal enterotoxin, tetrodotoxin, and trochothecene mycotoxins.

Introduction

The uses of biological substances as weapons pose a unique problem for the emergency response and public health communities. Unlike the consequences of a chemical attack or an explosion, which are essentially readily identifiable, in-your-face events, biological terrorism creates a slow-motion riot that builds with each hour after the event. The inability to quickly and immediately identify what has occurred allows the threat maturation process to continue while increasing the risk to a vulnerable population.

Biological terrorism is the use of etiological agents (disease) to cause harm or kill a population, food, and/or livestock. Biological terrorism includes the use of organisms such as bacteria, viruses, and the use of products of organisms—toxins.

Biological terrorism has recently become more threatening to the world. One only needs to consider the current state of technology, the future possibilities of biotechnologies, and what appears to be a readiness on the part of some individuals/countries to utilize this technology as a weapon.

Successful genetic engineering has arrived, and advances are being achieved almost daily. It requires a relatively easy process and only crude technology to manufacture a lethal organism/toxin in sufficient quantities. Some are specifically designed to be resistant to antibiotics for use as a horrible weapon. It has been said that "if you can make beer, you can make bugs (biological weapons)." This is an oversimplification, but it provides a vivid picture of what a motivated person with modern technology is capable of achieving. A recent phenomenon has emerged with the availability of equipment and the reduced costs associated with acquiring the same; it is referred to as "garage science." A simple Internet search easily reveals the extent of experimentation and activities that are associated with aspiring biology hobbyists. You can find individuals hacking DNA while others are conducting a variety of organic experiments—all interesting—but highly illustrious of the fact that technology can be exploited to help and hurt if the players are nefarious. Do-it-yourself biotechnology is now happening and encouraged by forums like *DIY Bio*, Biopunk, and others.

Biological weapons (BWs) have the potential to wreak considerable havoc and death among humans, resulting in a medical disaster. Moreover, should BWs be employed against livestock or vegetation, the results would be an economic disaster.

BWs are more deadly and financially efficient, pound for pound and dollar for dollar, than chemical agents or even nuclear weapons. It has been estimated that 10 grams of anthrax could kill as many people as a metric ton of the nerve agent sarin. BWs are relatively inexpensive and easy to manufacture, and dispersal devices can be disguised as agricultural or pest-control sprayers. A human carrying the disease is also a dispersal agent. Unfortunately for the law-abiding world, it is very difficult, if not impossible, for an intelligence service to detect research, production, or transportation of these agents for rogue intentions. It is equally hard to defend against these agents once they have been employed due to the inability to readily recognize delivery.

History of Biological Agents as Weapons

The use of biological agents as a warfare weapon has a long and deadly past. In fact, history has shown us that use of BWs occurred more than 2,000 years ago. Some examples of its employment include:

1. In the 6th century B.C., Assyrians poisoned enemy wells with rye ergot (U.S. Army, 1996); Solon used the purgative hellebore during the siege of Krissa (U.S. Army).
2. Persian, Greek, and Roman authors quote the use of animal cadavers to contaminate water supplies. In 1155, Barbarossa used the bodies of dead soldiers to poison the wells at the battle of Tortona.
3. The Scythian archers would dip their arrows in blood mixed with manure or in decomposing cadavers.
4. The Mongols in the 1300s catapulted plague victim corpses into the city of Kaffa to infect the defenders (U.S. Army). The besieged town was rapidly devastated by disease.
5. British and early American settlers gave American Indians blankets used by victims of smallpox. The resultant infection decimated the defenseless American Indian tribes.
6. In 1941, the Allies tested anthrax on Gruinard Island off the shore of Scotland (Bernstein, 1987). Starting in 1986, a determined effort was made to decontaminate the island, with 280 tons of formaldehyde solution diluted in seawater being sprayed over all 520 acres (2 km²) of the island, and the worst-contaminated topsoil around the dispersal site being removed. A flock of sheep was then placed on the island and remained healthy. On April 24, 1990, after 48 years of quarantine, junior defense minister Michael Neubert visited the island and announced its safety by removing the warning signs (Harrison, 2001).

7. During World War II, the Allies administered 235,000 doses of antitoxin to Allied troops and deliberately leaked this information to the Nazis. Simultaneously, they told the Nazis that the Allies were prepared to use BWs if they were employed in the war (Mobley, 1995).

8. During World War II, on the Pacific front, the Japanese tested BWs on prisoners of war in China, killing more than 1,000 people. In fact, it has been reported that the Japanese had "stockpiled 400 kilograms of anthrax to be used in specially designed fragmentation bombs" (U.S. Army, 1996).

9. Unclassified information from Central Intelligence Agency and Defense Intelligence Agency documents indicates that several rogue states such as Iran, Libya, and North Korea have or are pursuing BW programs (Horrock, 1997).

10. In September and October of 1984, followers of the Bhagwan Sri Rajneesh contaminated restaurant salad bars in Oregon. More than 750 people were intentionally infected with *Salmonella*.

11. In 1994, a Japanese sect of the Aum Shinrikyo cult attempted an aerosolized release of anthrax from the tops of buildings in Tokyo.

12. In 1995, two members of a Minnesota militia group were convicted of possession of *ricin*, which they had produced themselves for use in retaliation against local government officials.

13. In 1996, an Ohio man attempted to obtain *bubonic plague* cultures through the mail.

14. In 2001, anthrax was delivered by mail to U.S. media and government offices (**FIGURE 9-1A, 9-1B, and 9-1C).** There were five deaths. The first victim, Robert Stevens, worked at American Media Inc., in Boca Raton, Florida. Two were distribution clerks in the Brentwood postal facility in Washington, DC. Joseph P. Curseen, 47, died at the Southern Maryland Hospital Center in Clinton, Maryland, and Thomas L. Morris Jr., 55, died at the Greater Southeast Community Hospital in Washington, DC. Kathy Nguyen, 61, died October 31, 2001. She was a New York hospital worker who contracted inhalation anthrax. The last victim, Ottilie Lundgren, 94, died November 21, 2001, at Griffin Hospital in Derby, Connecticut.

In recent times, the military examined the possibility of biological actions against the United States. In the 1950s, *Serratia* and *Bacillus* species were released from ships in the San Francisco Bay area and caused at least one death (Cole, 1988). In the 1960s, military researchers introduced *B. subtilis* into New York City

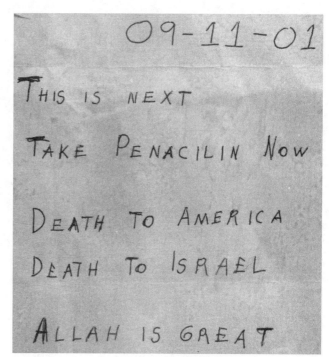

FIGURE 9-1A Anthrax letter sent to Tom Brokaw.

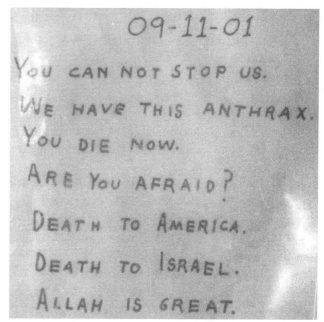

FIGURE 9-1B Anthrax letter sent to Senator Tom Daschle.

subway ventilator shafts. Both passengers and security guards were oblivious to the danger (Cole, 1985). The bacteria were rapidly spread to the ends of the subway system, successfully demonstrating the ability to exploit that environment with these substances.

The U.S. Office of Technology Assessment has estimated that a small private plane with 220 pounds of anthrax spores, flying over Washington, DC, on a

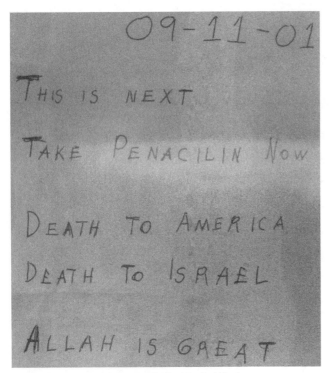

FIGURE 9-1C Anthrax letter sent to the *New York Post.*

windless night, could kill between 1 and 3 million people and render the city uninhabitable for years.

Other countries are certainly continuing to develop biowarfare capabilities. The Soviets and their allies employed a trichothecene mycotoxin dubbed "yellow rain" in Laos, Cambodia, and Afghanistan, and the former USSR and Iraq have independently developed anthrax species. In 1979, an outbreak of inhalational anthrax occurred in Sverdlovsk, Russia. This outbreak resulted from an accident at a Soviet biowarfare research facility.

Treaties

The Geneva Convention (1925) prohibited the use of biological and chemical warfare. In 1972, the United Nations Convention on the Prohibition of the Development, Production and Stockpiling of Bacteriological (Biological) and Toxin Weapons and on Their Destruction (a.k.a. the Biological and Toxin Weapons Convention) was executed with an implementation date of March 26, 1975. By June 2005, there were 171 signatories, and 155 of these had ratified the convention to stop development, production, and stockpiling of chemical and bacteriological (biological) weapons. Research for defensive purposes is still allowed and continues across the globe.

Treaties and multilateral agreements cannot completely rid the world of chemical weapons and BWs,

which are simple, inexpensive, and produced by widely available technology. Nor will they fully eradicate the threat of individuals who fervently desire to acquire and use them as weapons. Here are some recent examples:

Paris police, in 1984, raided a suspected safe house for the German Red Army Faction. During the search they found documentation and a bathtub filled with flasks containing *Clostridium botulinum* (Douglas, 1987).

Russia's biological warfare technology may be vulnerable to leakage to third parties through either theft or outright sale (like nuclear materials), as a result of the financial crises that exist. Open-source intelligence reports that army personnel and scientists have been known to sell off military equipment to get money to feed their families. In some cases, reports have been received that these individuals, in critical and sensitive positions, have not been paid in months, making them vulnerable to recruitment by rogue organizations or nations.

The Aum Shinrikyo cult members (famous for the sarin gas attack in Tokyo subways) were found to have anthrax and *botulinum* cultures when the Japanese national police conducted their raid of the Aum base camp at the foot of Mount Fuji. They had constructed dedicated laboratories and had purchased a helicopter equipped with a spraying apparatus. The Aum had also visited Zaire during the Ebola outbreak to collect specimens of Ebola virus (Flanagin & Lederberg, 1996).

In the town of The Dalles, Oregon, in 1984, more than 750 people became sick after eating in four different restaurants. The illness was traced to the Bhagwan Sri Rajneesh sect, which had spread salmonella on salad bars in the four restaurants (Cole, 1996). The intention of this group was to sicken many of the community to prevent them from going to the polls, thus interfering with the political process and manipulating a local election.

A U.S. microbiologist named Larry Wayne Harris fraudulently ordered three vials of bubonic plague cultures by mail in 1995 (Horrock, 1997). The ease with which he obtained these cultures prompted new legislation to ensure that biological materials are destined only for legitimate medical and scientific purposes. These products are often shipped via commercial delivery companies such as UPS and FedEx, which is perfectly legal.

In December 2002, six terrorist suspects were arrested in Manchester, England; their apartment was serving as a ricin laboratory. Among them was a 27-year-old chemist who was producing the toxin.

On October 15, 2003, a ricin-laced letter, addressed to the Department of Transportation in Washington,

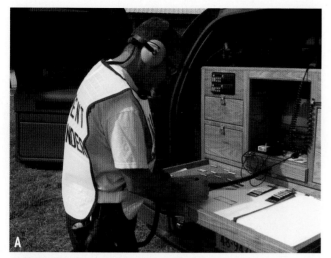

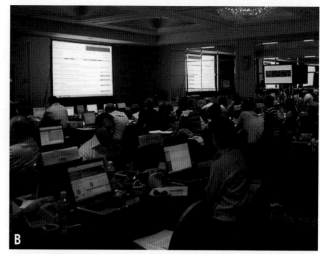

CP FIGURE 3-1 The National Response Framework can be used for both large and small scale incidents.

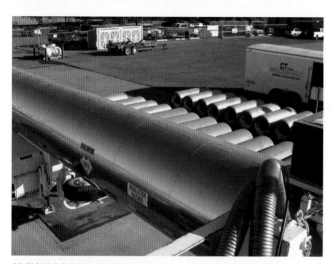

CP FIGURE 8-1 Chlorine is a common industrial chemical that is also an effective chemical warfare agent.

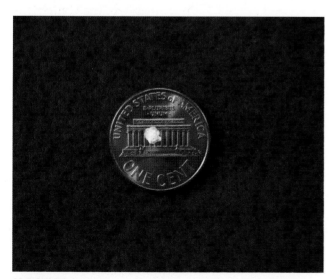

CP FIGURE 8-2 VX is the most toxic chemical ever produced. The dot on the penny demonstrates the amount needed to achieve the lethal dose.

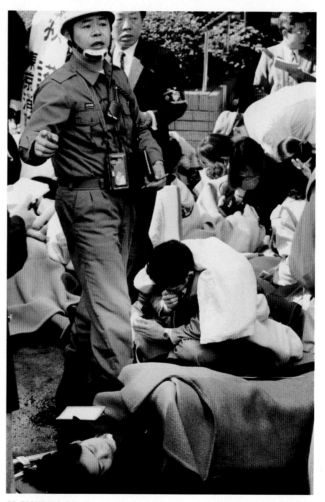

CP FIGURE 8-3 Sarin, a nerve agent, was used to attack the Tokyo subway system in 1995.

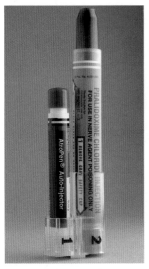

CP FIGURE 8-4 Items from a Mark 1 nerve agent antidote kit.

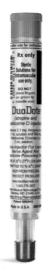

CP FIGURE 8-5 The DuoDote is intended as an initial treatment of the symptoms of organophosphorus insecticide or nerve agent poisonings.

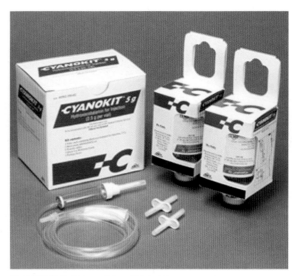

CP FIGURE 8-6 A cyanide antidote kit.

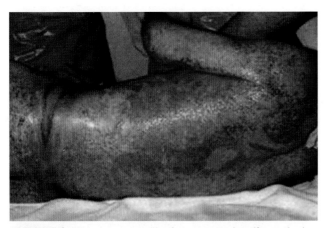

CP FIGURE 8-7 Skin damage resulting from exposure to sulfur mustard (agent H).

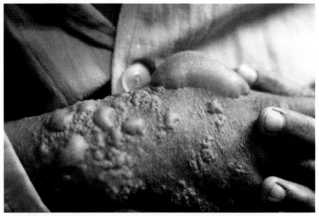

CP FIGURE 8-8 Typical effects of blistering agents, such as lewisite or sulfur mustard.

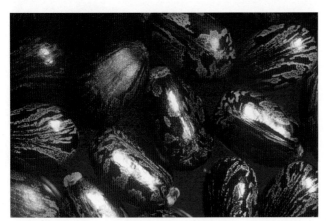

CP FIGURE 9-1 These seemingly harmless castor beans contain the key ingredient for ricin, one of the most potent toxins known to humans.

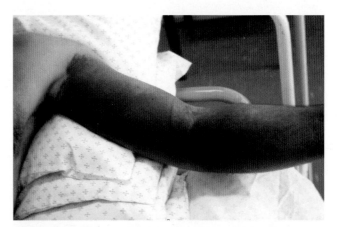

CP FIGURE 9-2 Viral hemorrhagic fevers cause the blood vessels and tissues to seep blood. The end result is ecchymosis, hemoptysis, and blood in the patient's stool. Notice the severe discoloration in this patient with Crimean-Congo hemorrhagic fever, indicating internal bleeding.

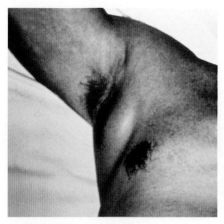

CP FIGURE 9-3A A plague buboe at a lymph node under the arm.

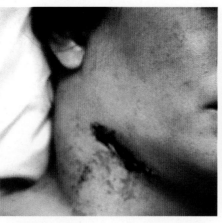

CP FIGURE 9-3B A plague buboe at a lymph node on the neck.

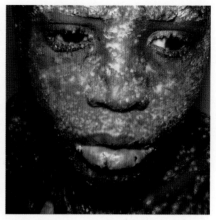

CP FIGURE 9-4 In smallpox, all of the lesions are identical in their development. In other skin disorders, the lesions will be in various stages of healing and development.

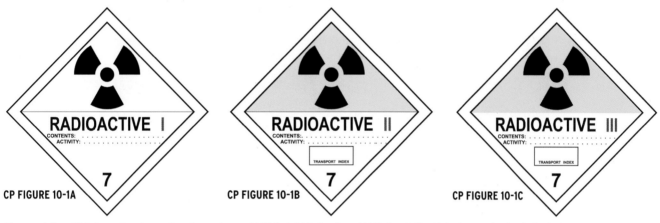

CP FIGURE 10-1A

CP FIGURE 10-1B

CP FIGURE 10-1C

Three varieties of labels are found on radioactive packages: (a) White I, (b) Yellow II, and (c) Yellow III (the highest amount). They indicate the lowest to highest amounts of radiation that can be measured outside of the package.

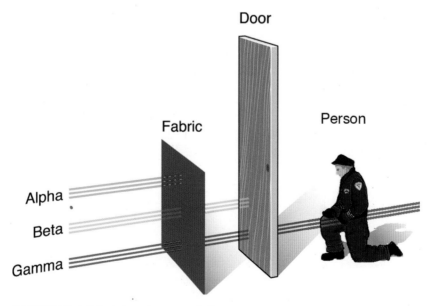

CP FIGURE 10-2 Alpha, beta, and gamma radiation.

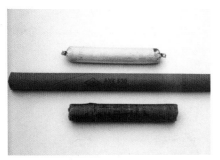

CP FIGURE 11-1 Every year, thousands of pounds of explosives, including dynamite, are stolen from construction companies and other legal owners.

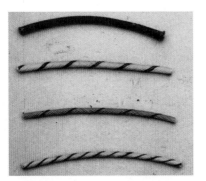

CP FIGURE 11-2 Included in the explosive train are detonating cords, which may look like rescue ropes to an uninformed responder.

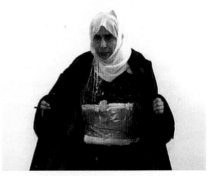

CP FIGURE 11-3 Suicide explosive devices can be concealed on an individual.

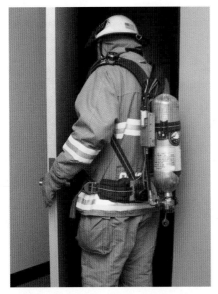

CP FIGURE 13-1 Self-contained breathing apparatus (SCBA) carries its own air supply, a factor that limits the amount of air and time the user has to complete the job.

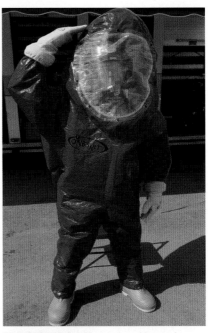

CP FIGURE 13-2 A Class 1 ensemble envelops the wearer in a totally encapsulating suit.

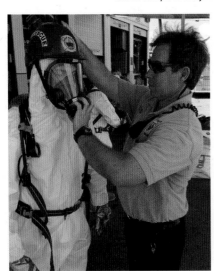

CP FIGURE 13-3 A Class 2 protective ensemble provides a high level of respiratory protection less skin protection.

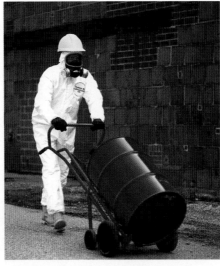

CP FIGURE 13-4 A Class 3 ensemble includes chemical-protective clothing and gloves as well as respiratory protection.

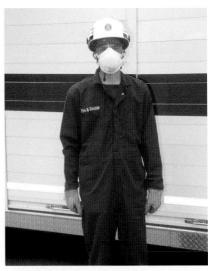

CP FIGURE 13-5 A Class 4 ensemble is primarily a work uniform that includes coveralls and provides minimal protection.

DC, U.S.A., was intercepted at a mail sorting facility in Greenville, South Carolina. The letter, which threatened future ricin attacks if the government didn't pass pending trucking legislation, was signed by Fallen Angel.

On February 3, 2004, three U.S. Senate office buildings were closed after the toxin ricin was found in the mailroom that serves Senate Majority Leader Bill Frist's office.

Threat Assessment

Although the conclusion that the United States is very vulnerable to a biowarfare attack or terrorism is indisputable, the BW programs of the 1950s and 1960s were appropriately criticized for the unethical exposure of unwitting test subjects. Despite the escalating BW threats and the experiences of the anthrax attacks of 2001, our level of preparedness is still insufficient given the potential harm and disruption that could be realized in the aftermath. With limited capacity to anticipate a biological attack, little or no ability to detect one if it occurs (unless the perpetrators decide to announce the release and take credit for their demonic acts), and a diminished ability to effectively manage the consequences if attacked, this problem poses a series of complex issues that need immediate review. There are a number of reasons for this unpreparedness, which will be discussed in the following sections.

Intelligence

When a BW manufacturing facility can be constructed in the area of a large garage, law enforcement/intelligence services are confronted with great difficulty in locating it. Accessing cultures is not nearly as expensive or tracked as well as nuclear material. BW culture processing requires equipment that would be considered suitable for a well-equipped hospital laboratory or academic research facility and is thus easily ordered and diverted. If this does not sound credible, please take some time to research the many events of missing samples from labs, black market activities, and incidents where individuals have exploited loopholes in the system to acquire samples under fraudulent terms (Harris & Paxman, 1982).

As the threat of terrorism has evolved over the years, so has the role of EMS in support of interagency operations. The importance of seamlessly integrating EMS representation into intelligence functions such as state, regional, and local intelligence fusion centers is a critical requirement to ensure the vertical and horizontal flow of essential information. For instance, tying in to the 911 dispatch data system to monitor call volume and activity with the ability to drill down on data from past years to quickly conduct a correlative analysis of activities for aberrancy is an important data node. Given that most EMS systems operate and staff on the margins, the sensitivity of call volume and the fragility of the system provide a source for rather quick alerts that something is not right. Drawing those EMS data along with emergency department activity data into a central location for the EMS representative to coordinate and collaborate on the end operations analysis with the public health representative could be that single, important clue that provides a community early notification of an incident. In the end, that early alert could mean the difference between quick response and control or expansion into a citywide/regional problem or worse.

Detection

Detection of biological agents occurs most often after a release. Quite simply, presently there are limited technologies that can detect the deployment of a bacterial agent in the civilian community under normal operating procedures. The only truly accurate means of detection is through the clinical presentation of patients, and that will be retrospective for most of the casualties. Some limited battlefield detection devices exist, but these are unusable in the majority of U.S. cities. These devices can be effective for special events such as the Olympics, a presidential inauguration, or where crowds are moderately constrained, but due to cost and availability, they have limited benefit to local emergency response organizations. When threat assessments are quite high and advance notice of the threat exists, use of these items through the National Guard civil support teams or through the Department of Defense is highly recommended.

Biological warfare agents are almost undetectable during transit. Likewise, there is no mechanism using routine customs, immigration, drug scan, or bomb search procedures to identify the agent. The only way to find it would be a physical search by a very well-trained and very lucky searcher (Mayer, 1995). Indeed, the agent could be simply sent using FedEx or a similar overnight carrier from one point to another. Even in an event where a package is broken and the product is leaked, law enforcement may have a high index of suspicion, but identification of the agent will usually take place at a laboratory, not in the field.

A bioterrorism threat might not be directly concentrated on actual humans. Livestock, crops, and water supply are strategic targets and vulnerable to attack. As an example, it is not inconceivable that a rogue individual or group could attempt to destroy all pork and pork products in the United States. Although this would not be a fatal blow for the United States on the whole, it would certainly not help the U.S. economy to have a porcine plague. Detection of this plague would be very difficult indeed prior to symptoms in a substantial number of the affected animals. (While they should for a number of strategic reasons, few communities include veterinarians in their biological surveillance plans.)

Control of Supplies

A military commander maintains the luxury of knowing that his troops are under threat of attack. The civilian emergency response chief does not usually have this warning and the targets for introduction of a biological agent are almost unlimited. To a large extent, the battlefield commander controls the food and water supply of his troops. To institute such control in the civilian sector would mean martial law, and this is unacceptable in a free society. This level of freedom is not without cost and it creates vulnerability for rogue groups to exploit.

Personal Protective Equipment

Biological terrorism is most likely to be executed covertly, and sick individuals may be the initial detector that an attack has occurred. If a biological agent is delivered effectively, a large number of casualties can be generated in a relatively short period of time depending on the etiologic agent utilized. In the midst of treating the casualties, the emergency responder and organization must not only provide effective care, but also protect themselves and their members.

This will be difficult most of the time due to the unknowing responders believing that they are operating at another sick job. After the release of a bioagent, there is an incubation period in the new host prior to its clinical manifestation. In some cases, this period may be more than 72 hours, and from some agents, it is 2 weeks or more.

One of the limiting factors of personal protective equipment (PPE) is that military issued gear is not certified by the Occupational Safety and Health Administration (OSHA). OSHA certification is a standard requirement for civilian use of any PPE. It has been only recently that some of this equipment is being considered for civilian use or "technology transfer," hence some testing for OSHA standard compliance is taking place (see Chapter 13, "Personal Protective Equipment").

Regardless, much of the civilian PPE that is available for bioagents is designed for use in the static environment of the laboratory and not the street. This, too, is another issue that will require a cooperative public/private working arrangement. Clearly, with the threat to the civilian responder escalating, continuing research for better and more functional PPE should be expected with the expertise of military, Homeland Security science and technology, academia, and private industry pooling talent and resources to create a successful resolution of this operational conundrum.

Even if the military or the Centers for Disease Control and Prevention (CDC) provide gear, it must be prepositioned and issued after either a significant threat or after the first casualties have been identified. In either case, there is a significant risk that many of the emergency services (including emergency physicians, nurses, paramedics, and EMTs) will be exposed and become unknowing casualties prior to the arrival of protective gear. Worst-case scenario is that these responders become additional disease vectors, further complicating the overarching response strategies.

Prophylaxis

The U.S. General Accounting Office found that at the beginning of the Gulf War in 1991, the U.S. Army's stockpiles of vaccine for anthrax and botulism had fallen far short of what was needed to protect U.S. troops. Indeed, the General Accounting Office felt that at least 20 percent and perhaps 40 percent of the military's biowar budget was not directed at diseases or toxins that were identified as threats by the military's own intelligence agencies (Horgan, 1994). Recently, heated discussions have again taken place at the Pentagon and in the media about the need to provide vaccinations to all uniformed service members as a provision of force protection in the face of these BW threats.

Protecting the armed forces against a biological attack is less challenging and complex than protecting the civilian population. Military personnel are a captive audience who have little choice regarding whether they will receive an immunization.

At present, we do not have sufficient emergency providers with enough immunizations to provide care for the population of a U.S. city (if attacked) without additional harm coming to the rescuers. These providers will be at the highest risk if an active agent is employed. On the positive side of this discussion, with recent advances in vaccinology, depending upon the threat being confronted, promising countermeasures are starting to be identified as is the ability to administer countermeasures after the exposure has occurred.

Training

Emergency responders might be called upon to know treatments for exotic diseases that they are unlikely to have ever encountered. Emergency service members must be aware of symptoms and epidemiological patterns that may indicate a biological attack, but many have never been taught these techniques of pattern identification. This creates a heavy reliance upon the expertise of the EMS medical director, the public health director, and the EMS training chief for guidance on next steps and real-time training.

EMS, the fire service, police, and even hospitals must purchase PPE and train employees for work in protective gear that has been found only in the military and specialized hazardous materials teams. Emergency service organizations must realize that they are significant targets for primary/secondary attacks and should conduct their routine operations appropriately while ensuring that the proper security measures are implemented.

Interagency Coordination and Public Perception

It is always difficult to balance the perceived needs of multiple population groups. Drawing the fine line between antiwar protesters who feel any research into biowar techniques should be forbidden and those who look for a threat around any corner is always difficult. When given the choice of where to spend defense money, it is easier to put it into real and visible tools such as guns, planes, and troops, playing the CNN factor to the max. In the past, cruise missiles shown on CNN are easier to sell to a congressional committee than protective garments for use in Bloomfield, New Jersey. Even in this post-September 11, 2001 world, we see reluctance on the part of some in Congress about really making the necessary sustainable investments in EMS, medical, public health, and other responder readiness. Hopefully, the momentum that has been attained regarding community bioterrorism and pandemic preparedness will continue to grow, and this view will change so a sustainable capacity can be achieved.

Likewise, control of a program that will spend millions of dollars brings a smile to many bureaucrats' faces. Will infighting between bureaucratic agencies dissipate any real effort to protect the United States? These issues require policy decisions with requisite directives to be issued in an effort to set the tone, from the top, ensuring that the process does not become mired in rivalry and competition. Perhaps we can start with a reexamination of the National Response Framework and refine this doctrine to incorporate an emergency support function that specifically addresses EMS and critical care medicine, while concurrently creating an agency that will have the responsibility for the same and be held accountable for seeing that readiness for this vital function is sustainably accomplished.

When a bioterrorism incident occurs, who will be in charge? Will it be local EMS, fire, police, or emergency management personnel? Will it be medical authorities from state, county, or local departments of health? Will it be medical authorities from the Department of Health and Human Services, CDC, or even military specialists from one of the biowar development centers at Dugway Proving Ground in Utah or Fort Detrick in Maryland? Will the Federal Bureau of Investigation attempt to assume control of the scene to preserve evidence? Will the Federal Emergency Management Agency attempt to usurp control of the incident? Will martial law be declared with the military in control of a city? With the recent H1N1 pandemic (2009) it was the secretary of the Department of Homeland Security who was front and center in the management of the federal response coordination. Even with the issuance of Presidential Decision Directive 39, these questions have not been fully and adequately answered.

Command and control issues are always best answered in advance of the incident, rather than during the emergency. Having a comprehensive emergency action annex to the existing community emergency management plan for bioterrorism incidents is strongly encouraged. Determination of issues such as these should be accomplished before "game day," not on the field of play. The latter will contribute to the chaos one can expect at this type of incident.

Deniability

The existence of naturally occurring or endemic agricultural pests or diseases and outbreaks will permit an adversary to anonymously use bioterrorism with completely plausible deniability. Such biological warfare attacks could be against the food supply or crops. The effects of such biological and economic warfare could bring devastation to the affected nation. The Russian wheat aphid has caused over $1 billion in losses in the western United States since it was first discovered/identified in Texas in 1986. What would a focused and deliberate release of a BW agent mean to the economics of the United States?

Response Time

Even if an astute emergency physician notes that an unusual number of patients brought in by EMS or as emergency department walk-ins have certain symptoms and contacts the CDC for help, and the crisis is immediately recognized as a bioterrorism event, and help is dispatched immediately, the lag time may be unwieldy. With some of the agents that have been identified, there is an incubation period that exceeds 3 days from time of agent distribution until the first cases occur and some agents carry as much as a 20-day period. A patient may be contagious during much of this incubation period with emergency personnel and hospital staff unaware of the jeopardy they are in. Some of the agents have mortality rates that approach 100 percent when symptoms go unrecognized.

Given an absolute best-case scenario from notification, it will take at least 2 hours for a qualified team of predesignated physicians and prehospital providers (paramedics and EMTs) to assemble (this best-case scenario occurs only if a community has had the foresight to convene a team prior to the event), ready gear, and respond to the deployment assembly point. It will take another few hours to assess the situation, draw appropriate clinical samples, and formulate an idea of what illness or toxin was employed. During this time, others will be exposed and potential carriers may be leaving the city, bound for other destinations.

When casualties exceed the available medical resources, additional resources must be identified and summoned, and either the patients must be transported to them or the providers and equipment transported to the patients. This scenario will warrant the deployment of federal assets in the form of National Disaster Medical System disaster medical action teams and military units such as the deployable medical teams, if available. All of this will take many hours or days.

If news services broadcast any warning, one can expect a panic-stricken response that may cause gridlock on the roads and further complicate any response team's travel to the area (and cause a spike in the standard 911 call volume). Essentially, we are looking at a regional, if not national or international emerging health crisis. This statement is very real. Consider the fact that in a conventional weapon attack such as the 1993 World Trade Center bombing, patients were tracked as far west as Pennsylvania and as far north as New Haven, Connecticut.

Response Strategies

In addition to the requisite response doctrine for protecting responders are support networks for responders' families and operational response and logistic sustainment tactics that the contemporary emergency response chief or executive must employ in response to a biological event. Given that the prevailing mantra for response to an infectious event is "social distancing and administration of countermeasures," we need to briefly examine the reality of this intervention.

The contemporary disaster response/planning doctrine involves bringing lots of people and resources to a location where an event has transpired and working our way out of it as quickly as possible. In the event of a bioterrorism incident or a pandemic, the reality of this strategy effectively being employed is questionable due to a number of issues, including but not limited to the scope of the event, limited resources, numbers of people affected, and the large geographic area that could be involved. Currently, conventional wisdom dictates that a social distancing response that is often bantered about translates into a concept we are all familiar with—shelter in place. It is important to note here that sheltering in place is a temporary, limited-duration tactic designed to protect individuals from an immediate pending event such as a gas leak, extreme inclement weather, or other hostile environment. Generally, these events can last a few hours to a day. As discussed previously, given that conventional responses and structures are neither designed nor configured to support hundreds if not thousands of individuals staying at home and servicing all of the affected people in disparate locations, the operationalization of the social distancing strategy becomes a complex problem that must be addressed sooner rather than later. Basically, we conduct emergency response operations daily in a "price club" manner, while the social distancing strategy will require us to refine and realign our response patterns and capacity to be more like Meals on Wheels—a retail approach rather than the standard wholesale scheme we utilize to conduct routine operations and run-of-the-mill disaster response.

It is important that the empowerment of the citizenry to become prepared for a disaster is achieved. Failure to take the necessary steps to create this environment could result in spontaneous and unnecessary evacuations of communities and failed or ineffective emergency response capacity.

Although highways leading from an attacked metropolitan area are most certainly attractive for citizens who feel they need to take matters into their own hands, they will likely be roads to nowhere, leaving citizens trapped and vulnerable. In most cases, remaining in homes or other safe havens in the community will provide the greatest personal security. This is true in terms of physical and emotional safety, because people make their best decisions when they are in stable, familiar environments, and make their worst decisions when in unstable, unfamiliar environments. A strategic concept and operational framework to address the emerging issues revolving around extended social distancing requirements has been developed out of the University of Virginia's Critical Incident Analysis Group. The presenting model is best described as "shelter in place on steroids" and looks at the series of complex and at times daunting requirements posed by needing to implement a coherent and supported social distancing strategy that will protect and support citizens.

<u>Community shielding</u> is a unique opportunity to engage individuals, communities, and government in a unified response to future acts of terrorism, in particular bioterrorism. The concept envisions an integrated, facilitated form of sheltering, wherein individuals and groups within a community employ a self-imposed isolation, or quarantine, within their natural and familiar surroundings, for a temporary period of time until a threat or danger abates. The success of community shielding depends upon the development of partnerships among government, business, the media, and the public, creating an integrated social infrastructure that facilitates a shelter-in-place response by providing essential resources to augment individual preparation for natural or unnatural catastrophic events.

Community shielding allows individuals to remain in their homes and communities, rather than evacuating an affected area in an attempt to avoid a threat or danger. Both a government-ordered, mandatory evacuation and a spontaneous evacuation of citizens in the absence of instructions to leave an area usually result in a chaotic response, mass movement of citizens on congested roadways to nowhere, and the entrapment of vulnerable citizens suffering from illness or in need of medical care. Gridlock of transportation systems in an affected area also hampers local first responders from reaching those most in need. By contrast, community shielding fosters empowerment and resilience in American citizens to remain at home in their communities and fight, rather than to flee, delivering a strong response to defeat the terrorist objective of disrupting and destroying American lives and the normal functioning of our society.

Just as individual cells in the body are nourished within organs, so too must places of refuge be supported through community shielding, a wider form of sheltering. When communities are deployed to provide necessary strategic support for sheltering in place, there is less chance for first responders to be overwhelmed by unnecessary and dangerous evacuation attempts.

A variety of survey outcome data sources demonstrates a significant increase in the willingness of citizens to participate in a community shielding strategy if their sheltering in place is augmented by the provision of resources until it is safe to leave their homes or communities (i.e., delivery of food, water, medications, and medical treatment; dissemination of reliable information as to the crisis, its duration, and the safety and well-being of family members; and a means to communicate within and outside the affected community). These findings strongly suggest that if local communities' emergency preparedness and response plans include bringing food, water, medications, and other necessities directly to citizens' homes and workplaces and providing assurances as to the safety and well-being of family members from whom they are separated, citizen response would be favorable and in support of community shielding.

Implementation of community shielding as part of emergency preparedness planning/response to future events will require continued efforts toward a national initiative to increase awareness of the concept and to gain support from key government and community leaders, as well as the American public. Public education will be necessary to enlist the citizens as significant participants in preparing for such future events, including the dissemination of information as to what steps to take to prepare, how notification of events will be provided, and how communication will be maintained during a crisis. Moreover, the fundamentals of how to respond to these challenges should be analyzed by the contemporary emergency response chief or executive now in order to allow for realignment of planning, training, and operational paradigms to effectively respond to a community in need with shielding implemented.

Realities and Costs

It is unlikely that a rational foreign government would risk potential military reprisals and the political/economic sanctions that overt use of biological warfare against the United States would bring (Lebeda, 1997). Covert action or deniable independent rogue factions and transnational terrorist organizations do not have the same constraints. Terrorist organizations operating in a civilian environment have freedom of movement and the ability to use commercially available equipment for development and discharge of their weapon. They are not constrained by a need for precise targeting or predictable results. A determined transnational organization or rogue individual may not be deterred, may escape detection and intelligence-gathering activities, and may succeed in releasing a biological agent in a susceptible target area. Lastly, transnational terrorist groups generally are not affiliated with one country or organization, and as such they have no return address, making a military retaliation very complicated if not impossible.

The effects of a bioterrorism incident are catastrophic. In a paper by researchers at the CDC, the projected economic impact alone ranges from $477 million per 100,000 people exposed to brucellosis to $26.2 billion in the case of anthrax (Kaufmann, Meltzer, & Schmid, 1997). Over 30,000 deaths were predicted if anthrax was used as the biological agent. The paper consistently used the lowest possible expense for all factors that affected costs, including the virulence of the disease. Costs of both preparedness and intervention were significant. It is clear that this would not be the case in a real disaster of this magnitude. Even so, the researchers concluded that reducing preventable losses has a significantly greater impact than reducing the probability of an attack through intelligence gathering and prevention strategies.

The authors also noted that the best possible measures to decrease both costs and deaths were those that would enhance rapid response to an attack. "These measures would include developing and maintaining EMS response operation and hospital critical care capacities, laboratory capabilities for both clinical diagnostic testing and environmental sampling, developing and maintaining drug medical counter-measure stockpiles, and developing and practicing response plans at the local level" (Kaufmann et al., 1997).

Possible Biotoxins

Until recently, toxins were of interest only to the toxicologist, the rare patient who ingested or was exposed to these toxins, and the even rarer writer who discussed toxicological environmental emergencies. Unfortunately, several simultaneous political and scientific events have moved these toxins to a more prominent medical and social position.

Discovery that some of these toxins have been used as agents in warfare or have been stockpiled to use in warfare has given the medical community an impetus to learn more about the effects and production of toxins for biological warfare. New uses for old toxins include *botulinum* therapy for spastic muscles and dystonia. For an overview of biological symptoms and treatments, refer to **TABLE 9-1**.

Botulinum Toxins

Botulinum neurotoxin is among the most potent toxins known. The mouse lethal dose is less than 0.1 nanogram per 100 grams. It is over 275 times more toxic than cyanide.

Mueller (1735–1793) and Kerner (1786–1862) in Germany first described botulism. They associated the disease with ingestion of insufficiently cooked blood sausages and described death by muscle paralysis and suffocation. In the early 1900s, botulism occurred commonly in the United States and nearly destroyed the canned-food industry (Meyer, 1956).

The major source of *botulinum* toxin is the organism *Clostridium botulinum*. There are seven serotypes produced by *clostridia* species. These serotypes are similar but do not cross-react to immune reactions. They are released as a single polypeptide chain of about 150,000 daltons, which is cleaved to generate two disulfide-linked fragments. The heavy fragment (histone 100,000 daltons) is involved in cell binding and penetration, while the light chain is responsible for the toxic intracellular effects.

Clinical Effects

Two natural types of poisoning occur. In the first type, food tainted with *clostridia* species is stored or processed in a way that allows the anaerobic organisms to grow and multiply. As they grow, they produce and release toxin. If the food is not subsequently heated to destroy the toxin, clinically significant amounts can be consumed. The toxin passes through the gut into the general circulation and is distributed throughout the body. In the second type, usually found in infants, the organisms colonize and produce their toxin in the gut. The clinical effects of the two types of botulism are the same.

After ingestion with *botulinum* toxin, the victim will develop diplopia and ptosis (difficulty speaking and swallowing), decreased bowel function, and muscle weakness that can progress to a flaccid paralysis. The patient will generally be awake, oriented, and afebrile. Development of respiratory failure may be quite rapid after initial symptoms develop. The hallmark sign is progressive, bilateral descending paralysis, which occurs usually within 24 hours of ingesting a contaminated product.

TABLE 9-1 Biological Agents: Symptoms and Treatment

	Signs and symptoms	Diagnosis	Treatment	Prophylaxis	Decontamination
Anthrax	Incubation period is 1-6 days. Fever, malaise, fatigue, cough, and mild chest discomfort are followed by severe respiratory distress with dyspnea, diaphoresis, stridor, and cyanosis. Shock and death occur within 36 hours of severe symptoms.	Physical findings are nonspecific. Possible widened mediastinum. Detectable Gram stain of the blood and by blood culture in the course of illness.	Although usually not effective after symptoms are present, high-dose antibiotic treatment with penicillin, ciprofloxacin, or doxycycline should be undertaken. Supportive therapy may be necessary.	A licensed vaccine for use in those considered at risk for exposure. Vaccine schedule is 0, 2, and 4 weeks for initial series, followed by boosts at 6, 12, and 18 months, and then a yearly booster.	Secretion and lesion precautions should be practiced. After an invasive procedure or autopsy is performed, the instruments and area used should be thoroughly decontaminated with a sporicidal agent such as iodine or chlorine.
Botulinum toxins	Ptosis, generalized weakness, dizziness, dry mouth and throat, blurred vision and diplopia, dysarthria, dysphonia, and dysphagia followed by symmetrical descending flaccid paralysis and development of respiratory failure. Symptoms begin as early as 24 hours, but may take several days after inhalation of a toxin.	Clinical diagnosis; no routine laboratory findings. Bioterrorism/warfare should be suspected if numerous collocated casualties have progressive descending bulbar, muscular, and respiratory weakness.	Intubation and ventilatory assistance for respiratory failure. Tracheostomy may be required. Administration of *botulinum* antitoxin (Investigational New Drug [IND] product) may prevent or decrease progression to respiratory failure and hasten recovery.	Pentavalent toxoid (types A, B, C, D, and E) is available as an IND product for those at high risk of exposure.	Hypochlorite (0.5% for 10-15 minutes) and/or soap and water. Toxin is not dermally active and secondary aerosols are not a hazard from patients.
Cholera	Incubation period is 1-5 days. Asymptomatic to severe with sudden onset. Vomiting, abdominal distention, and pain with little or no fever followed rapidly by diarrhea. Fluid losses may exceed 5-10 liters per day. Without treatment, death may result from severe dehydration, hypovolemia, and shock.	Clinical diagnosis. Watery diarrhea and dehydration. Microscopic exam of stool samples reveals few or no red or white cells. Can be identified in stool by dark field or phase contrast microscopy and can be grown on a variety of culture media.	Fluid and electrolyte replacement. Antibiotics such as tetracycline, ampicillin, or trimethoprim-sulfamethoxazole will shorten the duration of diarrhea.	A licensed, killed vaccine is available but provides only about 50% protection that lasts no more than 6 months. Vaccination schedule is at 0 and 4 weeks with booster doses every 6 months.	Personal contact rarely causes infection; however, enteric precautions and careful hand washing should be frequently employed. Bactericidal solutions such as hypochlorite would provide adequate decontamination.

(continues)

TABLE 9-1 Biological Agents: Symptoms and Treatment (continued)

	Signs and symptoms	Diagnosis	Treatment	Prophylaxis	Decontamination
Plague	Pneumonic plague: Incubation period is 2-3 days. High fever, chills, hemoptysis, toxemia, progressing rapidly to dyspnea, stridor, and cyanosis. Death results from respiratory failure, circulatory collapse, and bleeding diathesis. Bubonic plague: Incubation period is 2-10 days. Malaise, high fever, and tender lymph nodes (buboes); may progress spontaneously to the septicemic form, with spread to the central nervous system, lungs, and elsewhere.	Clinical diagnosis. A presumptive diagnosis can be made by Gram or Wayson stain of lymph node aspirates, sputum, or cerebral spinal fluid. Plague can also be cultured.	Early administration of antibiotics is very effective. Supportive therapy for pneumonic and septicemic forms is required.	A licensed, killed vaccine is available. Initial dose followed by a second smaller dose 1-3 months later, and a third 3-6 months later. A booster dose is given at 6, 12, and 18 months, and then every 1-2 years. This vaccine may not protect against aerosol exposure.	Secretion and lesion precautions with bubonic plague should be practiced. Strict isolation of patients with pneumonic plague. Heat, disinfectants, and exposure to sunlight render bacteria harmless.
Q fever	Fever, cough, and pleuritic chest pain may occur as early as 10 days after exposure. Patients are not generally critically ill, and the illness lasts from 2 days to 2 weeks.	Q fever is not a clinically distinctive illness and may resemble a viral illness or other types of atypical pneumonia. The diagnosis is confirmed serologically.	Q fever is generally a self-limiting illness even without treatment. Tetracycline or doxycycline are the treatments of choice and are orally administered for 5-7 days. Q fever endocarditis (rare) is much more difficult to treat.	Treatment with tetracycline during the incubation period may delay but not prevent the onset of symptoms. An activated whole-cell vaccine is effective in eliciting protection against exposure, but severe local reactions to this vaccine may be seen in those who already possess immunity.	Patients who are exposed to Q fever by aerosol do not present a risk for secondary contamination or reaerosolization of the organism. Decontamination is accomplished with soap and water or by the use of weak (0.5%) hypochlorite solutions.

	Signs and symptoms	Diagnosis	Treatment	Prophylaxis	Decontamination
Ricin	Weakness, fever, cough, and hypothermia about 36 hours after aerosol exposure, followed in the next 12 hours by hypotension and cardiovascular collapse.	Signs and symptoms noted above in large numbers of geographically clustered patients could suggest an exposure to aerosolized ricin. The rapid time course to severe symptoms and death would be unusual for infectious agents. Laboratory findings are nonspecific except for specific serum enzyme-linked immunosorbent assay. Acute and convalescent sera should be collected.	Patient management is supportive. Presently there is no available antitoxin. Gastric decontamination measures should be employed if the toxin is ingested.	Presently there is no vaccine or prophylactic antitoxin available for human use. Use of a protective mask (respirator) is currently the best protection against inhalation if an attack/exposure is anticipated.	Weak hypochlorite solutions and/or soap and water can decontaminate skin surfaces. Ricin is not volatile, so secondary aerosols are generally not a danger to healthcare providers
Smallpox	Clinical manifestation begins acutely with malaise, fever, rigors, vomiting, headache, and backache. About 2-3 days later, lesions appear, which quickly progress from macules to papules and eventually to pustular vesicles. They are more abundant on the extremities and face and develop synchronously.	Tests of electron and light microscopy are not capable of discriminating variola from vaccinia, monkeypox, or cowpox. The latest Polymerase Chain Reaction diagnostics techniques may be more accurate in discriminating between variola and other Orthopoxviruses.	At present there is no effective chemotherapy and treatment of a clinical case remains supportive.	Immediate vaccination or revaccination should be undertaken for all personnel exposed. Vaccinia-immune globulin is of value in postexposure prophylaxis of smallpox when given within the first week following exposure, and with vaccination.	Strict quarantine with respiratory isolation for a minimum of 16-17 days following exposure for all contacts. Patients should be considered infectious until all scabs separate.

(continues)

TABLE 9-1 Biological Agents: Symptoms and Treatment (continued)

	Signs and symptoms	Diagnosis	Treatment	Prophylaxis	Decontamination
Staphylococcal enterotoxin B	From 3-12 hours after aerosol exposure, sudden onset of fever, chills, headache, myalgia, and nonproductive cough. Some patients may develop shortness of breath and retrosternal chest pain. Fever may last 2-5 days, and cough may persist up to 4 weeks. Patients may also present with nausea, vomiting, and diarrhea if they swallow the toxin. Higher exposure levels can lead to septic shock and death.	Clinical diagnosis. Patient presents with a febrile respiratory syndrome without chest X-ray abnormalities. Large numbers of patients presenting with typical symptoms and signs of staphylococcal enterotoxin B pulmonary exposure would suggest an intentional attack with this toxin.	Treatment is limited to supportive care. Artificial ventilation might be needed for very severe cases and attention to fluid management is essential.	Use of protective mask. There is currently no vaccine available to prevent staphylococcal enterotoxin B intoxication.	Hypochlorite (0.5% for 10-15 minutes) and/or soap and water. Destroy any food that may have been contaminated.
Trichothecene mycotoxins (T2)	Exposure causes skin pain, pruritus, redness, vesicles, necrosis, and sloughing of epidermis. Effects on the airway include nose and throat pain, nasal discharge, itching, sneezing, cough, dyspnea, wheezing, chest pain, and hemoptysis. The toxin also produces effects after ingestion or eye contact. Severe poisoning results in prostration, weakness, ataxia, collapse, shock, and death.	Should be suspected if an aerosol attack occurs in the form of yellow rain with droplets of yellow fluid contaminating clothes and the environment. Confirmation requires testing of blood, tissue, and environmental samples.	There is no specific antidote. Superactive charcoal should be given orally if swallowed.	The only defense is to wear personal protective equipment during an attack. No specific immunotherapy or chemotherapy is available for use in the field.	Outer garments should be removed, and exposed skin should be decontaminated with soap and water. Eye exposure should be treated by copious saline irrigation. Once decontamination is complete, isolation is not required.

	Signs and symptoms	Diagnosis	Treatment	Prophylaxis	Decontamination
Tularemia	Ulceroglandular tularemia presents with a local ulcer and regional lymphadenopathy, fever, chills, headache, and malaise. Typhoidal or septicemic tularemia presents with fever, headache, malaise, substernal discomfort, prostration, weight loss, and a nonproductive cough.	Clinical diagnosis. Physical findings are usually nonspecific. Chest X-ray may reveal pneumonic process, mediastinal lymphadenopathy, or pleural effusion. Routine culture is possible but difficult. The diagnosis can be established by serology.	Administration of antibiotics with early treatment is very effective.	A live, attenuated vaccine is available as an investigational new drug. It is administered once by scarification. A 2-week course of tetracycline is effective as prophylaxis when given after exposure.	Secretion and lesion precautions should be practiced. Strict isolation of patients is not required. Organisms are relatively easy to render harmless by heat and disinfectants.
Venezuelan equine encephalitis	Sudden onset of illness with general malaise, spiking fevers, rigors, severe headache, photophobia, and myalgias. Nausea, vomiting, cough, sore throat, and diarrhea may follow. Full recovery takes 1-2 weeks.	Clinical diagnosis. Physical findings are usually nonspecific. The white blood cell count often shows a striking leukopenia and lymphopenia. Virus isolation may be made from serum, and in some cases throat swab specimens.	Supportive therapy only.	A live, attenuated vaccine is available as an investigational new drug. A second, formalin-inactivated killed vaccine is available for boosting antibody titers in those initially receiving the live vaccine.	Blood and body fluid precautions (body substance isolation) should be employed. Human cases are infectious for mosquitoes for at least 72 hours. The virus can be destroyed by heat (80°C [176°F] for 30 minutes) and ordinary disinfectants.
Viral hemorrhagic fevers	Viral hemorrhagic fevers (VHFs) are febrile illnesses that can be complicated by easy bleeding, petechiae, hypotension, and even shock, flushing of the face and chest, and edema. Constitutional symptoms such as malaise, myalgias, headache, vomiting, and diarrhea may occur in any hemorrhagic fevers.	Clinical diagnosis. Watery diarrhea and dehydration. Microscopic exam of stool samples reveals few or no red or white cells. Can be identified in stool by dark field or phase contrast microscopy and can be grown on a variety of culture media.	Intensive supportive care may be required. Antiviral therapy with ribavirin may be useful in several of these infections. Convalescent plasma may be effective in Argentine hemorrhagic fever.	The only licensed VHF vaccine is yellow fever vaccine. Prophylactic ribavirin may be effective for Lassa fever, Rift Valley fever, Crimean-Congo hemorrhagic fever, and possibly hemorrhagic fever with renal syndrome.	Decontamination with hypochlorite or phenolic disinfectant. Isolation measures and barrier nursing procedures are indicated.

Source: *Medical Management of Biological Casualties Handbook* (2nd ed.). (1996). Fredrick, MD: United States Army Medical Research Institute of Infectious Diseases, Ft. Detrick.

It is sometimes difficult to distinguish organophosphate nerve agent poisoning from botulism. The copious secretions of the nerve agent will be the significant clue to the differential. Isolated cases have a wider differential diagnosis including Guillain-Barré syndrome, myasthenia gravis, and tick paralysis.

Botulinum toxin penetrates into the cell and blocks release of acetylcholine, preventing neuromuscular transmission and leading to muscle weakness and paralysis (Jankovic & Brin, 1991). *Botulinum* toxin is thought to preferentially affect active neuromuscular fibers and has been shown in rats to have a greater affinity when nerve activity is greater (Hughes & Whaler, 1962). It may also affect the central nervous system (Hallett, Glocker, & Deuschl, 1994). The local injection of *botulinum* toxin has been used clinically to treat involuntary focal muscle spasms and involuntary dystonia.

Botulinum toxin was used to assassinate Reinhard Heydrich, a Nazi leader and probable successor to Hitler. The Czechoslovakian underground used a grenade impregnated with *botulinum* toxin made by English researchers in Porton Down near Wiltshire, England. Although Heydrich's wounds were relatively minor, he died unexpectedly several days after the attack (Mobley, 1995). *Botulinum* is a highly effective weapon of isolated assault. It is a one-shot weapon that is neither communicable or transmittable, but for assignation it can be highly effective.

Detection

Detection of *botulinum* may be done by mouse bioassay or by liquid chromatography. Uses of radioimmunoassay and radioreceptor assays have also been reported. A DNA probe has been designed for detection of *botulinum* toxin, which would markedly expedite diagnosis. An immunoassay has been developed by Environmental Technologies Group, Incorporated, in Baltimore, Maryland, to detect this toxin, ricin, and staphylococcal enterotoxin.

Survivors will probably not develop an antibody response due to the small amount of toxin required for lethality.

Prophylaxis and Treatment

Botulinum toxoid vaccine is available (Hanson, 1994; Hatheway, 1995; Wiener, 1996). The CDC provides a pentavalent vaccine that gives protection from toxin types A, B, C, D, and E but provides no protection against the F and G type toxins. The military believes that F and G type toxins are unlikely to be used in warfare because the strains of *Clostridium botulinum* that produce toxins F and G are difficult to grow in large quantities. If new techniques allow production of toxins F and G

in large quantities, the pentavalent vaccine will be useless. A heptavalent antitoxin against types A through G is available in limited supply at the U.S. Army Medical Research Institute of Infectious Diseases in Fort Detrick, Frederick, Maryland.

Treatment is supportive. Respiratory failure will require prolonged (weeks to months) ventilatory support. If ventilatory support is available, fatalities are likely to occur in less than 5 percent of the exposed population.

An equine antitoxin is available and may be of some help in both food-borne and aerosol botulism. This is available from the CDC and protects against A, B, and E toxins. It has been used for treating ingestion botulism and should be given as soon as the diagnosis is made. It is not without its own risks and it does not reverse paralysis, but does prevent progression of the disease. There is no human-based antitoxin currently available, but human-based antitoxin testing is now in progress. Obviously, it will not help in types C and D intoxication.

Although penicillin has been recommended, it is controversial because it may increase the release of toxin in the gut and may worsen neurological symptoms through lysis of bacterial cells in the gut or wound (Hatheway, 1995). It is also assumed to be ineffective if the toxin were to be inhaled in a direct toxin release.

Clostridium Toxins

Tetanus neurotoxin is secreted by *Clostridium* species in similar fashion to *botulinum*. The toxin is a single 150,000-dalton polypeptide that is cleaved into two peptides held together by disulfide and noncovalent bonds. The intoxication occurs at extremely low concentrations of toxin, is irreversible, and, like botulism, affects the activity of the nerve cell when toxicity occurs.

Clostridium perfringens also secretes at least 12 toxins and can produce gas gangrene (clostridial myonecrosis), enteritis necroticans, and *clostridium* food poisoning. One or more of these toxins could be produced as a weapon. The alpha toxin is a highly toxic phospholipase that could be lethal when delivered as an aerosol.

Clinical Effects

Where *botulinum* toxin causes a flaccid paralysis, tetanus causes spastic paralysis. The tetanus neurotoxin migrates retroaxonally (up the nerve fiber) and by transcytosis, it reaches the spinal inhibitory neurons, where it blocks neurotransmitter release and thus causes a spastic paralysis. Despite the seemingly different actions of tetanus and botulism, the toxins act in a similar way at the appropriate cellular level. The clinical effect in humans is well documented and includes twitches, spasms, rictus sardonicus, and convulsions.

Clostridium perfringens alpha toxin would cause vascular leaks, pulmonary damage, thrombocytopenia, and hepatic damage. In the case of an inhaled *clostridium perfringens*, severe respiratory distress would occur rapidly.

Detection
If *C. perfringens* is suspected, acute serum and tissue samples should be collected for further testing. Specific immunoassays are available for both *C. perfringens* and *C. tetani* species. As with most of these toxins and diseases, specific laboratory findings may be too late to be of clinical use.

Prophylaxis and Treatment
C. perfringens and tetanus are generally sensitive to penicillin, and this is the current drug of choice. There are some data that indicate treatment with either clindamycin or rifampin may decrease *C. perfringens* toxin production and give better results.

Every medical provider is aware of the schedule for tetanus immunizations. It is unlikely that there will be any use of this toxin in the United States due to widespread tetanus immunization (Lebeda, 1997). This may not be true in other countries, and in the United States there has been no published program about clinical syndromes of overwhelming amounts of tetanus toxin. Although the U.S. military apparently discounts this toxin, it is so easy to make and spread and so lethal that it would make a useful biological toxin.

There is no specific prophylaxis against most of the *C. perfringens* toxins. Some toxoids for enteritis necroticans are available for humans. Veterinary toxoids are in wide use.

Ricin
Ricin is a type II ribosome inactivating protein produced by the castor bean plant and secreted in the castor seeds (**CP FIGURE 9-1**). The toxin is a 576 amino acid protein precursor weighing 65,000 daltons. Once inside the cell, ricin depurinates an adenine from rRNA and thereby inactivates the ribosome, killing the cell.

Ricin is available worldwide by simple chemical process of the castor bean. Although ricin is only a natural product of the castor bean plant, ricin has been produced from transgenic tobacco using gene transfer principles. Large amounts of toxin could not be produced easily by this transgenic method (Sehnke, Pedrosa, & Paul, Frankel, & Ferl 1994).

Clinical Effects
The clinical picture of ricin poisoning depends on the route of exposure. Castor bean ingestion causes rapid onset of nausea, vomiting, abdominal cramps, coughing up blood, seizure activity, and severe diarrhea followed by vascular collapse. Death usually occurs on the third day. Inhalation of ricin will cause nonspecific weakness, cough, fever, hypothermia, and hypotension, followed by cardiovascular collapse about 24 to 36 hours after inhalation. Death will occur about 36 to 48 hours after inhalation. High doses by inhalation appear to produce severe enough pulmonary damage to cause death.

At least one fatality has been documented as a direct result of ricin employed in biowarfare. In 1978, ricin-impregnated pellets were fired from an umbrella at Georgi Markov and Vladimir Kostov. The pellets were coated with wax designed to melt at body temperature and release the ricin. Markov died as a result of the ricin attack, but Kostov survived. At least six other assassinations have used the same technique, according to intelligence sources.

Detection
<u>Enzyme-linked immunosorbent assay</u> for blood or histochemical analysis may be useful in confirming ricin intoxication. Ricin causes marked immune response and sera should be obtained from survivors for measurement of antibody response. An immunoassay technique has been developed by Environmental Technologies Group for ricin.

Standard laboratory tests are of little help in diagnosis of ricin intoxication. The patient may have some leukocytosis with neutrophil predominance. The pleomorphic picture of ricin intoxication would suggest many respiratory pathogens and may be of little help in diagnosis.

Prophylaxis and Treatment
There is no approved immunologic treatment or chemoprophylaxis for ricin poisoning at this time. Respiratory protection will prevent inhalation exposure and is the best prophylaxis currently available. Ricin has no dermal activity and is not transported through the skin.

There is ongoing effort to produce both active immunization and passive antibody prophylaxis suitable for humans. These techniques have been used in animals.

Treatment is supportive and includes both respiratory support and cardiovascular support as needed. If oral ingestion is suspected, lavage followed by charcoal is appropriate.

Saxitoxin
Saxitoxin is a dinoflagellate toxin responsible for paralytic shellfish poisoning. It is also found in several species of puffers and other marine animals and was originally discovered in 1927 (Sato et al., 1997). The toxin is very soluble in water, is heat stable, and is not destroyed by

cooking. The lethal dose is 1 to 2 mg. There are multiple related toxins with substitutions at key positions.

Clinical Effects

Saxitoxin is similar in effects and treatment to tetrodotoxin. Onset of symptoms is within minutes of exposure. Death may occur within 24 hours. If the patient survives, normal functions are regained within a few days.

Detection

A mouse unit is the minimum amount of saxitoxin that will kill a 20-gram mouse within 15 minutes. There is a standardized mouse assay for routine surveillance, and immunoassays are available.

Prophylaxis and Treatment

There is no antidote for saxitoxin, so symptomatic treatment is appropriate. Antibodies for tetrodotoxin will frequently protect against saxitoxin (Kaufman, Wright, Ballou, & Monheit, 1991).

Staphylococcal Enterotoxin

Staphylococcal food poisoning is familiar to most emergency practitioners. Although the disease is changed when the enterotoxin is delivered via aerosol, it will result in the common food poisoning syndrome. The organism that produces this agent is readily available and could be tailored to produce large quantities of the toxin.

Clinical Effects

Staphylococcal food poisoning begins 1 to 6 hours after exposure with the sudden onset of fever, chills, headache, myalgias, and a nonproductive cough. The cough may progress to dyspnea and substernal chest pain. In severe cases, pulmonary edema may be found. Nausea, vomiting, and diarrhea are common (as in the poisoning familiar to emergency physicians). The only physical finding of note is conjunctival injection.

In food-borne staphylococcal enterotoxin B, fever and respiratory involvement are not found, and the gastrointestinal symptoms predominate. Sickness may last as long as 2 weeks and severe exposures may cause fatalities.

Detection

The lab is not helpful in diagnosing staphylococcal enterotoxin poisoning. **Erythrocyte sedimentation rate** may be elevated, but this is a nonspecific finding. A chest X-ray is usually normal, but it may have increased interstitial markings and possibly pulmonary edema. An immunoassay has been developed by Environmental Technologies Group from Baltimore, Maryland, that is cost efficient and usable in the field environment.

Prophylaxis and Treatment

There is no significant treatment regimen available for staphylococcal enterotoxin. Therapy is entirely support-

ive. There is no current prophylaxis available, although experimental immunization has been reported.

Tetrodotoxin

Tetrodotoxin is a potent neurotoxin produced by fish, salamanders, frogs, octopus, starfish, and mollusks, notably the puffer (also called the globefish or blowfish) (Lange, 1990). The dangers of tetrodotoxin poisoning were known by the ancient Egyptians (2400 to 2700 B.C.). All organs of the freshwater puffer are toxic with the skin having the highest toxicity followed by gonad, muscle, liver, and intestine. In saltwater puffers, the liver is the most toxic organ. The lethal dose of tetrodotoxin is only 5 micrograms per kilogram in the guinea pig.

Puffer intoxication is a serious public health problem in Japan, and over 50 people each year are intoxicated. Raw puffer fish, commonly called fugu, is a delicacy in several Southeast Asian countries including Japan. Consumption of fugu causes mild tetrodotoxin intoxication with a pleasant peripheral and perioral tingling sensation. Improperly prepared fugu may contain a lethal quantity of tetrodotoxin. Fatalities have gradually decreased because of the increased understanding of the toxin and careful preparation of the puffer for food (Laobhripatr et al., 1990). Cooking the food will not dissipate the toxin. Tetrodotoxin is heat stable.

There are several microbial sources of tetrodotoxin including *Pseudomonas*, *Vibrio*, *Listonella*, and *Alteromonas* species. Although there is only one known bacteria that has produced tetrodotoxin toxicity in humans, there is a significant potential for genetic alteration of common species of bacteria to produce tetrodotoxin (Nozue et al., 1990).

Tetrodotoxin is well known for its ability to inhibit neuromuscular function by blocking the axonal sodium channels (Tambyah, Hui, Gopalakrishnakone, & Chin, 1994). Mortality from tetrodotoxin is thought to be due to hypoxic brain damage from prolonged respiratory paralysis.

Clinical Effects

The clinical symptoms and signs of tetrodotoxin poisoning are similar to those of the acetylcholinesterase poisons (Mackenzie, Smalley, Barnas, & Park, 1996). Clinical symptoms include nausea, vomiting, vertigo, perioral numbness, unsteady gait, and extremity numbness. Clinical symptoms begin within 30 minutes of ingestion. The speed of onset depends on the quantity of the toxin ingested. The symptoms progress to muscle weakness, chest tightness, diaphoresis, dyspnea, chest pain, and finally paralysis. Hypotension and respiratory failure are seen in severe poisonings. Patients will frequently complain of a sensation of cold or chilliness.

Paresthesias spread to the extremities with symptoms often more pronounced distally. Death can occur within 17 minutes after ingestion of tetrodotoxin.

Detection

Detection of tetrodotoxin is by mouse bioassay (Yasumoto, 1991) or by liquid chromatography. Use of radioimmunoassay and radioreceptor assays has also been reported. An in vitro colorimetric cell assay against a rabbit antiserum has been developed and may be more rapid than older methods, but it is not yet publicly available (Kaufman et al., 1991).

Prophylaxis and Treatment

At present, there is no known antidote for tetrodotoxin intoxication. There are numerous anecdotal treatments of survivors with supportive therapy alone. Certainly respiratory support and airway management will be life-saving for a majority of these patients. Gastric lavage will remove unabsorbed toxin from the gut and is used in puffer fish intoxication. Activated charcoal has been reported to effectively bind the toxin and may be employed in ingestions.

4-Aminopyridine has been used to treat tetrodotoxin intoxication in laboratory animals (Chang et al., 1996). 4-Aminopyridine is a potent potassium channel blocker and enhances impulse evoked acetylcholine release from presynaptic motor terminals. There have been no human studies of its use as an antidote. 4-Aminopyridine can cause muscle fasciculation and seizures in a dose-dependent phenomenon.

Naloxone has been proposed as a possible antidote against tetrodotoxin intoxication, because the opiates and tetrodotoxin have similar molecular configurations (Sims & Ostman, 1986). There are no reports of this in either laboratory or clinical use.

Active and passive immunization against tetrodotoxin has been demonstrated in laboratory animals, although there is no known available human immunization for tetrodotoxin (Fukiya & Matsumura, 1992). Tolerance does not develop on repeated puffer fish exposure. Monoclonal antibodies have been produced and protected laboratory animals against lethal doses of tetrodotoxin (Matsumura, 1995; Rivera, Poli, & Bignami, 1995).

Trichothecene Mycotoxins

The trichothecene mycotoxins are produced by fungi and achieved fame in the 1970s as the best candidates for the infamous yellow rain found in Laos, Cambodia, and Afghanistan. Naturally occurring trichothecenes have caused moldy corn toxicosis in animals.

Trichothecene mycotoxins are potent inhibitors of protein synthesis, inhibit mitochondrial respiration, impair DNA synthesis, and destroy cell membranes.

Clinical Effects

Consumption of trichothecenes causes weight loss, vomiting, bloody diarrhea, and diffuse hemorrhage. The onset of the illness occurs within hours, and death occurs within 12 hours. Inhalation adds respiratory distress and failure to the picture. Survivors have reported a radiation-sickness-like disease. This has included fever, nausea, vomiting, leukopenia, diarrhea, bleeding, and finally sepsis. Painful skin lesions also occur in survivors.

Detection

There is no readily available diagnostic test for trichothecenes, although reference laboratories may be able to help with gas-liquid chromatography. There are some polyclonal and monoclonal antibodies for detection in liquid or solid samples. Urine samples are most useful for this purpose because the metabolites can be detected as long as 28 days after exposure to the agent.

Prophylaxis and Treatment

Ascorbic acid has been proposed to decrease the lethality of trichothecenes. This has been studied in animals only, but because ascorbic acid has few side effects and is cheap, it should be used in all suspected cases.

Dexamethasone (1 to 10 mg intravenously) has also been shown to decrease lethality as late as 3 hours after exposure to these toxins.

In ingestions, charcoal or superactivated charcoal will absorb remaining toxin and decrease lethality.

Possible Live Bacteriological Warfare Agents

Possible live bacteriological warfare agents include only a few diseases that have been researched. Much of the information that is known to those in the field was obtained from *The United States Army Field Manual 8–9; Handbook on the Medical Aspects of NBC Defensive Operations* (FM 8–9) (U.S. Army, 1996; also available on the Internet at http://www.nbc-med.org/FMs). Other diseases have been proposed and researched as a result of multiple sessions with interested colleagues and this author's travels to the city of Sverdlovsk in the Union of Soviet Socialist Republics.

Although these diseases have been proposed by the U.S. military and others as possible biological warfare agents, there is no question that the list is neither exhaustive nor all-inclusive. Other diseases that have been considered include typhoid fever, Ebola virus, melioidosis, Rift Valley fever, epidemic typhus, Rocky Mountain spotted fever, scrub typhus, coccidiomycosis, histoplasmosis, Chikun-Gunya fever, Crimean-Congo fever, Lassa fever, dengue fever, eastern equine encephalitis, western equine encephalitis, Venezuelan encephalitis, Omsk hemorrhagic fever, Korean hemorrhagic fever, and many others (at least 60). The astute reader can recognize the potential for biowarfare in almost any disease that can possibly afflict humans. Numerous other diseases could be used as biowarfare agents against selected crops or livestock.

With the current level of gene manipulation, it is easy to foresee a chimera-tailored bacteria or rickettsia that has characteristics of one disease, with tailored resistance to all usual antibiotics, yet responsive to an unusual antibiotic that the designer has stockpiled. It is equally easy to think of a tailored virus that has unusual mortality for white Anglo-Saxon males, but has little mortality for Asian or African American people. One does not have to imagine an increase in lethality in order to find substantial biowarfare applications. A rapidly spreading upper respiratory illness—the common cold—that merely causes 3 days of cough, fever, rhinorrhea, and malaise could be incapacitating if an entire army caught it simultaneously. A city's police force would be unable to deal with terrorists effectively if over three-fourths of the entire city's population had uncontrollable diarrhea for a 2- or 3-day course.

Anthrax

Anthrax is caused by *Bacillus anthracis*. Under usual (nonwartime) conditions, humans become infected by contact with an infected animal or contaminated animal by-products. Anthrax is also known as wool-sorter's disease. This refers to the sheep shearers of the United Kingdom who frequently get the cutaneous form of the disease as part of the wool production process. There are three forms of anthrax: cutaneous, inhalation, and gastrointestinal. Almost all naturally occurring cases of anthrax are cutaneous or gastrointestinal.

Anthrax was proposed and investigated as a bioweapon by both the Allies in World War II and the Communists in the former Union of Soviet Socialist Republics. Indeed, an epidemic that caused 96 cases of human anthrax in the city of Ekatrinburg (formerly Sverdlosvk) in the spring of 1979 has been traced to an escaped Russian BW strain of anthrax. In these patients, the pathogen was airborne. Although medical records were confiscated by the Soviet State Security Committee known as the KGB, investigators have pieced together the epidemiology and the source of the epidemic (Meselson et al., 1994). Following the epidemic, thousands of citizens were immunized against anthrax, the exteriors of the buildings and trees were washed by local fire brigades, and several unpaved streets were asphalted. Notably absent in the public health response

was a military component. In 1992, Russian President Boris Yeltzin admitted that the military was the source of the outbreak. Perestroika and the downfall of the former Communist empire has led to greater release of information, but the staff of city hospital number 40, where the victims were cared for, remains quite sensitive in discussions about this event (Maniscalco, 2001).

In the case of weaponization of anthrax, it is likely to be disseminated as an aerosol of the very persistent spores. The incubation time is from 1 to 6 days, but as the Ekatrinburg incident showed, anthrax may have a prolonged incubation period of up to 2 months. The longer incubation periods are seen most frequently when partial treatment has been given. The spores can be quite stable, even in the alveolus, and as such frequently remain dormant, but very much alive for up to 3 months. The duration of the disease is between 2 and 5 days.

Presentation

The inhalation form of anthrax is particularly uncommon and particularly lethal. In its early presentation, inhalation anthrax could be confused with a plethora of viral or bacterial respiratory illnesses. The disease progresses over 2 to 3 days acting much like a common flu and then suddenly develops respiratory distress, shock, and death within 36 hours. Widening of the mediastinum on chest radiograph is common in the later stages of the disease and is due to the swollen and engorged lymph nodes within the mediastinum. Unfortunately the radiographic evidence is a late finding and does not bode well for survival of the patient. Evidence of infiltrates on the chest X-ray are uncommon. Other suggestive findings include chest wall edema, hemorrhagic pleural effusions, and hemorrhagic meningitis.

Diagnosis

Diagnosis can be made by culture of blood, pleural fluid, or cerebrospinal fluid. The blood culture is most often positive. In fatal cases, impressions of mediastinal lymph nodes or spleen will be positive. Anthrax toxin may be detected in blood by immunoassay.

The cases in Ekatrinburg were diagnosed on autopsy by a pathologist who noted a peculiar "cardinal's cap" meningeal inflammation typical in anthrax. Inhalational anthrax may be diagnosed at autopsy by the mediastinal inflammation that can also be observed on computerized tomography scan of the chest in the living patient.

Environmental Technologies Group, Incorporated, has developed an immunoassay for anthrax.

Therapy

Penicillin is considered the drug of choice for treatment of naturally occurring anthrax. However, penicillin-resistant strains do exist, and one could expect that anthrax used for a BW would be developed as penicillin resistant. Tetracycline and erythromycin have been used for patients who are allergic to penicillin. Induction of resistance to these antibiotics is an easy exercise for genetic manipulation, and warfare strains should be presumed to be resistant to these antibiotics until proven otherwise. Chloramphenicol, gentamycin, and ciprofloxacin would be appropriate choices for initial therapy. The U.S. military recommends oral ciprofloxacin or intravenous doxycycline for initial therapy (U.S. Army, 1996). This therapy is not appropriate for those under 18 years of age or for pregnant females. Supportive therapy for airway, shock, and fluid volume deficits is appropriate.

Prophylaxis

Two types of anthrax vaccine for human use are available in the United States and United Kingdom, albeit in totally insufficient quantities for a civilian biological warfare challenge. Both are based on the partially purified protective antigen of the *Bacillus anthracis* adsorbed to an aluminum adjuvant. The usual immunization series is six 0.5 mL doses over a span of 18 months. The military feels that a primary series of three 0.5 mL doses (at 0, 2, and 4 weeks) will be protective against both cutaneous and inhalation anthrax for about 6 months after the primary series. These immunizations were given to many coalition troops during the Gulf War in anticipation of Saddam Hussein's employment of this agent. Large quantities of antigen are presumed to be stockpiled for military use because this agent has been a recurring threat. Unless civilian immunizations start about 1 month prior to a terrorist attack, EMS and medical providers will be essentially unprotected.

Although minor reactions to the anthrax vaccine are common (occurring in 6 percent of the immunized population), major reactions are uncommon. Obviously, the vaccine is contraindicated for those who are known to be sensitive to it and for those who have already had clinical anthrax. The choice between immunization and some allergic reaction and no immunization in the face of a serious biowarfare threat presents a difficult clinical dilemma.

Live anthrax vaccine is used in Russia to immunize both livestock and human beings. It is a spore vaccine with both STI-1 and strain 3 mixtures. The Russians feel that this vaccine is superior at stimulating cell-mediated immunity (Shlyakhov & Rubinstein, 1994). There would be considerable resistance to use of the Russian vaccine in Western countries because of concerns over purity and residual virulence of a live vaccine.

There is no available evidence that these vaccines will adequately protect against an aerosol challenge. New vaccines with a highly purified protective antigen or designer attenuated strains have both been used in laboratories but are not commercially available (Coulson, Fulop, & Titball, 1994; Ivins et al., 1995).

Antibiotic prophylaxis with ciprofloxacin (500 mg orally twice day), or doxycycline (100 mg orally twice a day) is also recommended by the U.S. military for an imminent attack by a BW. Should the attack be confirmed as anthrax, then antibiotics should be continued for 4 weeks for all who are exposed. Those exposed should also be started on antianthrax vaccine with the standard schedule (if it is available) if they have not been previously immunized. Those who have received fewer than three doses of vaccine prior to exposure should receive a single booster injection. If vaccine is not available, antibiotics should be continued until patients can be safely and closely observed when the antibiotics are discontinued. Inhaled spores are not destroyed by antibiotics and may persist beyond the course of recommended antibiotics.

Brucellosis

Brucellosis is a zoonotic disease caused by small nonmotile coccobacilli. The natural reservoir is domestic herbivores such as goats, sheep, cattle, and pigs. There are four species: *Brucella melitensis*, *B. abortus* (cattle), *B. suis* (pigs), and *B. canis* (dogs). Humans become infected when they ingest raw infected meat or milk, inhale contaminated aerosols, or make contact with their skin. Human infection is also called undulant fever. Human-to-human transmission can occur only if serum is passed from an infected patient to another human, so it is extremely rare.

Brucella species have been long considered as biological warfare agents because of the stability, persistence, and ease of infection without human-to-human transfer. Brucellosis can be spread by aerosol spray or by contamination of food supply (sabotage). There is a long persistence in wet ground or food.

Presentation

The incubation period for brucellosis is about 8 to 14 days, but may be considerably longer. Clinical disease is a nonspecific febrile illness with headache, fatigue, myalgias, anorexia, chills, sweats, and cough. The fever can reach up to 105°F. The disease may progress and include arthritis, lymphadenopathy, arthralgias, osteomyelitis, epididymitis, orchitis, and endocarditis. Disability is pronounced, but lethality is only about 5 percent or less in usual cases. The disease may be followed by recovery and relapse. The duration of the disease is usually a few weeks, but brucellosis can last for years.

Diagnosis

Diagnosis of brucellosis is by blood culture, by bone marrow culture, or by serology. There are no other laboratory findings that contribute to a diagnosis of brucellosis.

Therapy

To treat brucellosis, the U.S. military recommends doxycycline (100 mg twice a day) plus rifampin (900 mg/day) for 6 weeks. These antibiotics are generally available in sufficient quantities in the United States. Alternative proposed therapy has been doxycycline (100 mg twice a day) for 6 weeks and streptomycin (1 g/day) for 3 weeks. Trimethoprim/sulfamethoxazole has been given for 4 to 6 weeks but is thought to be less effective. Relapse and treatment failure is common.

Prophylaxis

There is no information available about chemoprophylaxis for brucellosis. Human vaccines are not routinely available in the United States, but they have been developed by other countries. A variant of *B. abortus*, S19-BA, has been used in the former Union of Soviet Socialist Republics to protect occupationally exposed groups. Efficacy is limited and annual revaccination is needed. A similar vaccine is available in China. Neither of these two vaccines would meet Western requirements for safety and effectiveness (Corbel, 1997).

Cholera

Cholera is a well-known diarrheal disease caused by *Vibrio cholerae* acquired in humans through ingestion of contaminated water. The organism causes a profound secretory rice-water diarrhea by elaborating an enterotoxin.

Although cholera can be spread by aerosols, more likely terrorist or military employment would be contamination of food or water supplies. There is negligible direct human-to-human transmissibility. The bacterium does not have long persistence in food or pure water and is not persistent when applied by aerosols, thereby making it an ineffective bioweapon for mass distribution.

Presentation

Cholera can cause a profuse, watery diarrhea that causes hypovolemia and hypotension. Without treatment, cholera can rapidly kill adults and children alike from severe dehydration and resultant shock. The incubation period is 1 to 5 days and the course of the illness is about 1 week.

A patient with cholera may have vomiting early in the illness. There is little abdominal pain associated with the disease. The hallmark of the disease is rice-water diarrhea.

Diagnosis

Gram staining of the stool sample of a person with cholera will show few or no red or white cells. Renal failure may complicate severe dehydration. Electrolyte abnormalities are common with the profound fluid loss; generally hypokalemia predominates.

Rotavirus, *Escherichia coli*, and toxic ingestions such as staphylococcal food poisoning, *Bacillus cereus*, and even clostridia species can cause similar watery diarrhea. Bacteriological diagnosis of cholera diarrhea has been well studied for decades. Vibrio species can be seen and identified readily with dark field or phase contrast microscopes. Culture will prove the diagnosis but is not necessary for the treatment.

Therapy

Treatment of cholera is mostly supportive. Although most U.S. emergency physicians are used to treating significant hypovolemia with intravenous fluid replacement, it is unlikely to be readily available if an epidemic of cholera is caused by terrorist or enemy action. The World Health Organization (WHO) oral rehydration formula is appropriate but generally not stocked in sufficient quantities in most cities. Pedialyte and sport drinks such as Gatorade will provide interim oral hydration. If a cholera epidemic develops, intravenous fluids should be reserved for those patients who are vomiting and cannot tolerate oral rehydration, patients who have more than 7 liters per day of stool, and patients who have extensive hypovolemia and are in clinical shock.

Tetracycline and doxycycline have both been found to shorten the course of the diarrhea. Other effective drugs include ampicillin (250 mg every 6 hours for 5 days) and trimethoprim/sulfamethoxazole (1 tablet every 12 hours). Appropriate alteration of dosages should be used for pediatric patients.

Prophylaxis

The currently available vaccine for cholera is a killed suspension of *V. cholerae*. It provides incomplete protection and lasts for no longer than 6 months. It requires two injections with a booster dose every 6 months. Improved vaccines are being tested but are not yet available.

Ebola Virus

The Ebola virus is a member of a family of RNA viruses known as filoviruses commonly referred to as viral hemorrhagic fever (VHF) (CP FIGURE 9-2). When magnified several thousand times by an electron microscope, these viruses have the appearance of long filaments or threads. Ebola virus was discovered in 1976 and was named for a river in Zaire, Africa, where it was first detected (CDC, 2009).

Ebola virus has been covered significantly in the popular literature and in several books and movies (including *Outbreak*). Members of the Aum Shinrikyo cult visited Zaire to collect Ebola. This virus is highly contagious and easily spread by body fluids, particularly blood. It is quite dangerous for the healthcare provider because human-to-human contact will rapidly spread the disease. Ebola and all of the VHFs are capable of being aerosolized.

Use of this virus (with greater than 90 percent lethality) would be considered a doomsday operation by the military. There is no guarantee that this virus would be able to be contained if spread to a modern city. The persistence is low, but the transmissibility is so high that this is immaterial.

For example, the distribution of the virus might be effective by simply putting an infected individual on a plane that flies around the world and ensuring that he coughs repeatedly. The effect of this distribution plan could be extraordinary because the incubation period for overt illness is upwards of 14 days.

Presentation

Ebola virus is a viral hemorrhagic fever. It can be spread by blood and blood products, secretions, and by droplet nuclei or aerosol transmission (Jaax et al., 1995). It is highly lethal (more than 90 percent) with a rapid course.

Diagnosis

A diagnosis is made by detection of Ebola antigens, antibody, or genetic material, or by culture of the virus from these sources. Diagnostic tests are usually performed on clinical specimens that have been treated to inactivate (kill) the virus. Research on Ebola virus must be done in a special, high-containment laboratory to protect scientists working with infected tissues.

Therapy

Therapy is supportive only and involves extensive critical care medicine including artificial ventilation. A release of Ebola would significantly tax the overall healthcare system and require tremendous resources for each patient. Even then it is important that everyone understand that there is no known therapy for this disease.

Prophylaxis

There is no known prophylaxis for Ebola virus. Sera from survivors have been obtained, and it is possible that passive protection could be developed. A recent accidental exposure to live Ebola virus was successfully treated with convalescent antisera.

Plague

Plague is a zoonotic disease caused by *Yersinia pestis*. It is naturally found on rodents and prairie dogs and their fleas. Under normal conditions, the following three syndromes are recognized: inhalational (pneumonic), septicemic, and bubonic. Usually an initial infection is in the form of bubonic plague.

In 1994 defectors revealed that the Russians had conducted research on *Yersinia pestis*, the plague bacterium, to make it more virulent and stable in the environment. The plague can retain viability in water for 2 to 30 days, in moist areas for up to 2 years, and in near freezing temperatures for several months to a year.

Plague could be spread by either infected vectors such as fleas or by an aerosol spray. Person-to-person transmissibility is high and the bacterium is highly infective. The persistence is low, but the transmissibility is so high that this is immaterial.

Presentation

In bubonic plague, the incubation period is from 2 to 10 days. The onset is acute with malaise, fever (often quite high), and purulent lymphadenitis. The lymphadenitis is most often inguinal, but cervical and axillary nodes can also be involved, depending on where the flee bites occurred (**CP FIGURE 9-3A** and **CP FIGURE 9-3B**). As the disease progresses, the nodes become tender, fluctuant, and finally necrotic. The bubonic form may progress to the septicemic form whereby the plague bacterium infects the major organ systems systemically. Involvement of the lungs results in the pneumonic form and the patient becomes contagious through coughing and droplet nuclei. The course of the disease is 2 to 3 days, and the disease has a high mortality rate.

In primary pneumonic plague, the incubation period is 2 to 3 days. The onset is acute and fulminant with malaise, fever, chills, cough with bloody sputum, and toxemia. The pneumonia progresses rapidly to respiratory failure with dyspnea, stridor, and cyanosis.

In untreated patients, the mortality is over 50 percent for the bubonic and septicemic forms. In the pneumonic form, the mortality approaches 100 percent. The terminal events in septicemic plague are circulatory collapse, hemorrhage, and peripheral thrombosis. In pneumonic plague, the terminal event is often respiratory failure as well as circulatory collapse.

Diagnosis

A presumptive diagnosis of plague can be made by finding the typical safety pin bipolar staining organisms in Giemsa-stained specimens. Appropriate specimens are lymph node aspirate, sputum, or cerebral spinal fluid. Immunofluorescent staining is available and helpful if readily accessible. *Y. pestis* can be readily cultured from any of these sources.

Environmental Technologies Group, Incorporated, has developed an immunoassay for plague.

Therapy

Plague is readily contagious and strict isolation of patients is essential. Streptomycin, tetracycline, and chloramphenicol are all useful if they are given within the first 24 hours after symptoms of pneumonic plague begin. Supportive therapy of complications is essential.

Prophylaxis

Plague vaccine is available but has not been shown to be effective against an aerosol exposure and subsequent pneumonic plague. The plague vaccine is a whole cell formalin-killed product. The usual dose is 0.5 mL given at 0, 1, and 2 weeks.

Plague vaccines providing protection against aerosol exposure are not yet available but are under development (Oyston et al., 1995). Current whole-cell plague vaccines stimulate immunity against the bubonic form but are probably not effective for the pneumonic form (Meyer, 1970; Russel et al., 1995).

Q Fever

Q fever is a rickettsial zoonotic disease caused by *Coxiella burnetii*. The usual animals affected are sheep, cattle, and goats. Human disease is usually caused by inhalation of particles contaminated with *Coxiella*.

Presentation

Q fever is a self-limiting febrile illness of 2 days to 2 weeks. The incubation period is about 10 to 20 days. The patient is visually ill, but uneventful recovery is the rule. Q fever pneumonia is a frequent complication and may be noted only on radiographs in most cases. Some patients will have nonproductive cough and pleuritic chest pain. Other complications are not common and may include chronic hepatitis, endocarditis, meningitis, encephalitis, and osteomyelitis.

The value of this disease as a BW is in disruption of society. Mass distribution of the *C. burnetii* would cause significant societal disruption by overloading the healthcare system, creating fear, and causing mass social distancing, thereby disrupting the economy.

Diagnosis

Q fever's presentation as a febrile illness with an atypical pneumonia (characterized by a dry cough) is similar to a host of other atypical pneumonias, including mycoplasma, legionnaire's disease, chlamydia pneumonia, psittacosis, or hantavirus.

The diagnosis can be confirmed serologically and other laboratory findings are unlikely to be helpful. Most patients with Q fever will have slightly elevated liver enzymes. It is difficult to isolate rickettsia, and Q fever is no exception.

Therapy

As with other rickettsial diseases such as Rocky Mountain spotted fever, the treatment of choice for Q fever is tetracycline, doxycycline, or erythromycin. Although not tested, azithromycin and clarithromycin would be expected to be effective.

Prophylaxis

A formalin-inactivated whole cell vaccine is available as an investigational drug in the United States and has been used for those who are at risk of occupational infection with Q fever (Ackland, Worswick, & Marmion, 1994). One dose will provide immunity for an aerosol challenge within 3 weeks.

Skin testing is required to prevent a severe local reaction in previously immune individuals. A live attenuated strain (M44) has been used in the former Union of Soviet Socialist Republics (Genig, 1965).

Smallpox

Smallpox was used as a BW in the United States during the French and Indian War. Smallpox is an orthopox virus that affects primates, particularly man. The disease was declared eradicated in the world in 1977, and the last reported human case occurred in a laboratory in 1978. Theoretically, the virus exists in only two laboratories in the world, one in the United States and one in Russia. The virus can be transmitted by face-to-face contact, droplet nuclei, secretions, and aerosols. It is a durable virus and can exist for long periods outside the host. It is remotely possible that it is still living outside of the repository labs. A very closely related disease, monkeypox, cannot be easily distinguished from smallpox without significant evaluation of its RNA. A major concern of disaster medicine planners is/was the development of this virus as a war weapon by the former Soviet Union and the unknown amount of product produced at the time.

Release of this virus would have massive and extreme societal effects. Although much of world was vaccinated in the 1960s and 1970s, it is unknown whether those vaccinations would in fact protect an individual. Given that vaccinations were stopped by WHO in 1985, it is supposed that an entire generation could be totally unprotected and thus suffer massive mortality from the disease if it were to be released. Because of the virus's communicability, only one person need be infected to distribute this virus on an unsuspecting and unprotected world.

Presentation

Smallpox has a long incubation period of about 10 to 17 days. The illness has a prodrome of 2 to 3 days with malaise, fever, headache, and backache. Over the next 7 to 10 days, all of the characteristic lesions erupt, progress from macules to papules to vesicles to pustules and then crust and scarify (CP FIGURE 9-4). The lesions are more numerous on the extremities and face than on the trunk. The disease is fatal in about 35 percent of cases. Some patients will develop disseminated intravascular coagulopathy. Other complications include smallpox pneumonia, arthritis (a person who had smallpox may have permanent joint deformities), and keratitis (which may cause blindness).

Diagnosis

Like many viral diseases, the diagnosis of smallpox is best made by clinical impression. Routine labs are not helpful, although leukopenia is frequent. Clotting factors may be depressed and thrombocytopenia may be found. Diagnosis may be made with immunofluorescence, electron microscopy, or culture.

Clinical presentation would allow the diagnosis to occur rapidly in most healthcare settings. Much has been written and distributed about smallpox since the failed vaccination program of 2003. As a result, it is likely that any person presenting to most any healthcare clinic or emergency department would be identified rapidly.

Therapy

Therapy for smallpox is entirely supportive. Use of several antiviral medications has been proposed as possible amelioration treatment, but this is untested. It is understood by science that administration of the vaccination post–disease development will likely lessen the disease process and as a rule would be given to all patients, unless they are pregnant or immunocompromised.

Prophylaxis

Prophylaxis against smallpox has been available since the early 1800s when Dr. Edward Jenner developed a vaccine and is well documented. Because smallpox is presumed to have been eradicated worldwide, there is no recommendation or requirement for routine vaccination. Adequate stocks of smallpox vaccine are probably not available for exposure of large portions of the population. It is anticipated that if an outbreak were to occur, institution of a ring vaccination plan (similar to what eradicated the disease) would be immediately instituted, and this would limit the spread.

Objects in contact with a contaminated patient need to be cleansed with live steam or sodium hypochlorite solution.

Tularemia

Tularemia or rabbit fever is caused by *Francisella tularensis*, a gram-negative bacillus. Humans can contract this disease by handling an infected animal or by the bites of ticks, mosquitoes, or deerflies. The natural disease has a mortality rate of 5 to 10 percent. As few as 50 organisms can cause disease if inhaled.

Presentation

Like plague, tularemia has an ulceroglandular form, a pneumonic form, and a septicemic form. Two additional forms also occur with tularemia. Oculoglandular tularemia occurs when the inoculum is in the eye. Gastrointestinal tularemia occurs when tularemia bacilli are ingested. It may also infect the oropharynx.

The septicemic form can occur in 5 to 15 percent of natural cases. The clinical features include fever, prostration, and weight loss.

The pneumonic form may occur by inhaling contaminated dusts or by a deliberate aerosol. The resulting pneumonia is atypical and may be fulminant. Fever, headache, malaise, substernal discomfort, and cough are prominent. The cough is often nonproductive. A chest X-ray may or may not show a pneumonia.

Diagnosis

As noted, the diagnosis of pneumonic tularemia will be difficult clinically, with several types of atypical pneumonia as differential diagnoses. The laboratory is unhelpful early in this disease.

Therapy

Human-to-human spread of pneumonic tularemia is unusual and isolation is not required.

Treatment is streptomycin or gentamycin for 10 to 14 days. Tetracycline and chloramphenicol are also useful, but the military reports that there has been a significant relapse rate.

Prophylaxis

A live vaccine strain is available to U.S. military personnel. This vaccine is delivered intradermally and provides protection to an aerosol challenge by the third week postimmunization. Protection is dependent on the inhaled dose of tularemia, and inhalation of massive quantities of bacteria may overwhelm the protective effects of the vaccine (Hornick & Eigelsbach, 1966). Protection falls after 14 months, suggesting that a booster dose is appropriate. This vaccine is not available for civilian use.

Chapter Summary

As the emergency service community continues to be subjected to reports of escalating bioterrorism threats, the increase of media attention on the biothreat results in heightened fears and public questions of readiness. Events such as the West Nile virus outbreak immediately result in the press and public fearing that the event was a deliberate act rather than a naturally occurring event.

While the probability of a high-impact or widespread attack using BWs is low, the yield from such an event could be devastating. It is for this reason that being prepared to respond to the aftermath of a biological attack is critical. As highlighted in this chapter, there are many complex issues that nonmilitary responders are not familiar with that accompany the planning and response phases of a bioterrorism event. We strongly recommend that this matter be given the attention it deserves so that your members can be protected and the response effectiveness to your community can be maintained.

Remember that this type of incident can rapidly swell to a level that will overwhelm your EMS system as well as local healthcare resources. Incorporating the talents of your public health and hospital officials in the planning process will provide you with the ability to develop comprehensive and cohesive contingency plans.

Wrap Up

Chapter Questions

1. Define biological warfare. How is a biological attack different from other, more traditional forms of terrorism?
2. Briefly discuss the history of biological terrorism.
3. What are the major steps in a biological threat assessment?
4. What types of PPE are necessary for emergency responders in a biological event?
5. Discuss the clinical effects, detection, and prophylaxis/treatment for the following biological toxins:
   a. Ricin
   b. *Botulinum* toxin
   c. *Clostridium* toxin
6. Discuss the clinical effects and treatments for:
   a. Anthrax
   b. Ebola virus
   c. Tularemia
   d. Q fever

Chapter Project

Develop a comprehensive outline of a biological threat assessment for your jurisdiction or region. Consider key assessment elements from this chapter including detection, control of supplies, PPE, training, and prophylaxis.

Vital Vocabulary

Biological terrorism The use of etiological agents (disease) to cause harm or kill a population, food, and/or livestock.

Community shielding An effective and unique preparedness strategy to engage individuals, communities, and government in a unified response to disasters and future acts of terrorism, in particular bioterrorism. Originating from the University of Virginia's Critical Incident Analysis Group, this strategy is being adopted widely as a means of community and organizational resilience.

Enzyme-linked immunosorbent assay An immunological immunoassay technique for accurately measuring the amount of a substance, for example, in a blood sample.

Erythrocyte sedimentation rate Also called the sedimentation rate or Biernacki reaction, it is the rate at which red blood cells precipitate in a period of one hour; a common hematology test which is a nonspecific measure of inflammation. Anticoagulated blood is placed in an upright tube, known as a Westergren tube, and the rate at which the red blood cells fall is measured and reported in mm/h.

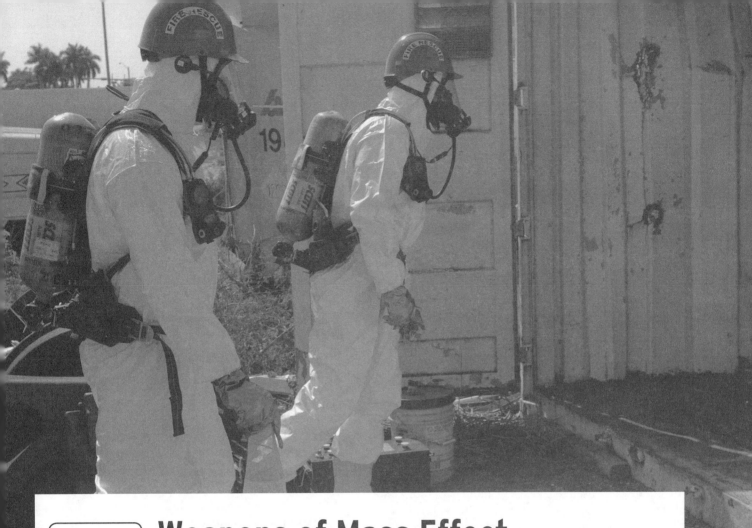

10 Weapons of Mass Effect– Radiation

Hank T. Christen
Paul M. Maniscalco
Harold W. Neil III

Objectives

- Describe the differences between a radiation incident and a traditional hazardous materials incident.
- Define the three types of radiation.
- Differentiate between the terms *dose* and *exposure*.
- Describe the distinction between acute and delayed effects of radiation exposure.
- Explain the difference between radiation exposure and contamination.
- Outline the first responder considerations in a radiological terrorism incident.

Introduction

Radiation is effective as a weapon of mass effect because of its long-term consequences and psychological effect on victims and the community. The word *radiation* immediately generates mental images of hideous and doomed casualties. This chapter provides an explanation of radiation and the types and hazards of radiation exposure. First responders need to understand the basics of radiation physics and protective measures to operate safely and effectively at a radiation attack or accident. Additional topics include the use of radiation as a terrorism weapon, the medical effects of radiation, and tactical considerations and critical factors related to an effective response to a radiation incident.

Radiation incidents are a special type of hazardous materials incident because of several common factors, including internal exposure pathways, contamination concerns, decontamination techniques, and personal protective equipment (PPE) requirements. These factors share commonality with chemical and biological threats.

Basic Radiation Physics

Radiation travels in the form of particles or waves in bundles of energy called **photons**. Some everyday examples are microwaves used to cook food, radio waves for radio and television, light, and X-rays used in medicine.

Radioactivity is a natural and spontaneous process by which the unstable atoms of an element emit or radiate excess energy in the form of particles or waves. These emissions are collectively called *ionizing radiation*. Depending on how the nucleus loses this excess energy, a lower energy atom of the same form results, or a completely different nucleus and atom are formed.

Ionization is a particular characteristic of the radiation produced when radioactive elements decay. These radiations are of such high energy that they interact with materials and electrons from the atoms in the material. This effect explains why ionizing radiation is hazardous to health and provides the means for detecting radiation.

An **atom** is composed of **protons** and **neutrons** contained in its nucleus. The only exception is the naturally occurring hydrogen atom, which contains no neutrons. Protons and neutrons are virtually the same size. **Electrons**, which are much smaller than protons and neutrons, orbit the nucleus of the atom. The chemical behavior of an atom depends on the number of protons, which are positively charged, and the number of electrons, which are negatively charged. Neutrons, which have no electric charge, do not play a role in the chemical behavior of the atom.

Special placards are required when transporting certain quantities or types of radioactive materials. In facilities that use radioactive materials, the standard radioactive symbol is used to label the materials for identification (**CP FIGURE 10-1**). Placard information is useful when responding to an accident involving radioactive materials. However, in a terrorist attack, there are no labels or placards to identify the hazards involved.

Alpha, beta, and gamma energy are forms of radiation (**FIGURE 10-1**). Because **alpha particles** contain two protons, they have a positive charge of two. Further, alpha particles are very heavy and very energetic compared to other common types of radiation. These characteristics allow alpha particles to interact readily with materials they encounter, including air, causing much ionization in a very short distance. Typical alpha particles travel only a few centimeters in air and are stopped by a sheet of paper.

Beta particles have a single negative charge and weigh only a small fraction of a neutron or proton. As a result, beta particles interact less readily with material than alpha particles. Beta particles travel up to several meters in air, depending on the energy, and are stopped by thin layers of metal or plastic.

Like all forms of electromagnetic radiation, the gamma ray has no mass and no charge. **Gamma rays** interact with material by colliding with the electrons in the shells of atoms. They lose their energy slowly in material and travel significant distances before stopping. Depending on their initial energy, gamma rays can travel from one to hundreds of meters in air and easily go through people. It is important to note that most alpha and beta emitters also emit gamma rays as part of their decay processes.

Radiation is measured in one of three units as noted. A **roentgen** is a measure of gamma radiation. A **radiation-absorbed dose (RAD)** is a measurement of absorbed radiation energy over a period of time. Radiation *dose* is a calculated measurement of the amount of energy deposited in the body by the radiation to which a person is exposed. The unit of dose is the **roentgen equivalent man (REM)**. The REM is derived by taking into account the type of radiation producing the exposure. The REM is approximately equivalent to the RAD for exposure to external sources of radiation. Detecting and measuring external radiation levels are critical at the scene of a radiation incident.

Radiation Measurements

It is equally important to develop an understanding of the dangers associated with different levels of exposure. Response agencies should develop policies regarding PPE and acceptable doses for emergency responders.

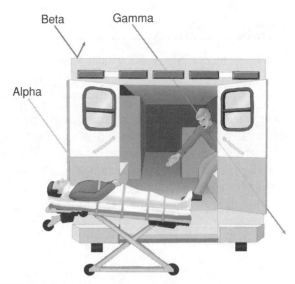

FIGURE 10-1 Alpha, beta, and gamma radiation.

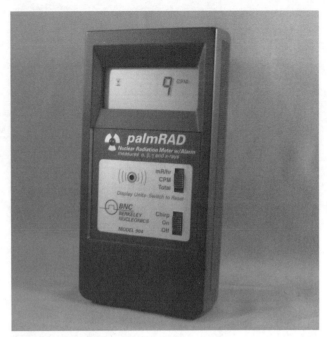

FIGURE 10-2 A radiation detection device.

These policies should be consistent with agency risk assessments and PPE standard operating procedures.

Radiation levels are measured with survey instruments designed for that purpose (**FIGURE 10-2**). Survey instruments usually indicate units of R/hr where *R* stands for either RAD or REM. The unit R/hr is an exposure (or dose) rate. An instrument reading of 50 R/hr means responders exposed for 1 hour will receive a 50-RAD dose. Dividing the unit determines the exposure for shorter or longer periods of time (e.g., a 30-minute exposure results in a 25-RAD dose). An exposure (or dose) rate can be compared to a speedometer. A speed of 80 miles per hour means traveling 1 hour to go 80 miles. Traveling for half an hour at that rate covers a distance of 40 miles.

Some instruments measure radiation dose over a period of time. These instruments are comparable to an odometer, which measures total miles traveled regardless of the speed. Handheld survey instruments may have this capability, but they are more useful in an emergency situation for measuring the exposure rate. Radiation **dosimeters** are useful for measuring the exposure received over time (**FIGURE 10-3**).

Responders must wear dosimeters during operations in any radiation hot zone or suspected radiation environment. Dosimeters should be checked frequently to determine the exposure received by on-scene first responders. Medical personnel should conduct final

CRITICAL FACTOR

It is critical that responders detect and measure radiation levels and exposure at an attack or accident.

dosimeter checks during postdecontamination medical evaluation.

Survey instruments and dosimeters have limitations because some instruments measure only beta and gamma radiation, not alpha radiation. The capability to measure alpha radiation is a requirement. It is important to develop a maintenance and inspection program that ensures instruments and dosimeters are properly functioning. Survey instruments, like all electronic devices, require inspection and recalibration by certified technicians at specified intervals. Survey instrument batteries must also

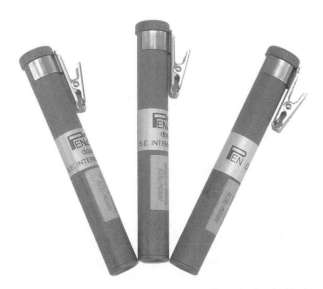

FIGURE 10-3 Dosimeters stay on the responder throughout an incident.

be checked and replaced when necessary. Dosimeters must be zeroed and checked on a regular basis.

Internal Radiation Exposure

For internal radiation exposure, the terms *RAD* and *REM* are not synonymous. It is important for first responders to know whether an internal exposure hazard exists and how to protect themselves by using PPE, including respirators. However, first responders should not be concerned with measuring internal radiation because internal exposure assessment is complicated due to the large number of factors involved. Some of these factors are the chemical form of the material, the type of radiation emitted, how the material entered the body, and the physical characteristics of the exposed person. Months of assessment may be required to determine an internal dose. Common methods for assessing internal exposure are sampling of blood, urine, feces, sweat, and mucus for the presence of radioactive material. Special radiation detectors measure the radiation emitted by radioactive materials deposited within the body. By considering the results of these measurements along with the characteristics of the material and the body's physiology, a measurement of radiation dose from internal sources is made.

Characteristics of Radiation

Despite the similarities to hazardous materials incidents, radiation incidents have a unique characteristic that first responders must understand. Namely, radiation exposure may occur without coming in direct contact with the source of radiation, which is a primary difference between chemical and biological incidents. A chemical or biological agent exposure occurs when a material or agent is inhaled, ingested, injected, absorbed through the skin, deposited on unprotected skin, or introduced into the body by some means.

Radioactive materials are naturally occurring or manufactured and emit particle radiation and/or electromagnetic waves. Contrary to popular science fiction, radioactive materials do not glow and do not have special characteristics making them readily distinguishable from nonradioactive materials. This means responders cannot detect or identify radioactive materials using the five human senses.

Radiation emitters may be liquid, solid, or gas. For example, radioactive cobalt, or cobalt-60, has the same chemical properties and appearance as nonradioactive cobalt. Radioactive water, known as tritium, cannot be readily distinguished from nonradioactive water. The difference lies in the atomic structure of the material, which is responsible for the characteristics of the material.

To understand the mechanism for radiation exposure, an explanation of **radiation** is necessary. Radiation is often incorrectly perceived as a mysterious chemical substance. Radiation is simply energy in the form of invisible electromagnetic waves or extremely small energetic particles. Waveforms of radiation are X-rays and gamma rays. Radiation is emitted by X-ray machines and similar equipment commonly found in medical and industrial facilities (**FIGURE 10-4**). Alpha, beta, and gamma are different types of radiation that have different penetrating abilities and present different hazards.

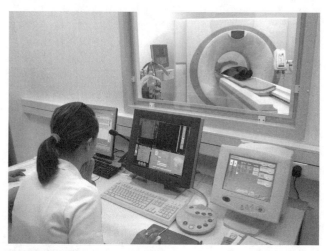

FIGURE 10-4 Radiation is emitted by medical equipment such as computed tomography scans.

Medical Effects of Radiation

Radiation energy can be deposited in the body during the exposure process regardless of the form or source. The amount of energy deposited in the body by a radiation source varies widely. It depends largely on the energy of the radiation, its penetrating ability, and whether the source of radiation is located outside or inside the body. Radiation exposure from a source outside the body is known as *external exposure*. Radiation exposure from a source within the body is known as *internal exposure*.

Consider the example of the radioactive cobalt, or cobalt-60, source discussed earlier. A person located within a few meters (the distance depends on the strength of the source) of the cobalt-60 source is exposed to the gamma radiation emitted from the source without directly touching the source. This is an external exposure. If the source becomes damaged, the cobalt-60 could leak from the container. In order to cause an internal exposure, the cobalt-60 has to enter the body via inhalation, ingestion, or some other means.

Another important concept involving radioactive materials is demonstrated with the cobalt-60 source. *Radioactive contamination* is the presence of radioactive material in a location where it is not desired. Radioactive contamination results from the spillage, leakage, or other dispersal of unsealed radioactive material. The presence of radioactive contamination presents an internal exposure hazard because of the relative ease of radiation entering the body. There may also be an external exposure hazard depending on the radioactive material involved. Any location where radioactive material is deposited becomes contaminated. The contamination spreads by methods including air currents, water runoff, and persons touching the source and cross-contaminating other objects and areas by touch or walking.

The effects of radiation exposure on responders vary depending on the amount of radiation received and the route of entry. Radiation can be introduced into the body by all routes of entry and through the body by irradiation. Victims can inhale radioactive dust from nuclear fallout or a dirty bomb, or they can absorb radioactive liquid through the skin. In the body, radiation sources irradiate the person internally rather than externally. Some common signs of acute radiation sickness are listed in **TABLE 10-1**. Additional injuries such as thermal and blast trauma, trauma from flying objects, and eye injuries occur from a radiological dispersal device (dirty bomb) detonation or a nuclear blast.

First responders should be aware of radiation's health effects and risks because a radiation incident presents both internal and external exposure hazards that may be significant. The fundamental question is how much radiation is too much? A substantial number of scientists and academics argue that any exposure is dangerous and extraordinary precautions are necessary to minimize exposure. At the other end of the spectrum, many scientists and academics argue that some radiation exposure is necessary to life and perhaps even beneficial. In essence, responders must have a healthy respect for radiation and its associated dangers.

High levels of radiation exposure cause serious health effects to occur. These effects are called *prompt* or *acute* effects because they manifest themselves within hours, days, or weeks of the exposure. Acute effects include death, destruction of bone marrow, incapacitation of the digestive and nervous systems, sterility, and birth defects in children exposed in utero. A localized high exposure can result in severe localized damage requiring amputation of the affected area. These effects are clearly evident at high exposures such as an atomic bomb detonation or serious accident involving radioactive materials. These effects are seen at short-term exposures of about 25 RAD and above. The severity and onset of the effect are proportionate to the exposure. Effects of radiation exposure that are not manifest within a short period of time are called *latent* or *delayed* effects. The most important latent effect is a statistically significant increase in the incidence of cancer in populations exposed to high levels of radiation.

The health effects of low exposures are not obvious and subject to debate in scientific and academic circles. Low exposures do not cause obvious bone marrow damage, digestive effects, nervous system effects, cancer, or birth defects. To minimize risks, occupational dose limits for persons working with radiation are 5 REMs per

TABLE 10-1 Common Signs of Acute Radiation Sickness	
Exposure	Effects
Low exposure	Nausea, vomiting, diarrhea
Moderate exposure	First-degree burns, hair loss, death of the immune system, cancer
Severe exposure	Second- and third-degree burns, cancer, death

year. This is not a dividing line between a safe and unsafe dose; it is a conservative limit set to minimize risk. This is why scientists and safety professionals advocate an approach based on a healthy respect for radiation.

Radiation Accidents

Most radiation accidents encountered by emergency medical personnel generally involve transported radioactive materials or radiation-emitting devices used in an industrial or institutional setting. Other incidents include the accidental or deliberate misuse of radioactive materials. Industrial accidents cover a range of situations from activities within nuclear power plants, isotope production facilities, materials processing and handling facilities, and the widespread use of radiation-emitting measurement devices in manufacturing and construction.

Institutional accidents generally involve research laboratories, hospitals and other medical facilities, or academic facilities. Generally, the victim was directly involved in handling the material or operating a radiation-emitting device. Transportation accidents occur during the shipment of radioactive materials and waste. However, due to stringent regulations and enforcement governing the packaging and labeling of radioactive material shipments, few of these incidents pose any serious threat to health and safety.

Commercial and private aircraft accidents may involve radioactive materials that are usually radio-pharmaceuticals carried as cargo or radioactive instrument components, but these sources seldom pose a serious exposure risk. Accidents involving military aircraft generally pose no increased risk because radioactive weapons are sealed, shielded, and protected against accidental detonation or accidental release.

There have been several international incidents where radioactive materials were unknowingly released by individuals who were unaware of the hazards. Improperly or illegally discarded radiation sources have been opened by scrap dealers and others, causing serious contamination and lethal exposure to many people.

EMS and fire/rescue agencies responding to a radiation incident must remember that expedient delivery of appropriate victim medical treatment, including transport to a hospital, is a priority. Treating the victim's medical condition is a priority.

Responders usually learn that radiation is involved by the following:

1. They are advised by dispatchers based on caller information.
2. They are advised on arrival by other responders such as police or fire officials that radioactive materials are present at the scene.
3. They are advised by victims that they were contaminated or exposed.
4. They determine from observations of the incident site that contamination or exposure is a possibility. Visual sources include signs, placards, or documents such as shipping papers.

Information regarding the source of the radiation, type of radioactive material, and exposure time is valuable data that should be gathered at the scene. It is important that EMS personnel consider the distinction between exposure and contamination. Responders should remember there is a minimal chance of encountering a radiological incident that is a serious threat to their health and safety. While accidents involving small amounts of radioactive material may occur in industry or commerce, incidents involving high levels or dangerous amounts of radiation are unusual and rarely occur outside the surveillance of qualified experts.

Contaminated victims should be treated using appropriate medical protocols. These victims are not radioactive, but they present a hazard to medical personnel if they are not decontaminated. EMS responders should take steps to minimize personal and vehicle contamination by using agency-approved decontamination procedures when radiation is known or suspected. Receiving medical facilities must also initiate appropriate decontamination procedures prior to the victim entering the emergency department to ensure that buildings and occupants are not contaminated.

External Radiation Exposure

Victims exposed to a high dose of radiation generally present no hazard to other individuals. The victim is not radioactive and is no different than a patient exposed to diagnostic X-rays. An exception to this rule is victims exposed to significantly high amounts of neutron radiation because persons or objects subjected to neutron radiation may become radioactive. Such activation is extremely rare and this is noted for information purposes only.

External Contamination

Externally contaminated victims present problems similar to encounters with chemical contamination. External

CRITICAL FACTOR...........................
Treating a victim's medical condition is a priority.

contamination usually means the individual has contacted unconfined radioactive material such as a liquid or powder or airborne particles from a radioactive source. Containment of the material to avoid spreading the contamination is important. People or objects coming in contact with radiologically contaminated victims or objects are considered contaminated until proven otherwise. Implementing isolation techniques to confine the contamination and protect personnel is a primary objective.

Internal Contamination

Externally contaminated victims may receive internal contamination by inhalation, by ingestion, or by absorption through open wounds. However, internal contamination is not usually a hazard to the individuals around the victim. The most common type of internal contamination is inhalation of airborne radioactive particles deposited in the lungs. Absorption through the skin of radioactive liquids or the entry of radioactive material through an open wound is also possible. There may be little external contamination, but the victim suffers the effects of exposure from the ingested or absorbed radioactive material. This means an injured person contaminated both internally and externally with radioactive material should be decontaminated, treated using universal precautions, transported, and evaluated for exposure by qualified medical experts.

External contamination may be eliminated or reduced by removing clothing and using conventional cleansing techniques on body surfaces, such as gentle washing and flushing that does not abrade the skin surface. However, internal contamination cannot be removed or treated at the incident scene.

Radiological Terrorism

The Oklahoma City federal building and World Trade Center bombings, the subway poison gas attack in Japan, the use of chemical and biological agents during the Gulf War, and other incidents highlight awareness of the potential for terrorist acts involving weapons of mass effect. The deliberate dispersal of radioactive material by terrorists is another potential source of contamination and/or exposure that must be considered.

> ## CRITICAL FACTOR.........................
> Victims must be decontaminated if they are externally contaminated by radioactive materials.

A weapon of mass effect incident in which chemical, biological, or radiological materials are released by explosives can cause significant numbers of casualties and create widespread panic. Such situations require that steps are taken to protect responders and facilities against unnecessary exposure. In any terrorist incident that produces mass casualties and extensive damage, the first consideration should be determining whether a chemical, biological, or radiological agent was involved. The presence of a hazardous material with the accompanying prospect of contamination and exposure drastically alters the approach that should be taken by medical service personnel.

A **radiological dispersal device** is any container that is designed to disperse radioactive material. Dispersion is usually by explosives, hence the nickname, "dirty bomb." A dirty bomb has the potential to injure victims by radioactive exposure and blast injuries. A radiological dispersal device creates fear, which is the ultimate goal of the terrorist. In reality, the destructive capability of a dirty bomb is based on the explosives used. The outcome may be long-term injuries and illness associated with radiation and long-term environmental contamination.

The destructive energy of a nuclear detonation surpasses all other weapons. This is why nuclear weapons are kept generally in secure facilities throughout the world. There are nations aligned with terrorists that have nuclear weapons. Yet the ability of some nations to deliver nuclear weapons such as missiles or bombs is debatable. Unfortunately, after the collapse of the former Soviet Union, the security of nuclear devices is questionable. Other nonfriendly nations such as Pakistan, North Korea, and Iran also have nuclear weapons.

Injured victims should be triaged, treated, monitored, and decontaminated, if possible, at the scene (**FIGURE 10-5**). The movement of contaminated or exposed victims to medical facilities poses the substantial risk of contaminating transportation resources, treatment facilities, and staff, which renders these resources unfit for treating other victims. EMS protocols should clearly outline the critical steps when there is notification of a terrorist incident involving a radioactive material. The considerations are the following:

- Dispatching on-shift and off-shift emergency staff to establish on-scene triage, treatment, and transport capabilities.
- EMS collaboration with local and regional medical facilities.
- Notification of the state warning point (usually the state emergency operations center) that a radiation attack or accident has occurred. This notification may initiate a federal response.

- Non–law enforcement responders must remember that a terrorist incident is a criminal act and interaction with law enforcement officials is an integral part of the response continuum. No physical evidence should be handled, moved, or discarded without authorization from law enforcement officials. All activities and observations should be carefully and thoroughly recorded because responders are potential witnesses in criminal proceedings.

Responder Tactical Actions

Refer to Chapter 13, "Personal Protective Equipment," and review local agency PPE procedures to ensure responders are adequately protected. Note that there are no protective ensembles designed to completely shield responders from radiation. Protective clothing with appropriate respiratory protection is effective for protection from alpha or beta radiation; however, there are no ensembles that provide shielding from gamma radiation. The most effective procedures for gamma protection are time, distance, and shielding such as concrete walls.

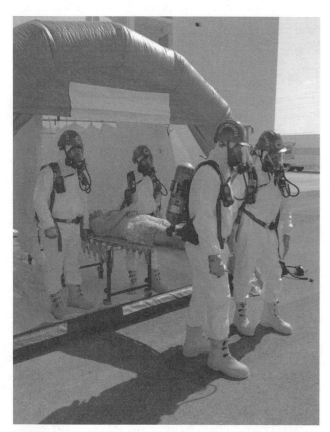

FIGURE 10-5 Victims should be triaged, treated, monitored, and decontaminated, if possible, at the scene.

Time
Radiation has a cumulative effect on the body over time. This means that reducing the time of radiation exposure reduces the overall exposure or dose. Every effort must be made to minimize working time in radiological hot zones.

Distance
Radiation travel is limited by distance. Doubling the distance from a radiation source reduces the effects to one quarter of the original exposure. For example, a gamma exposure of 100 REM/hr at 5 meters is reduced to 25 REM/hr at 10 meters. Increasing distance from the source is effective with alpha radiation because alpha particles do not travel more than a few centimeters.

Shielding
As discussed earlier, the path of all radiation can be stopped or reduced by specific objects called shields. Responders to a radiation incident should always assume they are exposed to the strongest form of radiation and use concrete shielding such as buildings or walls (if practical) to shield themselves. Remember that vehicles and traditional residential/commercial construction do not provide adequate shielding against gamma radiation (**CP FIGURE 10-2**).

Tactical Actions
Units responding to a suspected or confirmed radiation incident should initiate the following tactical actions:
1. Observe explosive protection procedures for radiological dispersion devices.
2. Don appropriate ensembles with respirator protection.
3. Use the principles of time, distance, and shielding for protection.
4. Notify the appropriate local and state agencies that a radiation incident is in progress.
5. Immediately establish a hot zone and enforce safe site entry and egress procedures.
6. Establish a decontamination corridor with medical surveillance for personnel exiting the hot zone.
7. Establish a security perimeter a safe distance around the incident scene.
8. Observe crime scene preservation procedures and collaborate with law enforcement efforts.

Chapter Summary

Radiation is effective as a weapon of mass effect because of its long-term consequences and psychological effect on victims and the community. Radiation travels in the form of particles or waves in bundles of energy called photons, and alpha, beta, and gamma energy are all forms of radiation. Survey instruments and dosimeters have limitations because some instruments measure only beta and gamma radiation, not alpha radiation.

Radiation is measured in one of three units. A roentgen is a measure of gamma radiation. A RAD is a measurement of absorbed radiation energy over a period of time. Radiation *dose* is a calculated measurement of the amount of energy deposited in the body by the radiation to which a person is exposed. The unit of dose is the REM.

Despite the similarities to hazardous material incidents, radiation incidents have a unique characteristic that first responders must understand. Namely, radiation exposure may occur without coming in direct contact with the source of radiation, which is a primary difference between chemical and biological incidents. Radiation exposure from a source outside the body is known as *external exposure*. Radiation exposure from a source within the body is known as *internal exposure*. High levels of radiation exposure cause serious health effects to occur.

The Oklahoma City federal building and World Trade Center bombings, the subway poison gas attack in Japan, the use of chemical and biological agents during the Gulf War, and other incidents highlight awareness of the potential for terrorist acts involving weapons of mass effect. It is important to remember that there are no protective ensembles designed to completely shield responders from radiation.

Wrap Up

Chapter Questions

1. How does a radiation incident differ from a traditional hazardous materials incident?
2. List and define the three primary types of radiation.
3. Define and differentiate the terms dose and exposure.
4. List and discuss at least five tactical actions at a radiation incident.
5. Discuss basic medical treatment procedures for each of the following radiation exposures:
   - External radiation exposure
   - External contamination
   - Internal exposure
6. Define the protection principles of time, distance, and shielding.

Chapter Project

There is a major international festival in your community with 50,000 attendees. A bomb detonation generates 95 trauma casualties. An immediate assessment by the hazardous materials team reveals the explosive device was combined with a radioactive material causing radiation exposure and contamination to 50 victims and 20 responders. Discuss the following questions in detail:

1. What emergency response operational procedures are in effect in your jurisdiction that address this scenario?
2. Based on this chapter, what protocols and operating procedure should be added to community response plans?
3. What role does hospital preparedness play in this incident? Consider that many victims will self-present at hospitals or immediate care centers, which circumvents the traditional EMS system.
4. What are the contamination issues in this incident?
5. What are the state and federal support agencies available for assistance to your locale in a major radiation incident?

Vital Vocabulary

Alpha particles Heavy and energetic radiation particles consisting of two protons; alpha particles interact readily with materials they encounter, including air, causing much ionization in a very short distance.

Atom The smallest unit of an element that contains a nucleus of neutrons and protons with electrons orbiting the nucleus.

Beta particles Negatively charged radiation particles that weigh a small fraction of a neutron or proton; beta particles travel up to several meters in air, depending on the energy, and are stopped by thin layers of metal or plastic.

Dosimeters Radiation measuring instruments that measure radiation over time.

Electrons Negatively charged particles that orbit the nucleus of the atom.

Gamma rays High-energy radiation rays that travel significant distances; gamma rays can travel from one to hundreds of meters in air and readily travel through people and traditional shielding.

Ionization A characteristic of the radiation produced when radioactive elements decay.

Neutrons Particles in the nucleus of an atom that are neutrally charged.

Photons Bundles of radiation energy in the form of particles or waves.

Protons Positively charged particles in the nucleus of an atom.

Radiation A natural and spontaneous process by which the unstable atoms of an element emit or radiate excess energy in the form of particles or waves.

Radiation-absorbed dose (RAD) Measurement of absorbed radiation energy over a period of time.

Radioactivity A characteristic of materials that produce radiation because of the decay of particles in the nucleus.

Radiological dispersal device A device using conventional explosives to physically disperse radioactive materials over a wide area.

Roentgen A unit of radiation exposure.

Roentgen equivalent man (REM) A radiation dose that takes into account the type of radiation producing the exposure and is approximately equivalent to the RAD for exposure to external radiation.

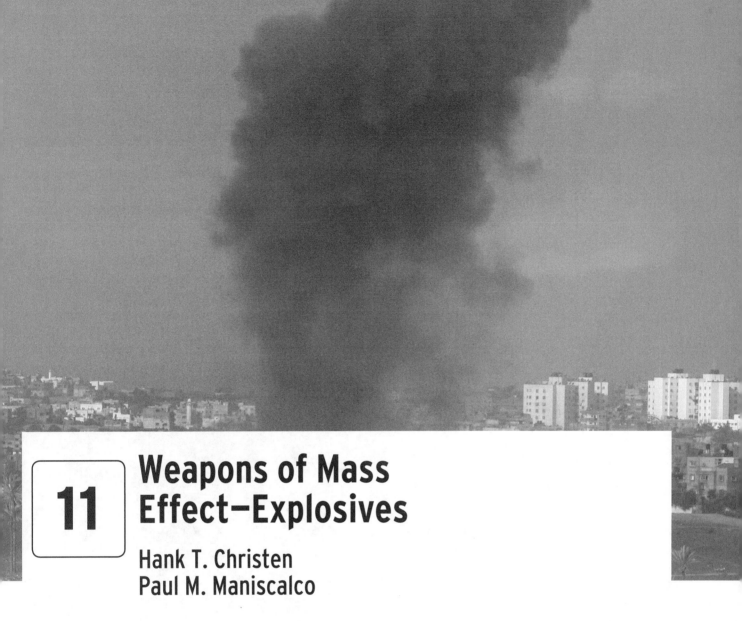

11 Weapons of Mass Effect–Explosives

Hank T. Christen
Paul M. Maniscalco

Objectives

- Discuss the significance of explosive devices in terrorism and tactical violence events.
- List the categories of explosives and their characteristics.
- Outline the basic elements in the explosive train.
- Describe the basic initiating elements in explosive devices.
- Outline the critical safety steps that must be utilized when operating in an environment where explosive devices are suspected or present.

Introduction

One of the first explosives, black powder, was invented by the Chinese in A.D. 600. History has not recorded the first use of explosives for terrorism, but there is little doubt that soon after the invention of black powder, someone used it as a weapon.

Today there are many types of explosives designed for industrial use, military operations, and entertainment. All of these explosives are available to people through various means (legal and otherwise) for clandestine use. Some explosives are made at home with common chemicals using recipes easily accessible to anyone seeking the information.

Explosive devices are effective as weapons of mass destruction or weapons of mass effect for the following basic reasons:

1. Explosives create mass casualties and property destruction.
2. Explosives are major psychological weapons because an explosion instills terror and fear in survivors and the unaffected population.
3. Secondary explosive devices increase the threat level at incidents and complicate law enforcement, medical, rescue, and suppression efforts.
4. The charges can be planted for timed or remote detonation.
5. Explosives are easy to obtain or manufacture.

There are many historical examples of the terrorist use of explosives. Factions throughout Europe, the Middle East, Asia, and Africa have initiated long-term bombing campaigns. The United States Bomb Data Center reported 2,772 explosive incidents, with 60 injuries and 15 fatalities in 2007. There are several detonations per week and numerous bomb-disarming incidents that are not covered beyond the local media. In the United States, responders experienced the horror of the abortion clinics, World Trade Center, and Oklahoma City explosions. The 1993 bombing of the World Trade Center in New York killed 6, injured 1,042, and caused $510 million in damage. The 1995 bombing of the Murrah Federal Building in Oklahoma City took the lives of 168 innocent people, injured 518 people, and caused $100 million in damage (**FIGURE 11-1**). Some bombers were able to elude police for years. Theodore Kaczynski, known as the "Unabomber," killed three

CRITICAL FACTOR

Explosives are very effective weapons for creating mass casualties and fear.

people and injured 22 others with 16 package bombs over a period of 18 years. Eric Rudolph, convicted for the Olympic Park bombing during the 1996 Olympic Games in Atlanta, eluded an intensive law enforcement manhunt until 2003.

There are indications that emergency responders in the United States may see an increase in explosive terrorism from international and domestic sources. The Internet abounds with information about simple explosives and timing devices that can be made at home. In addition, commercial explosives are readily available, and military explosives are accessible in world black markets.

Explosive Physics

How do explosives function? How do explosives differ? What causes some explosive devices to fail? The answers to these questions fall under the general category of explosives physics (the science of explosives). Explosive physics is important to emergency responders because

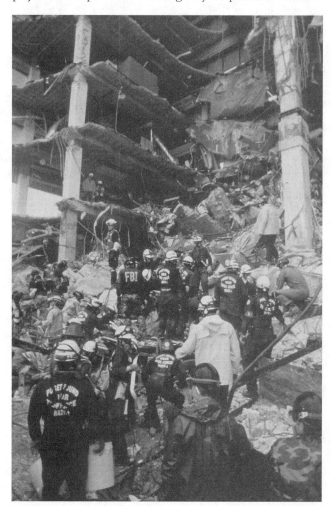

FIGURE 11-1 Search and rescue workers gather in the rubble at the Alfred P. Murrah Federal Building on April 26, 1995. The Oklahoma City bombing killed 168.

the laws of explosive physics kill and injure people and determine whether responders will survive an incident.

An explosive material is a substance capable of rapidly converting to a gas with an extreme increase in volume. This rapid increase in volume causes heat, noise, pressure, and shock waves that travel outward from the detonation. Chemists and physicists note that an explosion is not instantaneous. Academically, they are correct because explosives require several nanoseconds to develop. However, explosions appear as instantaneous to observers. More importantly, significant injury and property damage also occur instantly.

The most damaging by-product of an explosion is the **shock wave**. The shock wave is a supersonic wave of highly compressed air that originates at the origin of detonation, travels outward in all directions and dissipates with distance. It behaves much like ripples on the surface of water when a pebble is dropped into a pond. The wave travels the course of least resistance, reflects off hard objects such as strong walls or buildings, and becomes concentrated in spaces such as hallways or areas between buildings. Shock waves can be reflected back to the source.

The strength and characteristics of explosives are measured by the speed of the shock waves they produce. Shock wave is measured in feet per second (fps) or meters per second. For example, a shock wave traveling at 24,000 fps has a velocity exceeding 16,000 miles per hour. The velocity of detonation determines the dividing line between low explosives and high explosives. A more precise and scientific definition is that a low explosive is one that deflagrates into the remaining unreacted explosive material, at less than the speed of sound. A high explosive is an explosive that detonates into the remaining explosive material faster than the speed of sound. Confinement and initiation also affect explosive characteristics. For example, black powder, when burned in an open area, will not detonate. However, when black powder is confined in a container such as a pipe bomb, the outcome is very different. The same applies with the initiation of high explosives. When **C4** is ignited, it will burn without detonating, but if a shock is introduced to C4 via a blasting cap, there is an explosive detonation.

Explosive detonations also generate extreme heat near the point of origin called a **thermal wave**. Thermal temperatures are at 1,000 degrees Fahrenheit or more, depending on the type and quantity of explosives. Thermal waves do not travel long distances.

Some explosive shock waves produce a pushing effect. This pushing effect is caused by detonation or **deflagration**. Deflagration is a very rapid combustion that is less than the speed of sound. Deflagrating explosives push obstacles and are commonly used for applications such as quarrying, strip mining, or land clearing. Black powder, smokeless powder, and photoflash powders are examples of deflagrating or low explosives. A deflagrating effect or low explosive effect is analogous to the pressure felt when standing near deep bass speakers at full volume.

High explosives have a sharp, shattering effect. This shattering effect is called **brisance** and is comparable to an opera soprano's high-pitched voice that causes crystal glass to shatter. High explosives are very brisant and produce shock waves greater than the speed of sound. For example, military explosives such as C4 produce a shock wave of 24,000 fps (high brisance) with a very sharp and shattering effect. These explosives cause extensive damage with severe injuries and a high percentage of fatalities.

The devastating effect of land mines or Claymore mines (**FIGURE 11-2**) is a product of brisance. The shock wave literally pulverizes bone and soft tissue in the lower extremities. In improvised explosive devices (IEDs), the shock wave causes severe pressure injuries (barotrauma), major internal organ damage, head injuries, and traumatic amputations. A lethal secondary effect is fragmentation. Concrete, glass, wood, and metal fragments are expelled at ballistic speeds. The effect causes multiple fatalities and critical injuries.

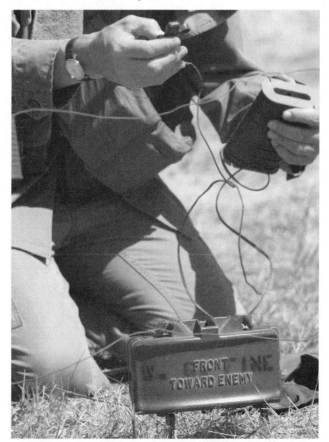

FIGURE 11-2 Claymore mines cause extensive damage through brisance, the shattering effect of shock waves that move faster than the speed of sound.

An explosive shock wave creates another effect called **blast overpressure**. Air in the vicinity of the explosion is compressed and expands, creating a pressure higher than atmospheric pressure. Blast overpressure causes barotrauma damage in the form of air embolisms and damage to tethered organs. Blast overpressure also causes severe structural damage to buildings. A blast pressure of 5 pounds per square inch does not sound high. However, the total impact force is 12,000 pounds on a door that is 30 by 80 inches. The impact force is 57,600 pounds on a wall that is 8 feet high and 10 feet long.

Explosive devices are often designed to produce shrapnel injuries by including objects such as nails, ball bearings, or nuts/bolts embedded in the IED. For example, nails were used in the Atlanta Olympics bombing to cause penetrating injuries. At detonation, these objects become high-speed projectiles causing severe injuries. Evidence of shrapnel injuries, especially from unusual metal objects, may be an indication that an explosion was intentional.

In summary, the physics of explosives explain the effects that kill people and severely damage property. The most damaging by-product is an unseen shock wave that travels very fast. The shock wave causes fragmentation, blast overpressure, and barotrauma injuries.

Types of Explosives

Explosives are designed to detonate with maximum power when initiated, yet be extremely stable when stored or transported. The invention of dynamite was a major breakthrough in explosive technology. Today, dynamite is the most widely known nonmilitary explosive. The prime ingredient in dynamite is nitroglycerin (nitro), an extremely unstable liquid that detonates violently with even minor shocks. In dynamite, the nitro is mixed with sawdust and other ingredients to stabilize the nitro.

Dynamite is a high explosive that generates a shock wave of 14,000 to 16,000 fps. It is readily available and legally procured in states that issue a blaster's permit. Quantities of dynamite are stored on construction sites and are frequently stolen (**CP FIGURE 11-1**). Dynamite is also used in agriculture for digging, land clearing, and stump removal. Dynamite is a popular choice for IEDs because of its availability, ease of use, stability, and explosive power.

Black powder and smokeless powder are also popular IED explosives. Powder explosives are easily purchased in small quantities in gun shops that cater to ammunition reloading hobbyists and are frequently used in pipe bombs. Black powder is a deflagrating explosive that detonates with extreme force when stored in a confined container. Pipe bombs were used in the Atlanta Olympics bombing and in many abortion clinic bombings.

Ammonium nitrate is another common civilian explosive. Ammonium nitrate fertilizer, when mixed with a catalyst, detonates with violent force. This explosive is frequently used in agricultural operations and was used in the Oklahoma City bombing.

Military explosives are extremely powerful, even in small quantities. C4 is the most well-known type of plastic explosive. It is soft, pliable, resembles a block of clay, and can be cut, shaped, packed, and burned without detonating. When detonated, C4 explodes violently and produces a very high-speed shock wave. A mere 2 pounds of C4 can totally destroy a vehicle and kill its occupants. C4 is not easily obtained but is illegally available on the black market. Similar plastic explosives are available on foreign markets. Semtex, a military explosive, was used to make the IED that caused the Pan American airplane crash in Lockerbie, Scotland. Other military explosives include trinitrotoluene, tritonal, RDX, and PETN.

All explosives (civilian and military) require an initial high-impact and concentrated shock to cause detonation. A small explosive device called an initiator produces this initiating shock. Initiators are a key step in a chain of events called the **explosive train** (also called explosive chain) (**CP FIGURE 11-2**). The most common type of initiator is a blasting cap.

The first step in the explosive train is a source of energy to explode the initiator. This source is usually electrical, but it can be from a thermal source, a mechanical source, or a combination of the three sources. The initiator contains a small amount of sensitive explosive such as mercury fulminate. The detonation of the initiator produces a concentrated and intense shock that causes a high-order detonation of the primary explosive. The explosive train is diagrammed as follows:

Initiating energy = initiator explosion = main explosive detonation

All elements of the explosive train must function properly for the detonation to occur. Any malfunction or separation of the elements breaks the explosive train, resulting in a failed detonation.

Improvised Explosive Devices

An **improvised explosive device (IED)** is an explosive device that is not a military weapon or commercially produced explosive device. In essence, IEDs are homemade devices that vary from simple to highly sophisticated.

When an IED is placed in a vehicle, it is sometimes referred to as a **vehicle-borne improvised explosive device**. IEDs and vehicle-borne IEDs are often sophisticated devices and should not be perceived as simple high school devices constructed from Internet bomb recipes.

Each year thousands of pounds of explosives are stolen from construction sites, mines, military facilities, and other locations. It is not known how much of this material is stolen by terrorists. They can also use commonly available materials, such as a mixture of ammonium nitrate fertilizer and fuel oil, to create their own blasting agents.

Most IEDs are made from smokeless powder or dynamite. Devices made from C4 or Semtex are rare and usually lead investigators to suspect foreign sources. A crucial element in an IED is a timing device. For many reasons, bomb makers do not want to be present when the device is initiated. Because of security and scope, this text does not cover timing devices in detail. Timers are chemical, electrical, electronic, or mechanical. Simple timers include watches or alarm clocks that close an electrical circuit at a preset time. Electronic timers operate in a similar fashion but are more reliable and precise. Some electronic timers or initiating devices are activated by radio signals from a remote site. In most cases, timers cause electrical energy to be routed from batteries to an initiator (usually an electric blasting cap).

Other devices have no timer and are designed to detonate when civilians or emergency responders trigger the detonation. These devices are called booby traps. A trip wire or mechanical switch initiates the detonation in simple booby trap devices. An explosion occurs when the wire is touched or the device is tampered with. In more sophisticated devices, an invisible beam is interrupted by people walking through it, causing the detonation. Other high-tech booby traps include light, sound, vibration, pressure, or infrared triggering systems.

Chemical, Nuclear, and Biological IEDs

An IED may be used to initiate a chemical, biological, or radiation event. In these cases, the improvised explosive is used to scatter a chemical, biological pathogen, toxin, or radiation source. The history of such devices is scarce, but increased use of these devices is anticipated. An especially dirty weapon is an **improvised nuclear device (IND)**. In an IND, conventional explosives are used to scatter radioactive materials (see Chapter 10). The device is considered dirty because the radioactive contamination renders an area radioactively hot for possibly thousands of years. An IND does not involve a nuclear explosion like a military nuclear weapon. Presently, there is no history of an IND incident, but the potential is there.

Pipe Bombs

The most common IED is the **pipe bomb**. A pipe bomb is a length of pipe filled with an explosive substance and rigged with some type of detonator. Most pipe bombs are simple devices made with black or smokeless powder and ignited by a hobby fuse. More sophisticated pipe bombs may use a variety of chemicals and incorporate electronic timers, mercury switches, vibration switches, photocells, or remote control detonators as triggers.

Pipe bombs are sometimes packed with nails or other objects to inflict as much injury as possible on people in the vicinity. A chemical, biological agent, or radiological material can be added to a pipe bomb to create a more complicated and dangerous incident.

Suicide Bombings

Suicide bombings are an effective terrorism tactic used throughout the world. Suicide explosive devices can be concealed in a vehicle (**FIGURE 11-3**) or on an individual (**CP FIGURE 11-3**). There is no common age or ethnic profile for suicide bombers. In recent years, women have joined their ranks. Precautionary suicide bombing surveillance and protective measures include:

1. Look for signs of suspicious behavior.
2. Note unusual dress such as coats in the summer.
3. Control vehicle entry into critical areas.
4. Avoid directly approaching suspicious people or vehicles—call for help.

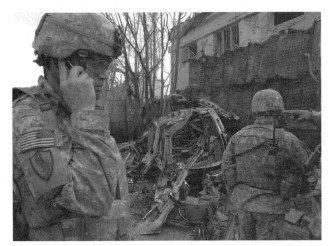
FIGURE 11-3 Members of the force protection team at Camp Eggers, Afghanistan, assess damage resulting from an explosion near the gate. A vehicle-borne improvised explosive device exploded near the German Embassy and a U.S. base.

Secondary Devices

High threats to emergency responders are secondary devices (review Chapter 6, "Terrorism Response Procedures"). **Secondary devices** are timed devices or booby traps that are designed and placed to kill emergency responders. The initial objective is to create an emergency event, such as a bombing or fire that generates an emergency response. After first responders arrive on the scene, the secondary device explodes and causes more injuries than the original event. A secondary device in a trash bin exploded after EMS, fire, and law enforcement responders arrived in one of the Atlanta abortion clinic bombings. In the Columbine High School shooting, multiple devices scattered throughout the school greatly restricted the tactical operations of EMS units and special weapons and tactics teams.

Secondary devices can be used to create an entrapment situation. Responders must beware of a situation that lures responders into narrow areas with only one escape route. A narrow, dead-end alley is a classic example. An incident such as a fire or explosion at the end of the alley is the initial event that causes emergency responders to enter the area. The secondary device (a booby trap or timed IED) is placed in the alley. When the IED detonates, there is only one narrow escape route that lies in the path of a concentrated shock wave.

A key to surviving an entrapment situation is to recognize the scenario by surveying the overall scene. A narrow focus (called tunnel vision) obscures the big picture. Responders should maintain situational awareness and not concentrate on a small portion of the incident

CRITICAL FACTOR................................

Beware of secondary devices. Avoid tunnel vision by carefully surveying the entire incident scene.

scene. Responders must look for trip wires, suspicious packages, and objects that appear to be out of place. Trash containers or abandoned vehicles may contain a secondary device. Responders should question bystanders familiar with the area if possible and enter suspicious areas by an alternate route.

Safety Precautions

Many of the safety precautions for explosive devices were discussed in Chapter 6. Several safety steps bear repetition, including the following:

1. Avoid radio transmissions within at least 50 feet of a suspected device. Electromagnetic radiation from radio transmissions can trigger an electric blasting cap or cause a sophisticated device to detonate. The 50-foot distance is based on U.S. Air Force procedures; local protocols may exceed this distance.
2. Avoid smoking within 50 feet (or further) from a suspicious device.
3. Do not move, strike, shake, or jar a suspicious item. Do not look in a suspicious container or attempt to open packages.
4. Memorize and later note clear descriptions of suspicious items.
5. Establish an outside hot zone of at least 850 feet around small devices and at least 1,500 feet around small vehicles (**TABLE 11-1**). (Large zones may not be practical in congested urban areas.) Maintain the required hot zone until bomb technicians advise otherwise.
6. Stay upwind from a device because explosions create toxic gases.
7. Take advantage of available cover such as terrain, buildings, or vehicles. Remember that shock waves bounce off surrounding obstacles.

CRITICAL FACTOR................................

Bomb technicians are the only personnel qualified to clear an area or remove/disarm an explosive device.

TABLE 11-1 Terrorist Bomb Threat Stand-off

Bomb Threat Stand-Off Distances

Threat Description		Explosives Capacity[1] (TNT Equivalent)	Building Evacuation Distance[2]	Outdoor Evacuation Distance[3]
	Pipe Bomb	5 LBS/ 2.3 KG	70 FT/ 21 M	850 FT/ 259 M
	Briefcase/ Suitcase Bomb	50 LBS/ 23 KG	150 FT/ 46 M	1,850 FT/ 564 M
	Compact Sedan	500 LBS/ 227 KG	320 FT/ 98 M	1,500 FT/ 457 M
	Sedan	1,000 LBS/ 454 KG	400 FT/ 122 M	1,750 FT/ 533 M
	Passenger/ Cargo Van	4,000 LBS/ 1,814 KG	600 FT/ 183 M	2,750 FT/ 838 M
	Small Moving Van/ Delivery Truck	10,000 LBS/ 4,536 KG	860 FT/ 262 M	3,750 FT/ 1,143 M
	Moving Van/ Water Truck	30,000 LBS/ 13,608 KG	1,240 FT/ 378 M	6,500 FT/ 1,981 M
	Semi-Trailer	60,000 LBS/ 27,216 KG	1,500 FT/ 457 M	7,000 FT/ 2,134 M

This table is for general emergency planning only. A given building's vulnerability to explosions depends on its construction and composition. The data in these tables may not accurately reflect these variables. Some risk will remain for any persons closer than the Outdoor Evacuation Distance.

Outdoor Evacuation Distance

Building Evacuation Distance

Preferred area (beyond this line) for evacuation of people in buildings and mandatory for people outdoors.

All personnel in this area should seek shelter immediately inside a building **away from windows and exterior walls**. Avoid having anyone outside—including those evacuating—in this area.[4]

All personnel must evacuate (both inside of buildings and out).

1: Based on maximum volume or weight of explosive (TNT equivalent) that could reasonably fit in a suitcase or vehicle.

2: Governed by the ability of typical US commercial construction to resist severe damage or collapse following a blast. Performances can vary significantly, however, and buildings should be analyzed by qualified parties when possible.

3: Governed by the greater of fragment throw distance or glass breakage/ falling glass hazard distance. Note that pipe and briefcase bombs assume cased charges that throw fragments farther than vehicle bombs.

4: A known terrorist tactic is to attract bystanders to windows, doorways, and the outside with gunfire, small bombs, or other methods and then detonate a larger, more destructive device, significantly increasing human casualties.

NCTC

000841ID 10-05

Courtesy of NCTC.

The search team searches from the floor to the ceiling. Often objects above or below eye level are unseen. Responders should make a floor-level sweep, followed by an eye-level sweep, and finally a high wall and ceiling sweep.

Searchers begin vehicle searches from the outside (just like buildings). If the driver is present, they assign one person to distract the driver from observing advanced search techniques. They leave the trunk and doors closed and concentrate on the outside. They must avoid touching the vehicle because touching can activate motion switches. Only trained technicians should open the vehicle. If the driver is present, he or she should open doors, the trunk, and dash compartments.

Responders must always emphasize the safety precautions previously discussed in this chapter. First, they must establish a hot zone and exercise effective scene control, and then wait for experienced bomb technicians before tampering with a device or searching the interior of a vehicle.

Basic Search Techniques

Emergency responders often conduct primary searches or assist bomb experts in conducting a thorough search for explosive devices. Remember that emergency responders are not trained to clear an area of explosive devices; only bomb technicians perform this function.

In building searches, responders always search from the outside in. Building occupants are an excellent source of information because they know what objects are supposed to be in a given location. Occupants can tell responders that a trash basket has always been there or that a paper bag is someone's lunch. Likewise, building occupants can state that the innocent looking newspaper machine was never there before. Custodians can assist in unlocking areas and pointing out obscure storage areas in building interiors.

Tactical Actions

- Call for immediate assistance and give a brief description of the device including location, general appearance, type/size and time/method of detonation if known. This information should be obtained only from a safe position and distance.
- Evacuate the area in accordance with evacuation guidelines in Table 11-1.
- Maintain a security perimeter.
- Never touch, remove, or examine a suspected explosive device.
- Do not touch or search suspicious vehicles.
- Maintain situational awareness; look for secondary devices from a distance.
- Follow instructions from bomb experts.

Chapter Summary

The use of explosives for terrorism goes back many centuries. Explosive devices are very effective weapons of mass effect. Bombings create mass fatalities and casualties. Bombs are also effective psychological weapons because they create fear in survivors and the community at large.

An explosive is a material that converts to a gas almost instantly when detonated. This detonation creates a shock wave, which is a measure of the explosive power of a given material. In a low-order detonation, a shock wave travels through the remainder of the unexploded material at a speed less than the speed of sound. High order explosives create shock waves greater than the speed of sound. High explosives have a sharp, shattering effect called brisance.

There are many types of explosives, with black powder being the earliest type. Black powder has considerable explosive force when confined in a device such as a pipe bomb. The first commercial type of explosive was dynamite, which produces a shock wave of 14,000 to 16,000 fps. Ammonium nitrate (fertilizer), when mixed with a catalyst, is a low-order explosive. Military explosives are extremely powerful and have high brisance, which creates shock waves as fast as 24,000 fps.

IEDs are homemade weapons that contain an explosive material, a power source, and a timer. The explosives are usually dynamite or black powder. The timing devices can be chemical, electrical, or electronic. Special devices called booby traps contain a triggering mechanism such as a trip wire. Booby traps are secondary devices designed to injure emergency responders.

Secondary devices are effective in entrapment situations where a device is concealed in a narrow area such as an alley with no escape route. A key prevention step is to survey the entire scene before entry and look for trip wires or other initiation devices.

Key safety steps in an unsecured area are:
- Avoid radio transmissions or smoking within 50 feet of a suspected device.
- Do not move, strike, or jar a suspicious item.
- Establish a hot zone 500 feet around a small device and 1,000 feet around a large device or vehicle. (These distances may not be practical in urban areas.)

Emergency responders often assist in searching an area for suspicious devices. Bomb disposal experts are the only personnel who can clear an area or safely remove an explosive device.

Wrap Up

Chapter Questions

1. Name three reasons why explosives are effective weapons of mass destruction or weapons of mass effect.
2. Define and discuss the most damaging product of an explosion.
3. What is blast overpressure? What are the injury and damage effects of blast overpressure?
4. Name and briefly describe at least three types of explosives.
5. List four types of explosive timers.
6. List and discuss safety precautions relating to secondary explosive devices.
7. What is the role of emergency responders in a basic search for explosive devices?

Chapter Project I

Research the previous year's history of explosive attacks in the United States. Ascertain trends in the types of explosives used and their effectiveness (casualties). Include the primary motives for major attacks. What was the number of explosive detonations in the United States last year? (Note—sources can include publications, news articles, or Web sites for the Bureau of Alcohol, Tobacco, Firearms and Explosives, Federal Bureau of Investigation, Department of Justice, and other law enforcement sources.)

Chapter Project II

Develop a standard operating procedure for an explosive device response for your agency. Include tactical procedures, safety, evacuation policies, and procedures for coordinating response actions with bomb disposal experts.

Vital Vocabulary

Ammonium nitrate A common civilian deflagrating explosive that detonates with great force when mixed with a catalyst.

Black powder A deflagrating explosive that detonates with extreme force when stored in a confined container.

Blast overpressure Air in the vicinity of an explosion is compressed and expands, creating a pressure higher than atmospheric pressure that causes barotrauma damage in the form of air embolisms and damage to tethered organs as well as structural damage to buildings.

Brisance A sharp and shattering effect produced by an explosive.

C4 A military explosive with high brisance.

Deflagration A very rapid combustion that is less than the speed of sound.

Dynamite A high explosive that generates a shock wave of 14,000 to 16,000 fps.

Explosive train A chain of events that initiate an explosion.

Improvised explosive device (IED) An explosive device that is not a military weapon or commercially produced explosive device.

Improvised nuclear device (IND) An improvised explosive used to scatter a chemical, biological pathogen, toxin, or radiation source.

Pipe bomb A length of pipe filled with an explosive substance and rigged with some type of detonator.

Secondary device Timed device or booby trap that is designed and placed to kill emergency responders.

Shock wave A supersonic wave of highly compressed air that begins at the origin of detonation, travels outward in all directions, and dissipates with distance.

Thermal wave A short-distance extreme heat wave near an explosive point of origin.

Vehicle-borne improvised explosive device An explosive device that is not a military weapon or commercially produced explosive device and is placed inside a vehicle.

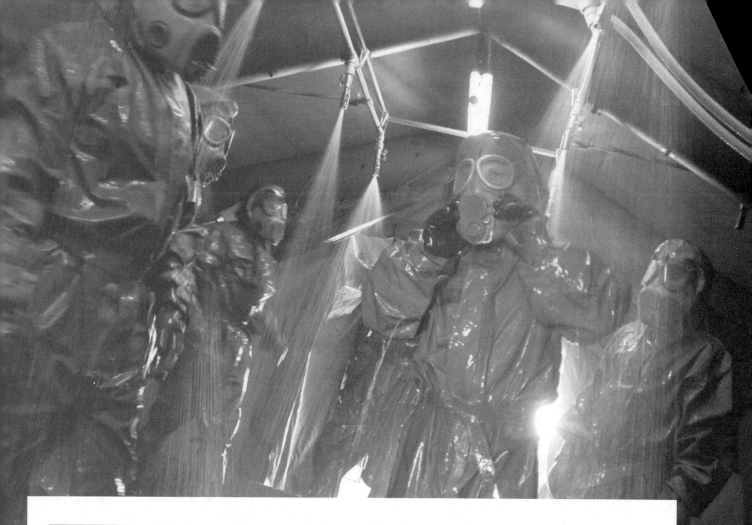

12 Mass Casualty Decontamination

Paul M. Maniscalco
Andrew Wordin
Hank T. Christen

Objectives

- List the four stages of decontamination.
- Describe several methods used by fire departments for gross decontamination.
- Recognize several considerations for setting up a decontamination area.
- Discuss the general principles of hospital decontamination.
- Outline the principles of mass casualty decontamination.
- Recognize the decontamination requirements for various agents.
- List features of biological agents that affect decontamination for biological agents.
- Describe weather factors that affect decontamination.
- Discuss considerations in local protocols for the establishment of triage procedures for contaminated victims.

Introduction

Decontamination is defined as the process of removing or neutralizing a hazard from the environment, property, or life form. According to the Institute of Medicine National Research Council, the purpose of decontamination is to prevent further harm and enhance the potential for full clinical recovery of persons or restoration of infrastructure exposed to a hazardous substance.

This chapter is an overview of the subject matter and provides emergency responders with a macroview of the decontamination strategies, science, and operational/tactical processes. Military decontamination principles are discussed because in many communities, emergency responders frequently train, exercise, and respond with military fire departments, the National Guard, and active military units. For example, in the Fort Walton Beach, Florida area, the Okaloosa County Special Operations Unit commonly responds with U.S. Air Force fire departments from Hurlburt Field and Eglin Air Force Base. It is important that civilian emergency responders understand the basic language and principles of military decontamination and the differences between military and civilian practices. It is also important to consider that the Environmental Protection Agency, and later the Occupational Safety and Health Administration, initially designed civilian decontamination standards as safe worksite procedures. Civilian procedures did not consider terrorism agents until NFPA 472, *Standard for Competence of Responders to Hazardous Materials/Weapons of Mass Destruction*, was adopted. Decontamination has evolved into an important and highly technical function that surpasses the old simple mantra of "the solution to pollution is dilution." Responders are advised that there are additional sources and educational opportunities that provide greater depth, cognitive ability, and operational competency for decontamination operations—especially at large incidents with unusual substances as the physical offender.

This chapter focuses on mass casualty decontamination and discusses these areas:

- The traditional decontamination process used by fire departments and hazardous material response teams
- The decontamination capabilities of hospitals or healthcare facilities

CRITICAL FACTOR.............................

Life-threatening medical conditions are priorities that should be addressed before decontamination when such treatment does not threaten the safety of medical practitioners.

- Military types of decontamination
- Methodology and principles applied to a mass casualty incident resulting from weapons of mass effect or an accidental release of a harmful substance
- Containment procedures
- Mass casualty decontamination, including decontamination requirements for victims with conventional injuries
- Site selection and environmental, weather, and responder requirements during the decontamination process

Basic Principles of Decontamination

The management and treatment of contaminated casualties varies with the situation and nature of the contaminant. Quick, versatile, effective, and large-capacity decontamination is essential. Responders must not force casualties to wait at a central point for decontamination. Decontamination of casualties serves two purposes; it prevents their systems from absorbing additional contaminants, and it protects healthcare providers and uncontaminated casualties from becoming cross-contaminated. Review of after-action reports and videotapes of the Tokyo subway incident in 1995 emphasizes this requirement.

The four types of decontamination, as defined in NFPA 472, are emergency, mass, gross, and technical. **Emergency decontamination** focuses primarily on the rapid removal of most of the contaminated material from an exposed individual. **Mass decontamination** is the emergency removal of contamination quickly from large numbers of victims. Commonly, fire fighters use fire-fighting hose lines or mounted appliances off an engine company to form a mass decontamination corridor and move victims into the flowing water to begin the washing process. This decontamination tactic is useful with large numbers of ambulatory victims. Ladder companies can also set up showers for large numbers of victims. Shower systems with provisions for capturing contaminated water runoff are commercially available and may provide a degree of victim privacy in a decontamination corridor. These systems also provide a method to decontaminate nonambulatory victims. **Gross decontamination** is performed in a decontamination corridor by trained and certified responders after emergency teams exit a hazardous environment. **Technical decontamination** (**FIGURE 12-1**) is part of the gross decontamination process and is a thorough cleaning procedure usually performed with cleaning materials and scrubbing equipment after individuals have been prewashed. Technical decontami-

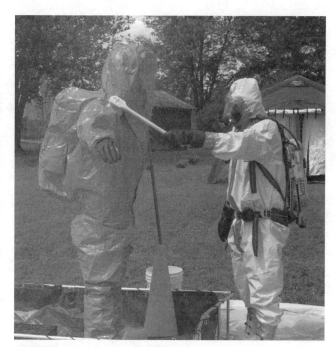

FIGURE 12-1 Technical decontamination is a more thorough cleaning process that often involves the use of specific tools and equipment including brushes and chemical-specific cleaning solutions.

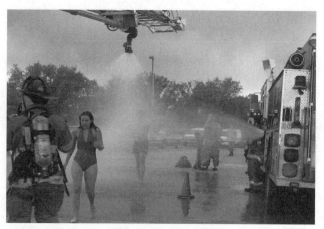

FIGURE 12-2 Fire departments are equipped and structured for rapid and effective emergency decontamination.

nation also involves the cleaning of equipment used by the entry teams. There are other forms of decontamination restricted to the hospital setting that are beyond the scope of this text.

Emergency decontamination is less common than gross decontamination because emergency decontamination is typically performed by first responders or hazardous material teams who encounter contaminated victims. Self-decontamination and team decontamination may be part of emergency or gross decontamination.

Note that the main limitations when performing decontamination are availability of equipment and personnel. For example, an effective decontamination corridor requires personal protective equipment (PPE) for the decontamination team, a water supply, victims' clothing bags, privacy facilities (if possible), cleaning materials, scrubbing equipment, and replacement clothing such as disposable garments or scrubs. Decontamination requires trained personnel to direct individuals to the decontamination corridor, perform decontamination procedures, and direct victims to other areas.

Fire departments are equipped and structured for rapid and effective emergency decontamination (**FIGURE 12-2**). In some communities, law enforcement and EMS agencies are also trained and equipped to perform decontamination. Many fire departments have developed procedures that use existing equipment to perform decontamination. A common practice is using two engines

parked 20 feet apart with an aerial ladder positioned over the top. The aerial ladder can have a water supply spraying from an overhead fog nozzle or it can have tarps suspended from the ladder for male and female separation and privacy. Hand lines, fog nozzles, and/or engine discharges are supplied with water with low pressure (60 pounds per square inch). This is important to avoid causing additional pain to victims or forcing chemicals into the skin from the water pressure. In most cities, common hydrant pressure is sufficient to supply water to the hand lines, fog nozzles, and side discharge gates. Decontamination crews do not commonly use engine pumps to boost pressure. Hydrant pressure is usually satisfactory. Additionally, engine pumps add unneeded noise to an already chaotic environment.

Stages of Decontamination

Mass Decontamination

Mass decontamination calls for the following steps:

1. Evacuate the casualties from the high-risk area (**FIGURE 12-3**). With limited personnel available to conduct work in the contaminated environment or hot zone, a method of triage needs to be established. First, decontaminate those victims who can self-evacuate or evacuate with minimal assistance to decontamination sites, then decontaminate individuals who require more assistance.

2. Remove the exposed person's clothing. It is estimated that the removal and disposal of clothing remove 70 to 80 percent of the contaminant (Cox, 1994); others estimate 90 to 95 percent (NATO, 1991).

3. Perform a 1-minute, head-to-toe rinse with water.

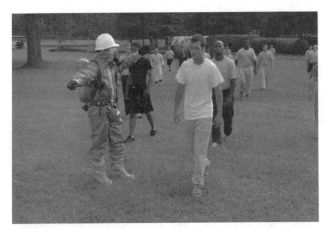
FIGURE 12-3 Direct victims out of the hazard zone and into a suitable location for decontamination.

Gross/Technical Decontamination

Gross decontamination requires the following steps:

1. Perform a quick, full-body rinse with water for nonwater-reactive contaminants (**FIGURE 12-4**). Remove water-reactive substances by dry decontamination using air pressure or dry wipes.
2. Wash rapidly with a cleaning solution from head to toe. A fresh solution (0.5 percent) of sodium hypochlorite is an effective decontamination solution for persons exposed to chemical or biologic contaminants. Undiluted household bleach is 5.0 percent sodium hypochlorite. Plain water is equally effective because of ease and rapidity of application. With certain biological agents, the sodium hypochlorite solution may require more than 10 minutes of contact. This is not possible in a mass casualty incident requiring rapid decontamination.
3. Rinse with water from head to toe.
4. Monitor the victim for signs of further contamination. If meter readings indicate contamination or victim symptoms are found or develop, have the

victim continue to secondary decontamination to ensure the contaminants are cleaned from the victim.

Definitive Decontamination

In definitive decontamination, complete the following steps:

1. Perform a thorough head-to-toe wash until the victim is clean. Rinse thoroughly with water.
2. Dry the victim and have him or her don clean clothes (**FIGURE 12-5**).

Methods of Initial Decontamination

A first response fire company can perform gross decontamination by operating hose lines or master streams with fog nozzles at reduced pressure. The advantage of this is that it begins the process of removing a high percentage of the contaminant in the early stage of an incident. The fire company must address methods to provide privacy and decontamination for nonambulatory casualties.

To set up decontamination procedures, considerations include:

1. Prevailing weather conditions (temperature, precipitation, etc.), which affect site selection, willingness of the individual to undress, and the degree of decontamination required.
2. Wind direction.
3. Ground slope, surface material, and porosity (grass, gravel, asphalt, etc.).
4. Availability of water.
5. Availability of power and lighting.

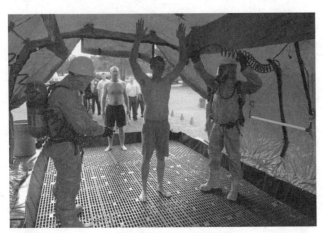
FIGURE 12-4 Flush victims with water from head to toe.

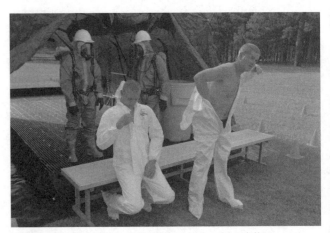
FIGURE 12-5 Dry victims and direct them to don clean clothes.

6. Proximity to the incident.

7. Containment of runoff water if necessary or feasible. The Department of Mechanical and Fluid Engineering at Leeds (U.K.) University has determined that if a chemical is diluted with water at the rate of approximately 2000:1, pollution of water courses will be significantly reduced (Institute of Medicine Research Council, 1998). Examples of containment devices or methods include children's wading pools, portable tanks used in rural firefighting, hasty containment pits formed by tarps laid over hard suction hoses or small ground ladders, and dikes with loose earth or sandbags covered with tarps. Remember that NFPA 472 does not mandate material containment at emergency incidents.

8. Supplies, including PPE and industrial-strength garbage bags.

9. Clearly marked entry and exit points with the exit upwind and uphill, away from the incident area.

10. A staging area at the entry point for contaminated casualties. This is a point where casualties can be further triaged and given self-decontamination aids, such as spray bottles with a 0.5 percent solution of sodium hypochlorite or a solution of fuller's earth.

11. Access to triage and other medical aid upon exit, if required.

12. Protection of personnel from adverse weather.

13. Privacy of personnel. (Decontamination is a media-intensive event where clothing removal by victims occurs in public, such as the B'nai B'rith incident, Washington, DC, 1997).

14. Security and control from site setup to final cleanup of the site.

Decontamination and Triage

In a mass casualty event, decontamination of chemically exposed victims must be prioritized before triage is performed. The objective is to first decontaminate salvageable victims who are in immediate need of medical care. Deceased victims should not be immediately decontaminated. Victims who are ambulatory and nonsymptomatic are the lowest decontamination priority. Again, the primary objective is to immediately decontaminate exposed, salvageable victims.

CRITICAL FACTOR..........................

First decontaminate victims who are severely exposed, yet salvageable.

The U.S. Army Soldier and Biological Chemical Command (SBCCOM) published a guide in January 2000 called *Guidelines for Mass Casualty Decontamination During a Terrorism Chemical Agent Incident*. The SBCCOM guidelines suggest that casualties are determined using several factors when assigning decontamination and triage priorities. First, casualties closest to the point of release should be top priority. Second, casualties exposed to vapor or aerosol should be next priority. Those with liquid deposition on their clothing or their skin are the third priority. Finally, casualties with conventional injuries should come last. Note that life-threatening medical conditions are treated before decontamination and remember that civilian responders are not subject to the SBCCOM guide.

The major factor in triage in hazardous environments is the criteria for determining where or when not to treat/decontaminate a nonambulatory victim who is symptomatic. Emergency response agencies must adopt a local protocol that should be based on the following issues:

- *The nature of the incident.* Severe exposure to nerve agents with major symptoms usually results in death.
- *Sufficiency of antidotes available.* For example, nerve agents require very high doses of atropine and valium (for seizures).
- *Available personnel for moving and treating mass numbers of nonambulatory victims.* A single nonambulatory victim requires two to four responders.
- *Ambulatory victims who are symptomatic or were severely exposed.* These victims should be immediately decontaminated.
- *Ambulatory victims who are nonsymptomatic.* These victims should be moved to the minor treatment area for possible clothing removal and medical evaluation.
- *Nonambulatory victims.* These victims should be evaluated in place while further prioritization for decontamination occurs.
- *Victims in respiratory arrest, grossly contaminated with a liquid nerve agent, having serious symptoms, or failing to respond to atropine injections.* These victims should be considered as critical (red triage level) and closely monitored for changes in status. If one of these victims dies on the scene, the victim's triage tag is updated (red to black) to reflect deceased.
- *Extreme cases that require treating a victim in a hot zone prior to decontamination.* Treatment usually consists of immediate antidote administration

and airway maintenance. Clothing removal is the only expedient method of field decontamination, with decontamination by showering or flushing later, if appropriate.

Hospital Decontamination Standards

The Joint Commission on Accreditation of Healthcare Organizations requires hospitals to be prepared to respond to disasters including hazardous materials accidents. The majority of hospitals that have decontamination capabilities utilize existing indoor infrastructure and do not have the ability to expand to accommodate mass casualties. Outside the standard universal protection procedures followed by the medical community, required protective equipment and trained personnel are limited in most hospital systems.

A common hospital practice, especially in suburban or rural areas, is to call the fire department for a hazardous materials response. Some hospitals may have in-house decontamination teams that do not require fire department assistance. Due to the stress placed on the response system mitigating the effects of a large incident, hazardous materials teams will not be available. Hospitals that depended on fire departments are at risk when the response system is stressed to the point that victims start self-referring or independent sources deliver victims to the hospital.

The military has identified two types of decontamination—personnel and equipment. It has divided personnel decontamination into two subcategories—hasty and deliberate. Specialized units within the military (U.S. Marine Corps Chemical Biological Incident Response Force and the National Guard's Civil Support Teams) have further subdivided deliberate decontamination to encompass ambulatory and nonambulatory personnel.

Hasty decontamination is primarily focused on the self-decontaminating individual using the M258A1 skin decontamination kit. This kit is designed for chemical decontamination and consists of wipes containing a solution that neutralizes most nerve and blister agents. Another type of kit, the M291 decontamination kit, uses laminated fiber pads containing reactive resin, which neutralizes and removes the contaminant from a surface by mechanical and absorption methods. These kits require user training and are not usually available for civilian emergency response organizations.

CRITICAL FACTOR ....

The Joint Commission, an entity for hospital accreditation, requires hospitals to have decontamination procedures and equipment.

The procedure of removing and exchanging (donning and doffing) personal protective clothing is also considered a component of hasty decontamination. **Deliberate decontamination** is required when individuals are exposed to gross levels of contamination or for individuals who were not dressed in personal protective clothing at the time of contamination. The established process is to completely remove the individual's clothing, apply a decontamination solution (0.5 percent sodium hypochlorite or water) followed by a fresh water rinse, then use a chemical agent monitor (CAM) to detect the presence of nerve and blister agents or M8 paper to validate the thoroughness of the decontamination process. If the CAM or M8 paper detects the presence of a chemical agent, the victim must be put through the decontamination process again. At the end of this process, the individual is provided replacement clothing and PPE if appropriate. If the individual presents symptoms, he or she will be processed through the healthcare system.

Decontamination Site Setup

The decontamination site should be established with the following considerations:
1. Upwind from the source of contamination
2. On a downhill slope or flat ground with provisions made for water runoff
3. Water availability
4. Decontamination equipment availability
5. Individual supplies
6. Healthcare facilities
7. Site security

Mass Casualty Decontamination

Specialized military units have developed rapidly deployable personnel decontamination facilities that process large numbers of contaminated personnel, both ambulatory (**FIGURE 12-6**) and nonambulatory (**FIGURE 12-7**). These systems are portable and capable (agent dependent) of processing up to 200 ambulatory or 35 nonambulatory personnel per hour depending upon the agent(s) involved. The facilities are incorporated in tents or inflatable enclosures that utilize a shower system that sprays a decontaminant, followed by a rinse.

Step one of this process is removal of the victim's clothing. Ambulatory victims use a process similar to that used by military personnel during their doffing procedures. Nonambulatory casualties' clothing is cut off by decontamination specialists.

Step two is to place clothing into disposable bins, which are sealed.

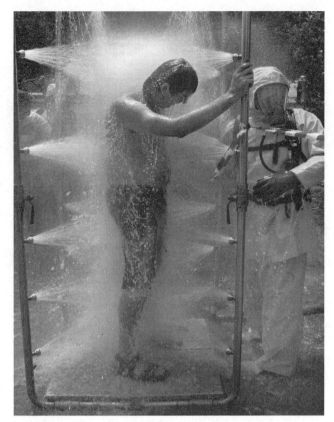

FIGURE 12-6 A mass decontamination configuration for an ambulatory victim.

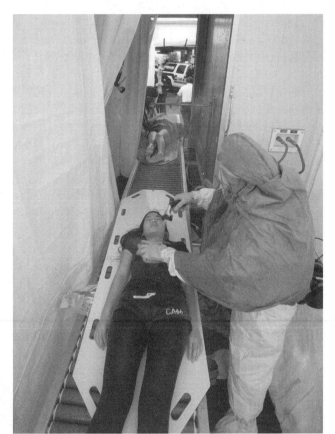

FIGURE 12-7 A mass decontamination configuration for a nonambulatory victim.

Step three is to remove personal effects, tag them, and place them into plastic bags. Disposition of the personal effects will be determined later. These items may be crime scene evidence.

Step four is to apply a decontamination solution. For ambulatory casualties, this is done through a shower system. Nonambulatory casualties are rinsed and sponged down.

Step five is for individuals to use brushes to clean themselves or for a decontamination specialist to do so for nonambulatory victims. This step aids in the removal of the contaminant and allows for a 3-minute contact time for the decontaminating solution.

Step six is a freshwater rinse.

Step seven is to monitor for the agent or contaminant. This is conducted using a CAM or M8 paper for chemical agents, or using a radiation meter for radiation.

Step eight is to don dry clothing.

Step nine is medical monitoring. Individual documentation is developed.

Step ten provides for individuals' release or transport to a medical facility.

Both ambulatory and nonambulatory victims follow these steps, but while ambulatory victims can complete most steps unassisted, nonambulatory victims are moved along a series of rollers and cleaned by decontamination specialists. Care must also be taken at the nonambulatory site to decontaminate the roller surface with a 5 percent solution of sodium hypochlorite between victims. These sites are self-contained, require a water source, and provide the following:

- Heated water (if required; warm water opens the pores of the skin and could accelerate dermal exposure)
- Water runoff capture
- Decontamination solution
- Protection from the elements
- Privacy
- Continuous medical monitoring during the decontamination process
- Postdecontamination checks
- Clothing
- Site control

The specialized decontamination assets just described are from prepositioned military units and are not usually available for rapid response to civilian incidents. These units are highly competent and professional, but they are limited by numbers and location. The military refers to them as low-density, high-demand assets. The U.S. Public Health Service has developed a similar capability resident in the Metropolitan Medical Response System and the National Disaster Medical Response Teams.

Radiation Decontamination

Radiation injuries do not imply that the casualty presents a hazard to healthcare providers. Research has demonstrated that levels of intrinsic radiation present within the casualty from activation (after exposure to neutron and high-energy photon sources) are not life threatening. If monitoring for radiation is not available, responders must conduct decontamination for all casualties. Removal of the casualty's clothing reduces most of the contamination, with a full-body wash further reducing the contamination.

Wearing surgical attire or disposable garments such as those made of Tyvek reduces the potential exposure of healthcare providers. Inhalation or ingestion of particles of radioactive material presents the greatest cross-contamination hazard. Responders must minimally don filter respirators to mitigate this inhalation and ingestion threat. They must take care to capture runoff or retrieve the material. Industrial vacuum cleaners are commonly used. The vacuum cleaner should use a high-efficiency particulate air filter to prevent rerelease of the material into the air.

Decontamination Requirements for Various Agents

Decontamination requirements differ according to the type of chemical agent or material to which individuals were exposed. Water is the accepted universal decontaminant for nonwater-reactive materials. The importance of early decontamination cannot be overemphasized due to the mechanism of injury with organophosphorous compounds (nerve agents). Nerve agents are absorbed through any surface of the body. Decontamination of the skin must be accomplished *quickly* to limit effects of the agent. Liquid agents may be removed using fuller's earth. Persistent nerve agents pose the greatest threat to healthcare providers. Once a victim is decontaminated or the agent is fully absorbed, there is a limited risk of cross contamination to responders.

Responders do not always notice exposure to a vesicant (blister agent) immediately because of the latent effects of the agent. This may result in delayed decontamination or failure to decontaminate at all. Mucous membranes and eyes are too sensitive to be decontaminated with normal skin decontaminant solutions. Vesicants have an oily consistency and are persistent

---

CRITICAL FACTOR ....

Early decontamination is critical for severe exposure to nerve agents.

CRITICAL FACTOR ....

Vesicant contamination may not be immediately noticed.

---

in the environment. Affected sensitive surfaces should be flushed with copious amounts of water, or, if available, isotonic bicarbonate (1.26 percent) or saline (0.9 percent). Physical absorption, chemical inactivation, and mechanical removal should decontaminate skin. Chemical inactivation using chlorination is effective against mustard and lewisite and ineffective against phosgene oxime. If water is used, it must be used in copious amounts. If the vesicant is not fully removed, the use of water will spread it.

Choking agents do not remain in liquid form long due to their extremely volatile physical properties. Decontamination is not required except when used in very cold climates. Choking agents are readily soluble in organic solvents and fatty oils. In water, choking agents rapidly hydrolyze into hydrochloric acid and carbon dioxide.

Blood agents do not remain in liquid form very long due to their extremely volatile physical properties. Decontamination is not required.

In the case of incapacitants, responders complete total skin decontamination with soap and water at the earliest opportunity. Symptoms may appear as late as 36 hours after a percutaneous exposure, even if the individual is decontaminated within 1 hour of exposure.

Responders should move personnel exposed to riot control agents to fresh air, separate them from other casualties, facing into the wind with their eyes open, and tell them to breathe deeply. Exposed individuals should remove their clothes, which should be washed to preclude additional exposure from embedded residue.

Biological Agents

Biological agents are unique in their ability to inflict large numbers of casualties over a wide area by virtually untraceable means. The difficulty in detecting a biological agent's presence prior to an outbreak; its potential to selectively target humans, animals, or plants; and the difficulty in protecting the population conspire to make management of casualties (including decontamination) or affected areas particularly difficult. The intrinsic features of biological agents that influence their potential use and establishment of management criteria include virulence, toxicity, pathogenicity, incubation period, transmissibility, lethality, and stability.

If a dermal exposure is suspected, it should be managed by decontamination at the earliest opportunity. Exposed areas should be cleansed using the appropriately diluted sodium hypochlorite solution (0.5 percent) or copious quantities of plain soap and water. The victim's clothing should also be removed as soon as possible.

Secondary contamination of medical personnel is a concern and is avoided by strict adherence to universal medical precautions. Biological agents, for the most part, are highly susceptible to environmental conditions, and all but a few present a persistent hazard.

Anthrax is a very stable agent; however, in a nonaerosolized state it presents only a dermal (requiring breaks or cuts in the skin) or ingestion hazard. The strategy recommendations for potential exposure to anthrax are:

1. Gather personal information from the potentially exposed individual(s).
2. Explain the signs and symptoms of the disease.
3. Give victims a point of contact to call if they show symptoms.
4. Send victims home with the following instructions: remove clothing and place it in a plastic bag, securing it with a tie or tape. Shower and wash with soap for 15 minutes.
5. Inform exposed individuals of the lab analysis results of the suspected agent as soon as possible. If results are positive, the correct medical protocol will be administered.

Effects of Weather on Decontamination

Weather impacts the manner in which an agent will act in the environment and will have an impact on decontamination requirements. A release of chemical agents or toxic industrial materials always has the potential to cause injuries to unprotected people proximal to the point of release. Strong wind, heavy rain, or temperatures below freezing may reduce effects. Weather is of importance for the respiratory risks expected at different distances from the point of release. Weather conditions also influence the effect of ground contamination.

High wind velocity implies a short exposure time in a given area, reducing the number of casualties in an unprotected population. Low wind velocity increases the exposure time, increasing the number of casualties, and may cause effects at a greater distance.

CRITICAL FACTOR ....

Weather is an important determination in the effectiveness of a chemical attack.

To a high degree, the gas/aerosol concentration in the primary cloud depends on the air exchange or turbulence of the atmosphere. In clear weather, at night, the ground surface is cooled and inversion is formed (stable temperature stratification). Inversion leads to weak turbulence, resulting in the presence of a high concentration of material. Unstable temperature stratification occurs when the ground surface warms, resulting in increased turbulence. The effect is decreased concentration, particularly at increased distances from the point of release.

The concentration in the primary cloud may also decrease in cold weather, particularly at temperatures below −20°C (−4°F), due to a smaller amount of agent(s) evaporating during dispersal. However, this will increase ground contamination at the point of release. Precipitation also reduces concentration but can increase ground contamination.

Low temperatures will increase the persistency of some agents. Some agents may cease to have an effect at very low temperatures due to their freezing point; however, they present a problem when temperatures increase or if they are brought into a warm environment.

Biological agents are potential weapons of mass destruction and generally have the following characteristics: they are odorless and tasteless, difficult to detect, and can be dispersed in an aerosol cloud over very large downwind areas. Ideal weather conditions for dispersal include an inversion layer in the atmosphere, high relative humidity, and low wind speeds. Incubation periods can be as long as several days; therefore, wind speed and direction are a primary weather concern to determine the exposed population and predict the effects upon that population. Ultraviolet light has a detrimental effect on many biological agents, making periods of reduced natural sunlight the optimal time for release.

Most biological agents will not survive in extremely cold weather and it is difficult to aerosolize live biological agents in freezing temperatures. Toxins are less affected by cold weather; however, cold weather tends to provide a temperature inversion that prolongs the integrity of an aerosolized cloud.

Chapter Summary

A common-sense, well-informed approach to decontamination should be adopted. The following are additional considerations for decontamination operations in a mass casualty setting:

1. Establish a local protocol for decontamination and triage.

2. Decontaminate as soon as possible to stop the absorption process.
3. Establish multiple decontamination corridors including one for men, one for women, and one for families.
4. Establish security and control measures to contain contaminated casualties and prevent noncontaminated individuals/nonresponders from entering the affected area.
5. Decontaminate only when it is required.
6. Decontaminate as close to the point of contamination as possible (100 m or 328 ft outside, if the point of contamination was inside a building; 1 km (0.6 miles) for an outside release.

7. Involve the victim in the process, allowing as much self-decontamination as possible.
8. Use existing infrastructure as needed.
9. Continuously monitor the victims throughout the process.
10. Provide privacy if possible with use of tents, available facilities, and/or removal of the media.

Organizations that have potential requirements to provide decontamination support for a mass casualty incident should focus on existing inherent capabilities. With modifications and enhanced training, a good, thorough decontamination system can be effectively implemented.

Wrap Up

Chapter Questions

1. List and discuss the three stages of decontamination.
2. Discuss at least five considerations for setting up a decontamination area.
3. Discuss lockdown procedures for controlling entry of contaminated victims at medical facilities.
4. Outline the 10 steps in mass casualty decontamination.
5. Outline triage procedures for mass casualty decontamination.
6. What factors determine the severity or effectiveness of a given biological agent?
7. How do the following weather elements influence the effects of a weapon of mass effect agent?
   - Wind direction and speed
   - Temperature
   - Atmospheric stability

Chapter Project

1. Develop a mass decontamination procedure for your community. Consider training, equipment, protocols, and triage procedures.
2. Develop a mass decontamination plan for a medical facility. Consider security and lockdown, training, equipment, and control of contaminated vehicles.

Vital Vocabulary

Decontamination The process of removing or neutraizing a hazard from the environment, property, or life form.

Deliberate decontamination Type of decontamination that is required when individuals are exposed to gross levels of contamination or for individuals who were not dressed in personal protective clothing at the time of contamination.

Emergency decontamination Actions taken by first responders to establish and perform decontamination operations for victims in a field setting.

Gross decontamination The process of removing clothing and flushing the affected area with water as quickly as possible to reduce contamination by a chemical or infectious agent.

Hasty decontamination Type of decontamination that is primarily focused on the self-decontaminating individual using the M258A1 skin decontamination kit; this kit is designed for chemical decontamination and consists of wipes containing a solution that neutralizes most nerve and blister agents.

Mass decontamination Type of decontamination for large numbers of victims exposed to unknown chemicals or infectious agents.

Technical decontamination A process performed by hazardous materials teams to clean the members of the entry team once the members have entered a contaminated environment. The process involves a thorough cleaning of personnel and equipment that often involves the use of brushes and chemical-specific cleaning solutions.

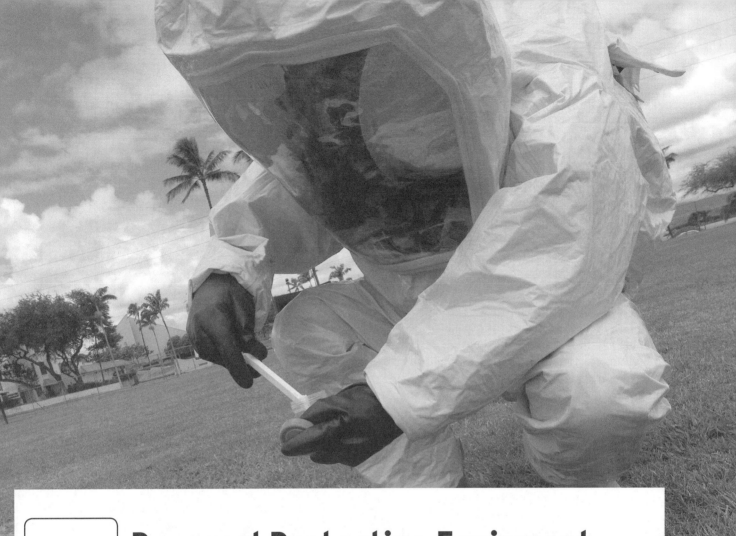

13 Personal Protective Equipment

Hank T. Christen
Paul M. Maniscalco

Objectives

- Determine the proper respiratory protection and ensemble based on the chemical, biological, radiological, and nuclear (CBRN) agent and concentration.
- Summarize the intent of NFPA Standard 472, 2008 edition, and explain how the changes in this standard apply to emergency response disciplines.
- Classify the major levels of respiratory protection and compare the strengths and weaknesses of each level.
- Identify and describe four classes of protective ensembles.
- Summarize the key elements in a personal protective equipment (PPE) training program.
- Outline an effective employee exposure control plan.

Introduction

In the 21st century, especially in terrorism incidents and technological accidents, chemical, biological, radiological, and environmental hazards may confront emergency responders. These threats are generally referred to as CBRN. There is a growing concern that most emergency response disciplines do not have the training or protection programs to protect members in CBRN environments. Respiratory protection and protective ensembles are primary examples. Most law enforcement officers have only their work uniform and body armor, which offers no protection. Traditional law enforcement riot masks are not suitable for protection in oxygen-deficient atmospheres or chemical releases, or for nerve gas exposure, radiological, or biological exposure. Fire fighters have high levels of respiratory protection, but traditional firefighting turnout gear offers little or no protection in CBRN environments (**FIGURE 13-1**). Many emergency response agencies such as EMS, public health, and public works have no CBRN respiratory protection or protective ensembles (**FIGURE 13-2**).

Upgrading levels of protection presents many challenges to emergency response agencies. First, there is added expense. Higher levels of PPE require costly respiratory protection and protective ensembles that may not be in the current equipment inventory. Second, members must be trained on how to properly select and wear PPE. This includes respirator face piece testing/fitting and ongoing training to ensure proficiency is

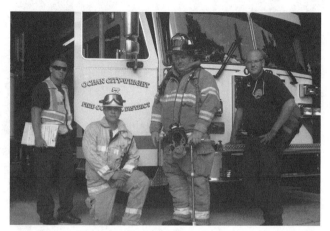

FIGURE 13-2 Traditional firefighting and medical protective ensembles are unsuitable for operations in the CBRN environment.

maintained. Third, maintenance is a consideration. Equipment must survive long periods of storage—frequently in a car trunk or vehicle compartment—yet be tested, calibrated, and maintained in working order. Last, equipment must be replaced if it is damaged or its recommended service life is exceeded.

This text is a focused review and is not a reference source for protective equipment standards, training, or compliance. It is important that emergency responders meet CBRN protection challenges to ensure safety and compliance with national safety standards. This chapter is an overview of national standards and exposure control procedures including their intent and compliance requirements. Because there is prolific literature on ballistic and blood-borne pathogen protection, these subject areas are not elaborately discussed. Our intent is to explore general categories of threats and summarize the PPE requirements for the threat categories.

New Standards

New standards related to hazardous materials and terrorism incidents have major implications for the emergency response community. Previously, law enforcement, EMS, and support agencies were considered first responders, which required training only at the awareness level in accordance with Occupational Safety and Health Administration (OSHA) workplace safety standards. There was an assumption that law enforcement and EMS units would remain outside the hot zone in a defensive posture and not be engaged in operational activities that directly exposed them to CBRN agents. This assumption is now unrealistic and is replaced with a proactive response philosophy that aligns with proper training, equipment, and incident management.

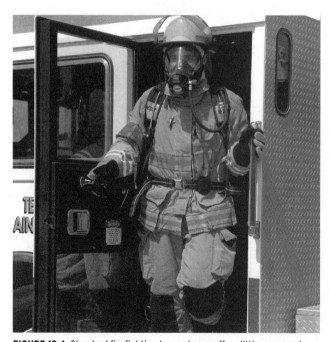

FIGURE 13-1 Standard firefighting turnout gear offers little or no protection in CBRN environments.

The National Fire Protection Association Standard 472 (NFPA 472, 2008 edition), *Standard for Competence of Responders to Hazardous Materials/Weapons of Mass Destruction Incidents,* is no longer a fire service–only standard; NFPA 472 now applies to *all* disciplines that respond to hazardous materials or CBRN incidents. It is interesting to note that the NFPA 472 technical committee included representatives from the Federal Bureau of Investigation's Hazardous Materials Unit, the National Tactical Officers Association, the National Bomb Squad Commanders, and the U.S. Capitol Police. NFPA 473, *Standard for Competencies for EMS Personnel Responding to Hazardous Materials/Weapons of Mass Destruction Incidents*, applies to medical personnel not directly involved in on-scene operations. NFPA 472 has overarching implications for the emergency response community and support disciplines because it means that individuals responding to a hazardous materials or CBRN incident—including law enforcement, EMS agencies, and special teams—are now classified as operations-level responders. In essence, anyone who responds to a hazardous materials or CBRN incident is now subject to the requirements and competencies in NFPA 472.

NFPA 472 is divided into core and mission-specific competencies for operations-level responders. Core competencies apply to *all* operations-level responders who are likely to be exposed to a high-threat CBRN environment. Mission-specific requirements are additional competencies applying to all emergency response agencies or disciplines that have a specified mission. These competencies include hazardous materials technicians, agent-specific categories such as radiological or biological categories, and container categories that include tank cars, cargo tanks, or intermodal containers. There are also operations management competencies for hazardous materials branch officers, hazardous materials branch safety officers, and incident commanders.

Most law enforcement officers require core competency training. Specialized law enforcement teams such as special weapons and tactics, bomb squads, and forensic units are subject to high levels of hazardous exposure and require mission-specific training. Drug lab operations are an example of mission-specific high exposure environments for law enforcement agencies.

CRITICAL FACTOR ....

Fire/rescue departments, law enforcement, EMS, and any agency that responds to a CBRN incident are subject to the requirements and competencies of NFPA 472.

It is important that training officers and supervisors from all agencies and disciplines be familiar with NFPA 472 and develop training, operational policies, and incident management systems accordingly. This applies to the fire service, law enforcement, and EMS, and includes any agency that may perform operations in a hazardous materials or CBRN environment.

Respiratory Protection

Proper respiratory protection for emergency responders in hostile atmospheres is critical. In an environment with high levels of chemical or nerve agents, respiratory exposure can cause unconsciousness and death within minutes. In lesser concentrations, hazardous atmospheres can cause physical and mental impairment with possible long-term effects. An example is the long-term respiratory problems suffered by many rescuers and workers from the 2001 World Trade Center attack. Fire/rescue departments and hazardous materials teams are equipped with self-contained breathing apparatus (SCBA); traditional law enforcement and EMS units do not usually have this level of protection.

CBRN hazardous agents are chemical terrorism agents, biological terrorism agents, and radiological particulate terrorism agents and are defined by the National Institute for Occupational Safety and Health (NIOSH) as:

1. CBRN terrorism agents—Chemicals, biological agents, and radiological particulates that could be released in a terrorist attack, disease outbreak, or technological accident.
2. Chemical terrorism agents—Liquid, solid, gaseous, and vapor chemical warfare agents and industrial chemicals that could be used to cause death or injury in terrorist attacks.
3. Biological terrorism agents—Biological toxins or pathogens in liquid or particle form used to cause death or injury in a terrorist attack.
4. Radiological particulate terrorism agents—Particles emitting hazardous levels of ionizing radiation that are used to cause death or injury in a terrorist attack.

Self-Contained Breathing Apparatus

A **self-contained breathing apparatus (SCBA)** has an internal air supply that provides breathing air in hostile or oxygen-deficient atmospheres (**CP FIGURE 13-1**). SCBA offers a major advantage because it is the *only* type of respiratory device that offers protection in CBRN environments where the concentration is at or above the **immediate danger to life or health (IDLH)** level.

NIOSH sets certification standards for SCBA and requires that all devices have a positive pressure face piece. Positive pressure ensures that during face piece leakage, air in the mask will flow into the contaminated atmosphere instead of outside air flowing inward and harming the user.

SCBA devices have several deficiencies. Breathing apparatus use may negatively affect unaccustomed users who are prone to claustrophobia. Air supplies are finite and require frequent air cylinder changes during prolonged operations. In high-stress and heavy-exertion situations, it is not unusual for a 30-minute cylinder to last only 15 minutes. SCBA users must have a fitted face mask and meet yearly competency standards. SCBA devices may cost several thousand dollars and require frequent testing, maintenance, and calibration. For these reasons, few agencies and disciplines outside of the fire service use SCBA devices for respirator protection.

Powered Air-Purifying Respirators

Respirators rely on filters to protect users from particulate exposure. Filter cartridges that meet the protection standards for particulates that the user is exposed to must be used. These devices are not suitable in oxygen-deficient atmospheres or cases involving hazardous vapors. It is critical that the type and concentration of hazardous agent(s) are known before **powered air-purifying respirators (PAPR)** are used. The PAPR filters must also be certified and appropriate for the specific agent to which the user is exposed.

PAPR devices use a battery-powered unit to pump air into the face mask. This unit creates a positive pressure in the mask that offers leakage protection and makes breathing less labored than a nonpowered device. The pressurized air also has a cooling effect within the face piece. PAPRs are less expensive than SCBAs and offer greater mobility because of small size and light weight. Filters do not have to be changed as frequently as SCBA air cylinders. PAPR batteries and pressure units must be maintained and periodically tested.

Air-Purifying Respirators

An **air-purifying respirator (APR)** is a face mask with protective filtering canisters (**FIGURE 13-3**). The canisters must be certified to meet the requirements for known agents and concentrations and are not suitable in oxygen-deficient atmospheres. Air from the outside atmosphere is drawn through the filtering canisters and into the face piece when the user inhales; APRs are not pressurized like PAPRs are. The advantage of APR devices is they are lightweight, inexpensive, and simple to operate. The primary disadvantage, compared to PAPRs, is that outside air enters a leaking face piece during inhalation.

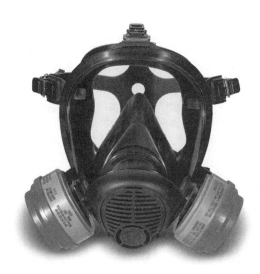

FIGURE 13-3 Air-purifying respirators offer some degree of protection against airborne chemical hazards.

Because the face piece is not pressurized, inhalation is more labored compared to that of someone wearing a PAPR or SCBA.

It is critical that the agent and concentration are known, and one must know the environment is not oxygen deficient before utilizing an APR for respiratory protection. The APR filters must also be certified for the specific agent to which the user is exposed.

Protective Ensembles

An ensemble is defined in NFPA Standards 1991 (NFPA, 2005) and 1994 (NFPA, 2007) as an interrelated system including garments, gloves, and footwear, with respiratory protection, that is certified as a protective system. Ensembles are categorized as class 1, 2, 3, and 4. A class 1 ensemble offers the highest level of protection; a class 4 ensemble provides the lowest level of protection. Class 2, 3, and 4 ensembles are disposable after a single use.

NFPA 1991 and 1994 ensembles are not suitable for firefighting. The ensembles do not provide protection from open flames, flash fires, radiated heat, molten metals, electric shock or arcs, hot liquids, or steam.

Previously, protection levels were defined by the OHSA Hazardous Waste Operations and Emergency Response Standard (HAZWOPER) as levels A, B, C, and D. Level A was a fully encapsulated system that provided the highest level of protection and was utilized when hazards and/or concentrations were unknown. Level B incorporated the highest level of respiratory protection with a reduced level of skin protection. Level C was used when agents and concentrations were known and APRs were appropriate. Level D was essentially traditional clothing or work uniforms with an optional escape mask.

HAZWOPER levels of protection were essentially descriptions of the desired ensemble without formal scientific performance standards. For example, Level A was described as being fully encapsulating for vapor protection, without specifications and standards for permeation resistance for materials, seams, zippers, or fittings. Training programs, procedural manuals, or agency policies that refer to A through D protection levels are outdated and should be revised to reflect proper terminology—namely Class 1–4 ensembles. Many entities have not adopted the Class 1–4 terminology and continue to use Level A–D terminology.

Class 1 Ensembles

Class 1 ensembles (similar to Level A) are encapsulating suits with SCBA that provide vapor, liquid, and permeability protection (**CP FIGURE 13-2**). The protective suit covers the breathing apparatus and includes protective boots and gloves. Outer boots and gloves are required for additional protection.

All seams and closures must provide protection from vapors and liquids. The intent is an ensemble that has gas-tight integrity (**FIGURE 13-4**). NFPA 1991 also provides provisions for CBRN protection that are addressed specifically in NFPA 1994.

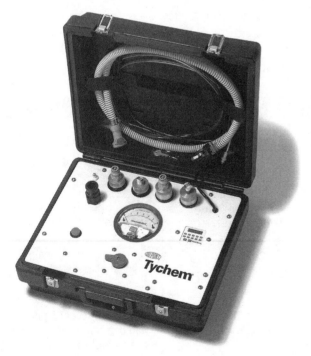

FIGURE 13-4 Level A suits are required to be periodically pressure tested with suit-testing kits.

Class 1 ensembles are used by specially trained and certified hazardous materials technicians on government or private-sector hazardous materials teams. Safe entry procedures require that members in Class 1 ensembles operate in teams, with a backup or safety team immediately available and partially suited to provide rescue if needed. Teams utilizing Class 1 ensembles must also have dedicated communications, a team leader, safety officer, and a decontamination team, along with an incident commander and operational procedures beyond the scope of this text. Reduced mobility, heat stress, low dexterity, and the limited duration time of SCBA are factors that severely inhibit the capabilities of teams using Class 1 ensembles.

Class 1 Ensemble Example

Consider a scenario in an underground rail station where masses of people are overcome by an unknown gaseous chemical agent. There appears to be a high concentration. Because the type of agent and concentration are unknown, a hazardous materials team enters the affected area with monitors to determine the type, concentration, and origin of the agent. Class 1 ensembles are used because the agent is unknown and the highest level of vapor protection is required. In this case, the Class 1 ensemble provides complete skin protection from gaseous and/or liquid contact and SCBA respiratory protection.

Class 2 Ensembles

Class 2–4 ensembles are governed by NFPA 1994 and are disposable after a single use or exposure. A **class 2 ensemble** (similar to Level B) is suitable when the agent is known and liquid or particulate hazards are at a concentration at or above the IDLH (**CP FIGURE 13-3**). This ensemble is intended for IDLH environments where skin exposure does not result in severe health risks. NIOSH CBRN-compliant SCBA is required with the Class 2 ensemble when an agent is at or above the IDLH concentration—the SCBA is worn outside the ensemble. The ensemble is tested for resistance to mustard gas, soman nerve agents, and liquid or gaseous common industrial chemicals.

Class 2 Ensemble Example

After responding to a minor fire in a garage, fire fighters discover that the facility is a methamphetamine lab. Identified chemicals include acetone and benzene;

CRITICAL FACTOR ....

A Class 1 ensemble is required when the specific agent and concentration are unknown.

monitors indicate concentrations near IDLH levels. Because there is a need for respiratory and liquid exposure protection, cleanup teams and evidence collection officers enter the area in Class 2 ensembles with SCBA. The ensembles are properly discarded after use.

Class 3 Ensembles

Class 3 ensembles (similar to Level C) are suitable for use in incidents with low levels of vapor, liquid, chemical, or particulate hazards with concentrations below the IDLH threshold (**CP FIGURE 13-4**). Respiratory protection can be PAPRs or APRs that are NIOSH CBRN compliant. The Class 3 ensemble includes a garment with attached or separate gloves and footwear or booties with outer boots. All components must be certified as a complete system similar to Class 2.

Class 3 ensembles are used after an initial release or at locations distant from the initial release where there is a low threat of liquid or vapor contact. Examples of class 3 missions include treatment and transport of exposed patients or law enforcement scene control or off-site search operations.

Class 3 Ensemble Example

In the Class 2 ensemble example, entry teams must be decontaminated after leaving the hot zone work area. Decontamination teams at the decontamination corridor (warm zone) are working in an environment that involves low levels of vapor and liquids—concentrations of acetone and benzene are below the IDLH threshold. For these reasons, a Class 3 ensemble with an APR or PAPR respirator that is NIOSH CBRN certified with appropriate filters is an acceptable level of protection for the decontamination teams.

Class 4 Ensembles

Class 4 ensembles (similar to level D) are used when biological or radiological particulate hazards are below IDLH levels; APR or PAPR respiratory protection is permitted (**CP FIGURE 13-5**). Class 4 ensembles do not provide protection against chemical vapors or liquids and are designed for particulate protection only. These ensembles are also tested for resistance to blood-borne pathogens using a bacteriophage viral penetration test. The advantage of a Class 4 ensemble is the protective garment system is lightweight and places less physical stress on the wearer than the higher levels of protection. Operations teams can work for longer periods with a higher level of comfort and lower level of heat stress when they wear Class 4 ensembles.

Class 4 Ensemble Example

A high-profile political campaign office receives a package of suspicious powder that is dispersed throughout the office area when the package is opened. Emergency responders on the scene determine there is a high probability the material is anthrax. Forensic teams must enter the area to collect evidence. Because there is no vapor or liquid hazard, teams are able to operate safely using Class 4 ensembles with PAPRs for respiratory protection.

TABLE 13-1 provides an overview of PPE ensemble classifications.

Employee Exposure Control Plan

Emergency response agencies and support entities should have a formal employee exposure control plan (ECP). The primary intent of an ECP is to ensure that employees and team members end their duty shift safe and uninjured.

TABLE 13-1 PPE Ensemble Classifications

Level	Specific use for which this level of PPE is designed	Example of situation requiring this level of PPE	Limitations
Class 1 ensemble	Unknown gaseous chemical agent	Underground rail station filled with unknown gaseous agent	Mobility limitations; high heat stress
Class 2 ensemble	Known liquid or particulate hazard with a concentration at or above the IDLH level.	Methamphetamine lab with known chemicals	Does not protect against gaseous chemical agents
Class 3 ensemble	Low levels of vapor, liquid, chemical, or particulate hazards with concentrations below the IDLH threshold.	Decontamination	Does not protect against high levels of vapor, liquid, chemical, or particulate hazards
Class 4 ensemble	Biological or radiological particulate hazards are below IDLH levels, APR or PAPR respiratory protection is permitted.	Anthrax or suspicious powder investigation	Does not protect against liquid or vapor hazards; not suitable in oxygen-deficient areas

The Centers for Disease Control and Prevention and NIOSH have developed a model for a blood-borne pathogens exposure control plan called *Protect Your Employees with an Exposure Control Plan.* This model is easily expandable to a comprehensive exposure control plan that includes PPE guidelines and procedures for CBRN threats and hazards.

Formal Plan

An ECP should be a stand-alone document that is written and formal; exposure control procedures should not be dispersed throughout a myriad of policy, operations procedures, and training documents. The plan must be comprehensive, yet brief and written in an understandable language; compliance with national standards is essential. The ECP should be updated annually through a process that includes appropriate stakeholders. Stakeholders may include unions or employee groups, human resource specialists, safety and protection specialists, legal advisors, training officers, and managers. The ECP should be approved by the chief executive of the agency or jurisdiction.

ECP Accessibility

The ECP must be visible and accessible to all members within an agency or organization. A plan that gets lost on a bookshelf is a paper plan that seldom transcends into the real world of tactical operations. It is important that members are aware of the ECP and that it is visible at every workplace.

ECP Oversight

Although the ECP is a team effort with many stakeholders, a single manager should be ultimately responsible for the development, implementation, and ongoing revision of the ECP. This management structure ensures responsibility and accountability in the ECP effort.

Employee Exposure Determination

The ECP should include a list of agency or organizational job titles and tasks where it is anticipated that members may be exposed to blood-borne pathogens, ballistic threats, hazardous environments, or CBRN exposure.

Exposure Controls

The ECP should include specific practices and controls that reduce or eliminate exposure to hazardous threats or environments. Controls are a broad area and include practices such as vaccinations, environmental assessment and monitoring, establishment of hazard zones, scene entry procedures, protective devices, tactical operations, and decontamination. Individuals responsible for exposure controls should have defined roles and be identified.

PPE Selection

The ECP should specify what types and/or levels of PPE are required for each type of hazard, threat, or CBRN environment. The type or level of PPE can be as simple as medical gloves and eye protection or as complex as class 1 ensembles worn by a hazardous materials team.

Postexposure Evaluation and Follow-up

The ECP should include procedures for medical evaluation immediately after an exposure to any form of hazardous environment. Formal medical records should be maintained with follow-up medical care and evaluation if appropriate.

Chapter Summary

The modern CBRN environment is dangerous and presents new protective equipment challenges for law enforcement officers. NFPA Standard 472, originally a fire service standard, now applies to law enforcement, EMS, and any agency that has operational capabilities during a hazardous materials or terrorist incident. The 2008 edition of NFPA 472 redefines law enforcement, EMS, and other agencies that respond to a CBRN incident as operations-level responders and specifies core and mission-specific competencies.

Respiratory protection is a major concern for all operations-level agencies and responders. The highest level of respiratory protection is SCBA, followed by PAPR and APR. All respiratory devices must be NIOSH CBRN certified.

An ensemble is a garment, glove, and footwear system certified in accordance with NFPA Standards 1991 and 1994. Class 1 ensembles are used by hazardous materials teams. Class 2, 3, and 4 ensembles are the most likely protection systems used by law enforcement, EMS agencies, and cleanup teams.

It is important that all members who are likely to respond to a CBRN incident or hazardous materials event be trained to the core and mission-specific competencies as specified by NFPA 472 to ensure compliance, safety, and operational proficiency. It is equally important that

> **CRITICAL FACTOR** ....
>
> Emergency response and support agencies should have a formal and comprehensive ECP to ensure employee safety from blood-borne pathogen and CBRN exposures.

emergency response agencies are equipped with certified NIOSH CBRN certified respiratory devices and NFPA 472 compliant protective ensembles.

CBRN response agencies should have an ECP. The ECP is a formal and written plan developed by stakeholders that serves as a guide for managing exposures to high-threat environments. The ECP should be visible and accessible to all members and assigned to a manager to ensure accountability and responsibility. The core of the ECP is guidelines that prescribe the respiratory protection and ensembles required for CBRN threats and exposures. After an incident, all members should be required by the ECP to be medi-cally evaluated with periodic medical follow-up when warranted.

Agencies should use the Interagency Board Selected Equipment List (SEL) as a guide for determining what respiratory and ensemble systems meet NIOSH, OHSA, NFPA, and other personal protection certification standards. The SEL defines CBRN and ballistic threats and aligns them with a table of federal and consensus-based standards that respirators and ensembles must comply with to provide adequate CBRN and hazardous materials protection. The SEL is electronically available on the Department of Homeland Security responder knowledge base at www.rkb.us.

Wrap Up

Chapter Questions

1. Compare SCBA with respirators. What are the advantages and disadvantages of SCBA, PAPR, and APR?
2. What are the major elements of NFPA 472, and how do they apply to emergency response agencies?
3. Name at least three mission-specific competencies addressed in NFPA 472.
4. Describe a Class 1 ensemble. What threats or environments require a Class 1 ensemble?
5. Briefly define Class 2, 3, and 4 ensembles. What are the advantages and disadvantages of each class?
6. Define an exposure control plan and outline the critical elements that should be included in an effective plan.

Chapter Project

You have just been hired as a consultant to develop a CBRN PPE program for a third service EMS agency with 175 members. The agency director's objective is compliance with NFPA 472 within 1 year. What type of respirators and ensembles will be most effective and why? What levels of core and mission-specific training will be required?

Vital Vocabulary

Air purifying respirator (APR) A face mask with protective filtering canisters certified to meet the requirements for known agents and concentrations. Air from the outside atmosphere is drawn through the filtering canisters and into the face piece when the user inhales. APRs are not suitable in oxygen-deficient atmospheres.

Class 1 ensemble Encapsulating suit with SCBA that provides vapor, liquid, and permeability protection. The protective suit covers the breathing apparatus and includes protective boots and gloves. Outer boots and gloves are required for additional protection. All seams and closures must provide protection from vapors and liquids.

Class 2 ensemble A protective ensemble with SCBA that is worn outside the protective garment and utilized when the agent is known and liquid or particulate hazards are at a concentration at or above the immediate danger to life and health.

Class 3 ensemble A garment with attached or separate gloves and footwear or booties with outer boots utilized in incidents with low levels of vapor, liquid, chemical, or particulate hazards with concentrations below the IDLH threshold. Respiratory protection can be PAPRs or APRs.

Class 4 ensemble Lightweight garment certified for protection against blood-borne pathogens and utilized when biological or radiological particulate hazards are below IDLH levels; APR or PAPR respiratory protection is permitted. Class 4 ensembles do not provide protection against chemical vapors or liquids and are designed for particulate protection only.

Immediate danger to life or health (IDLH) The maximum hazardous substance concentration allowable for escape without a respirator within 30 minutes and without impairment or irreversible health effects.

Powered air-purifying respirator (PAPR) A face mask with protective filtering canisters certified to meet the requirements for known agents and concentrations that uses a battery-powered unit to pump air into the face mask, creating a positive pressure that offers leakage protection and makes breathing less labored than a nonpowered device. PAPRs are not suitable in oxygen-deficient atmospheres.

Self-contained breathing apparatus (SCBA) A respiratory device with an internal air supply that provides breathing air in hostile or oxygen-deficient atmospheres. Certification standards require that devices have a positive-pressure face piece to ensure that during face piece leakage, air in the mask flows into the contaminated atmosphere instead of outside air flowing inward and harming the user.

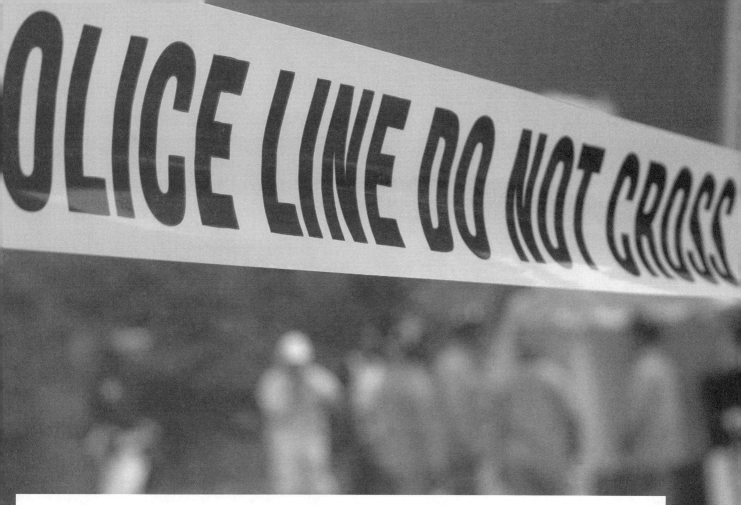

14 Crime Scene Operations

Neal J. Dolan
Paul M. Maniscalco

Objectives

- Define a crime scene.
- Recognize the value and importance of physical evidence.
- Understand the evidence theory of exchange.
- Recognize the evidence classification of objects, body material, and impressions.
- List key crime scene observations that initial responders should make.
- Understand the key steps for emergency responders in preservation of evidence.
- Understand the concept of *chain of custody*.

"Wherever he steps, whatever he touches, whatever he leaves, even unconsciously, will serve as silent evidence against him. Not only his fingerprints or his footprints, but his hair, the fibers of his clothing, the glass he breaks, the tool-marks he leaves, the paint he scratches, the blood or semen that he deposits or collects—all these and more bear united witness against him. This is evidence that does not forget. It is not confused by the excitement of the moment. It is not absent because human witnesses are. It is factual evidence. Physical evidence cannot be wrong; it cannot be wholly absent. Only its interpretation can err. Only human failure to find it, study and understand it, can diminish its value." (Kirk, 1974)

Introduction

The significance of physical evidence at a crime scene cannot be overestimated. Proper training and technique are necessary to maintain the integrity and value of evidence. Every day, emergency personnel respond to incidents to render aid, many times as the result of a criminal act. These responders shoulder a formidable burden to accomplish their mission and cause no further harm to the people or the incident scene. Crime scenes are exciting, chaotic, and dangerous places. They are replete with hidden clues that hold the answer to the question, "Who committed this crime?"

Emergency responders often carry out their duties in conflict with important crime scene procedures. It is important that emergency responders focus on the preservation of life and recognize that the preservation of evidence is secondary to life-sustaining efforts. Yet, evidence should be preserved whenever possible. Responders may not be aware that a shooting victim's clothing that medics are removing may contain valuable evidence to solve the crime (**FIGURE 14-1**). As another example, at an explosion scene, fire fighters may be employing legitimate firefighting techniques that destroy evidence that identifies who committed the offense. It is possible to carry out an emergency response mission without creating more problems for the crime scene. This act of evidence preservation is accomplished through training and awareness of potential crime scenes and through efforts to minimize damage to the area and its contents.

The Crime Scene–Physical Evidence

A **crime scene** is any specified area in which a crime may have been committed. It is anywhere the criminal was during the commission of the crime and the egress from the scene. The exact dimensions of the scene will be determined by the nature and type of crime (**FIGURE 14-2**).

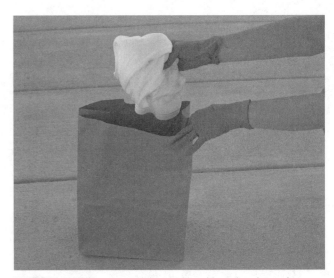

FIGURE 14-1 Clothes may contain valuable evidence to solve a crime.

For example, a shooting crime scene could be as large as the room or building where the victim was discovered. A terrorist incident could be several blocks or even miles in diameter. At the Murrah Federal Building incident in Oklahoma City, a 20-block perimeter was established and a critical piece of evidence, the crankshaft from the rented Ryder truck, was found 2 blocks from the explosion site. A similar extended perimeter was established for a long period of time in lower Manhattan after both the 1993 and 2001 World Trade Center attacks.

Awareness of what constitutes physical evidence is the key to uncovering the vast amount of information and

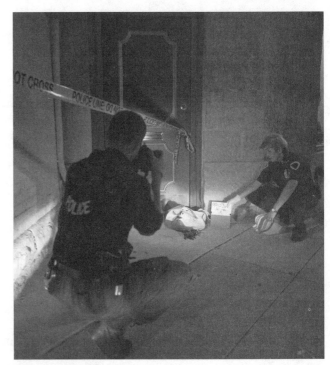

FIGURE 14-2 The exact dimensions of the scene will be determined by the nature and type of the crime.

physical evidence present at the crime scene. **Evidence** is something legally submitted to a competent tribunal as a means of ascertaining the truth in an alleged matter under investigation. **Physical evidence** is one form of evidence. It is defined as anything that was used, left, removed, altered, or contaminated during the commission of a crime by either the victim or the suspect (**FIGURE 14-3**).

The benefits of physical evidence are best summarized in the opening paragraph by the issuing judge in the case of *Harris v. United States* (1947). Physical evidence does not lie, forget, or make mistakes. It has no emotional connection to anyone or anything. It is demonstrable in nature and not dependent on a witness. It is the only way to establish the elements of a crime.

In order to heighten responder awareness, it is necessary to explain how physical evidence evolves at the scene. Forensic scientists propose the *theory of exchange* to describe this process. Whenever two objects come in contact with each other, each will be altered or changed in some way. When a rapist comes in contact with a victim, numerous substances will be exchanged. The suspect or the victim could deposit or remove skin

traces, blood, body fluids, carpet fibers, soil, and many other items. Bombing victims may have chemical traces on their clothing or fragments of evidence embedded in their bodies that may prove to be important in the investigation and prosecution of the perpetrators. These evidence sources have been invaluable to law enforcement investigators in the past, including high-profile cases such as the bombing of a Pan Am airliner arriving in Honolulu, Hawaii, from Narjita, Japan, in 1982, as often taught by forensics expert Rick Hahn (retired from the Federal Bureau of Investigation). Changes in the objects may be microscopic and require detailed examination to establish the variations. However, responders should be cognizant that exchanges will take place and are not always noticeable to the naked eye (**FIGURE 14-4**).

(A)

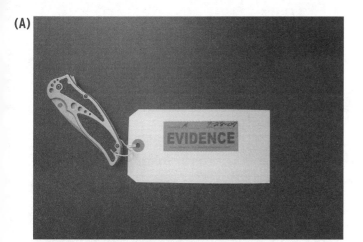

(B)

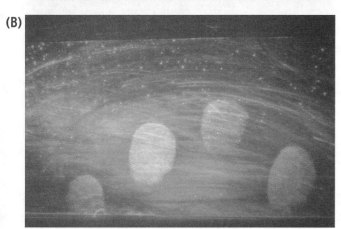

FIGURE 14-3 Physical evidence can range from something that has been used **(A)** to something that was left behind **(B)** by either the victim or the suspect.

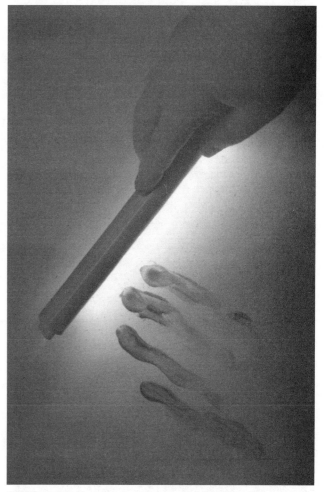

FIGURE 14-4 Evidence may not always be visible to the naked eye.

A pristine crime scene is altered whenever one or more people enter the area, and responders must understand that they always bring contamination to a crime scene.

Physical evidence can be almost anything. **TABLE 14-1** gives some examples of items that could be encountered by responders working at a potential or actual terrorism/crime scene.

Being aware of potential hazards at a scene is not new to EMS, fire fighters, emergency managers, or hazardous materials responders. Scene safety, sizing up the scene, or just taking a minute to examine the environment of a scene can minimize the impact of costly mistakes of overzealous responders.

Actions of First Arriving Units

Literature in the EMS, emergency management, and fire/rescue fields stresses initial scene evaluation. However, few texts elaborate on the importance of viewing an event as a crime scene and analyzing the hot zone accordingly. First arriving units are usually overwhelmed because the scene is chaotic and dynamic. Observations at this early stage are very important to law enforcement investigators.

Several key observations are important for initial responders. There is no time to write anything; responders should just remember key crime or evidence observa-

CRITICAL FACTOR..........................

An initial scene evaluation should include a basic crime scene evaluation.

tions and report them to the incident manager or the law enforcement branch as soon as possible. Important observations include:

- Chemicals on the scene that would not normally be present
- Damage, debris fields, and fragmentation that indicate an explosion
- Suspicious people (people hiding or running)
- Statements issued by bystanders
- Unusual odors at the scene
- Evidence of gunfire (shell casings, bullet holes, or gunshot wounds)
- Weapons in the area
- Suspicious casualties (patients may be terrorists)
- Multiple fires that appear to be from separate sources
- Suspicious devices

TABLE 14-1 Possible Items of Evidence at a Crime Scene		
Objects	**Body material**	**Impressions**
Weapons	Blood	Fingerprints
Tools	Semen	Tire traces
Firearms	Hair	Footprints
Displaced furniture	Tissue	Palm prints
Notes, letter, papers	Sputum	Tool marks
Matchbooks	Urine	Bullet holes
Bullets	Feces	Newly damaged areas
Shell casings	Vomit	Dents and breaks
Cigarette or cigar butts		
Clothes		
Shoes		
Jewelry		
Bomb fragments		
Chemical containers		
Mechanical delivery systems		

Evidence Preservation by Emergency Responders

What do we do with physical evidence when we find it? There are several answers. Observations should be written down on a notepad or in an electronic device as soon as it is practical to do so (**FIGURE 14-5**). Admittedly, this step may take place hours later. Observations of weapons, suspects, or devices must be communicated to the incident commander or law enforcement branch immediately. Other observations should be conveyed when emergency response tasks are completed (put out the fire and treat the patients first).

There are several important rules in preserving physical evidence, including the following:

- Unless critical to life safety, do not touch or move evidence. Law enforcement knows how to photograph, document, package, and remove evidence.
- If evidence must be moved for tactical reasons, note the original location and report it to law enforcement investigators. If possible, place a mark on the ground near the original location of the evidence.
- If possible, photograph evidence removal during tactical operations. Forensic photographers will photograph normal evidence removal during an investigation.
- Avoid evidence contamination caused by walking through the scene. Stretch a rope or scene tape into the crime scene area and instruct personnel to walk along the established path.
- Minimize the number of personnel working in the area.

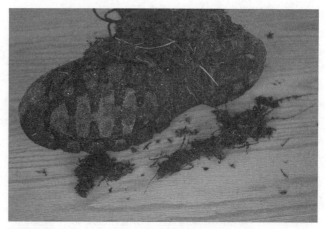

FIGURE 14-6 Check the soles of boots or shoes when personnel exit the crime scene because fragments or fibers may be embedded.

- Check the soles of boots or shoes when personnel exit the crime scene because fragments or fibers may be embedded (**FIGURE 14-6**).
- Check the tires of response vehicles for embedded objects in the tire treads.
- Consider clothing or personal effects removed from victims as evidence. Ensure that law enforcement personnel practice biohazard safety procedures when examining red-bagged evidence or clothing.

Emergency responders can also become victims (**FIGURE 14-7**). A classic case was the sarin gas attack in the Tokyo subway system. This incident was considered to be a normal call until emergency physicians realized they were dealing with a nerve agent as the cause of the sickness. The importance of preparation procedures and the use of protective equipment is paramount. Every day, police, fire fighters, and EMS personnel encounter dangerous situations during the normal course of performing their services. However, the potential for lethal hazards and long-term effects that result from terrorist incidents is much greater (Burke, 2000).

Another unique hazard of terrorist incidents is the probability of a secondary device targeting the responders

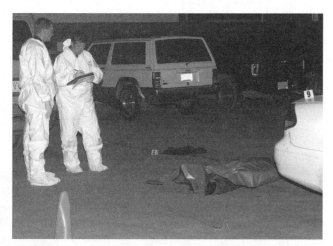

FIGURE 14-5 Although it may take place hours after emergency responders first arrive to a crime scene, observations should be written down on a notepad or in an electronic device as soon as it is practical to do so.

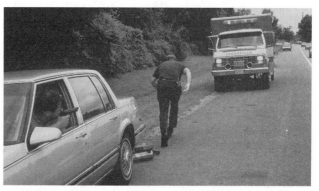

FIGURE 14-7 Emergency responders can also become victims.

to the incident. Remember that the goal of the terrorist is to create chaos and fear, and what better way to accomplish this than to turn the responders into victims? Past bombing incidents offer examples of this scenario, such as the events in Atlanta, Georgia, and Birmingham, Alabama. In both cases, secondary devices were detonated.

Emergency responders must be alert, aware, and suspicious of their surroundings when responding to incidents that have the potential to be terroristic in nature. Terrorists have used different types of tactics, techniques, and procedures in carrying out attacks. Responders must keep up to date on the current terrorist tactics to maintain situational awareness and ultimately responder safety when responding to suspected terrorist incidents.

Crime Scene Analysis

The thorough analysis of a crime scene consists of the identification, preservation, and collection of physical evidence as well as the recording of testimonial evidence. Without adherence to this basic assertion during the initial stages of a crime scene investigation, the potential to disrupt the integrity of the evidence is great. Hawthorne states that this could result in the evidence being challenged by the defense in a court of law, which, in turn, could lead to dismissal of the charges or the finding of a lesser offense against the criminal defendant (Hawthorne, 1999). More often than not, the proper collection of physical evidence from a crime scene is the definitive portion in the resolution of a criminal offense. Admissible physical evidence has the potential to (1) establish that a crime has occurred; (2) place a suspect in contact with the victim and/or the scene; (3) establish the identity of those associated with the crime; (4) exonerate the innocent; (5) corroborate the victim's testimony; and (6) cause a suspect to make admissions or to confess (Fisher, 2000).

Responders should approach the crime scene as if the first entrance to the scene will be the only opportunity to gather the physical evidence that is present (Department of Justice, 2000). Those collecting the evidence should initially direct their attention toward observing and recording the information present at the crime scene, rather than taking action to solve the crime immediately (Hawthorne, 1999). They should also give careful consideration to other case information or statements from witnesses or suspects.

This chapter was prepared with the intention of providing the reader with rudimentary principles of crime scene investigation, from the initial approach of the crime scene to final disposition of physical evidence found at the crime scene. Although the methods initially used to approach a crime scene are virtually universal in terms of application of use, it should be noted that at some point the investigation takes on unique characteristics that may be atypical or unorthodox in nature. Therefore, it is impossible to propose a single, step-by-step procedure that ultimately resolves every type of crime scene (Department of Justice, 2000).

However, regardless of the unique nature of a crime scene, thorough crime scene analysis, effective interviews and interrogations, and common sense make it less likely that evidence is overlooked or improperly collected or preserved or that mistakes are made (Adcock, 1989).

A review of the literature reveals that a common set of generalized categories for crime scene procedures exists. These procedures are:

1. Protect the crime scene
2. Identify evidence
3. Document evidence
4. Collect evidence
5. Mark evidence
6. Package evidence
7. Transport evidence

Law Enforcement Responsibilities

Upon initial arrival at the scene of a crime, the first responders have a great responsibility. It is their task to set the foundation for what Hawthorne termed the *process of analyzing a crime scene*. The basic elements of the process are: (1) approach and mitigate any hazards as well as provide for safety of victims and responders, (2) render medical aid, (3) identify additional victims or witnesses, (4) secure the crime scene and physical evidence, and (5) make appropriate notifications. While adhering to these principles, the first law enforcement responders provide subsequent investigators and technicians with a sound foundation for conducting a comprehensive analysis of the crime scene.

When approaching a crime scene, the first law enforcement responder must maintain professional composure regardless of the often overwhelming factors associated with the task to be completed (Hawthorne, 1999). Officers must be vigilant and able to recognize anything, whether it be animate or inanimate, that has a connection to the crime committed. Furthermore, officers should note the relationship of items to other items at the crime scene in terms of the distances and the angles that separate them. First arriving law enforcement responders must be objective in their initial approach to a crime scene and resist the temptation to form conclusions about what occurred.

Upon arrival at a crime scene, the paramount concern should be the preservation of human life and/or the prevention of additional injuries. Life preservation always trumps evidence preservation. The first law enforcement responders must provide adequate first aid and/or request professional medical assistance if medical professionals are not on the scene. According to Hawthorne, if law enforcement responders are providing medical assistance and the crime scene or physical evidence becomes contaminated, altered, or lost, that is a price that must be paid. The preservation of life outweighs the preservation of evidence at a crime scene.

After satisfying the immediate medical issues, the search for additional victims or witnesses should commence. The reasons for an aggressive search include: (1) additional victims may need medical assistance requiring additional medical personnel; (2) victims may provide needed information that aids law enforcement responders in determining the extent of the crime, the crime scene, and any physical evidence; and (3) victims corroborate what happened and provide needed information to establish the elements of the crime, suspect descriptions, vehicle descriptions, and avenue of escape. If there is more than one witness, law enforcement responders should make arrangements to separate witnesses to prevent collaboration. There is the possibility that the witnesses collaborated before the law enforcement responders' arrival. Law enforcement responders should take all possible steps to ascertain if collaboration occurred. After obtaining all the facts from additional victims and/or witnesses, law enforcement responders have the knowledge to enable them to implement the security of the scene and/or any physical evidence (Hawthorne, 1999).

It is the task of the first law enforcement responder to coordinate with emergency responders in properly identifying and securing the crime scene and its contents. The first law enforcement responder must continually question the scope of the crime scene and not limit the scope of his or her investigation. All possibilities must be considered regardless of their degree of improbability. Once the crime scene is established, an account of personnel coming into and leaving the scene must be maintained through the use of a crime scene log. The crime scene log lessens the possibility of unauthorized personnel entering and contaminating the crime scene (Hawthorne, 1999). This log must be coordinated with the EMS/fire personnel accountability system.

The final step in Hawthorne's process is making notification. Notification entails notifying supervisors as well as investigators or detectives who are handling the case and those people who are ultimately responsible for documenting the scene and collecting the evidence.

The first law enforcement responders must be prepared to make split-second decisions on arrival at a crime scene. These decisions can have a lasting impact on victims, witnesses, the accusatory process, and even the community in which the crime occurred. For these reasons and others, the first law enforcement responders must be well trained in the significance of crime scene preservation, enabling the crime scene to be analyzed with as little disruption as possible. When this task is done properly, a successful investigation and conclusion of the case can be achieved (Hawthorne, 1999). The advanced technology and expertise at the disposal of law enforcement may potentially be rendered useless if proper crime scene preservation is not maintained in accordance with professional standards.

Processing of Crime Scene/Physical Evidence

To achieve the maximum benefit from physical evidence, investigators must not only be skilled in evidence identification, preservation, and collection, but they must know how to handle and care for the evidence beyond the time of collection. These actions preserve evidence for the development of leads, laboratory examination, and/or presentation in court. Effective handling and care involves documenting and storing the evidence to retain the integrity of the item in its original condition (as nearly as possible), maintaining a chain of custody for the item to ensure responsibility, and ensuring its evidentiary value and its disposition when it is no longer of evidentiary value (Schultz, 1977).

The proper processing of a crime scene begins with properly documenting the evidence found within its boundaries. The investigator who first receives, recovers, or discovers physical evidence must be able to identify such evidence positively, at a later date, as being the specific article or item obtained in connection with a specific investigation (Fox & Cunningham, 1973). This is best accomplished by utilizing various proven techniques of recording the nature of the scene and its contents when they are obtained or collected (Schultz, 1977). This process entails providing pertinent data about the evidence as it relates to a particular crime scene investigation.

Chain of Custody

In order for physical evidence collected from a crime scene to be considered admissible in a court of law, a valid chain of custody must be established (Hawthorne, 1999). The chain of custody, which ensures continuous accountability, comprising all people who had custody of the evidence since its acquisition by a law enforcement agency. It begins when the item is collected and is maintained until its disposition. People in the chain of custody are responsible for the safekeeping and preservation of an item of evidence while it is under their control. Because of the sensitive nature of evidence, an evidence custodian often assumes responsibility for the item when it is not in use by the investigating officer or other competent authority involved in the investigation (Schultz, 1977).

Once the evidence from a crime scene is properly identified, collected, and stored, it must be processed by a multitude of professionals who analyze the evidence until its evidentiary value is no longer of use. At this point the evidence may be considered for disposal. To determine when an item of evidence should be disposed of, the evidence custodian consults with the investigator who originally produced it, and any other investigator who has an official interest, to ensure the item is no longer needed as evidence (Schultz, 1977).

Chapter Summary

Law enforcement history shows that when mistakes are made, they predominantly occur during the initial stages of an investigation or at the crime scene (Adcock, 1989). Many cases are lost or unresolved because the crime scene was not processed properly.

Further, there are numerous incidents where police officers were careless and valuable evidence was not identified, not collected, or lost, resulting in a poor follow-up by the investigating officers. Worse, in some situations, this carelessness lost the only evidence that proves or disproves that a crime was committed and identifies the perpetrator.

The critical nature of evidence cannot be ignored (Hawthorne, 1999). The responsibility of ensuring this does not happen belongs to all of those involved, from the first law enforcement responder to the investigators and technicians. Everyone within the system needs to know the importance of the crime scene and how it should be processed (Adcock, 1989).

Wrap Up

Chapter Questions

1. Define a crime scene.
2. Discuss the theory of exchange in the evidence process.
3. What are the three major classifications of evidence? List several examples in each category.
4. List and discuss at least four crime scene observations that should be made by emergency responders.
5. List and discuss five key steps for first responder preservation of evidence.
6. Discuss the concept of chain of custody.

Chapter Project

Research law enforcement manuals, books, articles, or training modules for information about evidence preservation and collection. Examine their standard operating procedures for evidence preservation and recovery. Based on your findings, write a comprehensive on-scene procedure for an emergency response agency relating to crime scene preservation.

Vital Vocabulary

Crime scene Any area in which a crime may have been committed as well as anywhere the criminal was during the commission of the crime and the egress from the scene.

Evidence Something legally submitted to a competent tribunal as a means of ascertaining the truth in an alleged matter under investigation.

Physical evidence Anything that has been used, left, removed, altered, or contaminated during the commission of a crime by either the victim or the suspect.

References

Ackland, J. R., Worswick, D. A., & Marmion, B. P. (1994). Vaccine prophylaxis of Q fever: A follow-up study of the efficacy of Qvac (CSL) 1985–1990. *Medical Journal of Australia, 160,* 704–708.

Adcock, J. M. (1989). *Crime scene processing.* JMA Forensics.

Arquilla, J., & Ronfeldt, D. (Eds.). (2001). *Networks and netwars: The future of terror, crime and militancy.* Santa Monica, CA: Rand.

The Associated Press. (2004, September 9). Nurses fired or suspended for not working hurricane. Retrieved December 21, 2009 from http://www.accessmylibrary.com/coms2/summary_0286-13300902_ITM

The Associated Press. (2005, September 29). New Orleans police may have participated in looting. *USA Today.* Retrieved December 21, 2009 from http://www.usatoday.com/news/nation/2005-09-29-police-looting_x.htm

Asst. Secretary of Defense. (1998). Weapons of mass destruction response team locations announced. Washington, DC: Armed Forces News Service, No. 512-98.

Barnes, J., & Newbold, K. (2005, November). *Humans as a critical infrastructure.* IEEE Critical Infrastructure Protection Conference, Darmstadt, Germany.

Bernstein, B. J. (1987, June). The birth of the U.S. biological-warfare program. *Scientific American, 256*(6):116–121.

bin-Laden, Osama. (1998, February 23). Fatwa—Declaration of the World Islamic Front for Jihad against the Jews and the Crusaders. *Al-Quds Al-Arabi News.*

Blair, D. (2009). Testimony of the director of national intelligence: The annual threat assessment of the intelligence community for the Senate select committee on intelligence. Washington, DC. Retrieved December 10, 2009 from http://www.dni.gov/testimonies/20090212_testimony.pdf

Burke, R. (2000). *Counter terrorism for emergency responders.* Boca Raton, FL: Lewis Publishers.

Butler, F. (1996). *Combat casualty care* [Department of Defense briefing]. Washington, DC: Department of Defense.

CBWInfo.com. (2005). Nerve agent: GB (sarin). Retrieved December 21, 2009 from http://cbwinfo.com/Chemical/Nerve/GB.shtml

Centers for Disease and Control and Prevention, National Center for Infectious Diseases. (2009). Ebola virus hemorrhagic fever: General information. Retrieved December 21, 2009 from http://www.cdc.gov/ncidod/dvrd/spb/mnpages/dispages/ebola.htm

Chang, F. T., Bauer, R. M., Benton, B. J., Keller, S. A., & Capacio, B. R. (1996). 4-Aminopyridine antagonizes saxitoxin and tetrodotoxin induced cardiorespiratory depression. *Toxicon, 34,* 671–690.

CNN. (2001). Real IRA guerrillas back to haunt London. Retrieved December 21, 2009 from http://archives.cnn.com/2001/WORLD/europe/UK/03/04/britain.irish.blast.01.reut/

Cohen, W. S. (1998, May 22). *National Guard rapid assessment elements.* Washington, DC: Armed Forces News Service.

Cole, L. (1996). The specter of biological weapons. *Scientific American, 275*(6), 60. http://search.ebscohost.com.proxy1.nyu.edu

Cole, L. A. (1985). Operation bacterium: Testing germs on the A train. *Washington Monthly, 17*(6-7), 38–45.

Cole, L. A. (1988). Cloud cover: The army's secret germ warfare test over San Francisco. *Common Cause Magazine, 14,* 16–37.

Convention on the Prohibition of the Development, Production and Stockpiling of Bacteriological (Biological) and Toxin Weapons and on Their Destruction. (1972). http://www.opbw.org/convention/conv.html

Corbel, M. J. (1997). Vaccines against bacterial zoonoses. *Journal of Medical Microbiology, 46,* 267–269.

Coulson, N. M., Fulop, M., & Titball, R. W. (1994). *Bacillus anthracis* protective antigen expressed in *Salmonella typhimurium* SL 3261, afford protection against spore challenge. *Vaccine, 12,* 1395–1401.

Covello, V. T., & Allen, F. (1998). *Seven cardinal rules of risk communication.* Washington, DC: Environmental Protection Agency.

Covello, V. T., & Sandman, P. (2004). *Risk communication: Evolution and revolution.* Retrieved November 30, 2009 from http://www.petersandman.com

Cox, R. D. (1994). Improving civilian medical response to chemical or biological terrorist incidents: Interim report on current capabilities. *Annals of Emergency Medicine, 23,* 761–770.

Critical Incident Analysis Group (CIAG). (2009). University of Virginia, Charlottesville, VA *Community shielding.* Retrieved November 30, 2009 from http://www.healthsystem.virginia.edu/internet/ciag/programs/community_shielding/index.cfm

Crumpton, H. (2006, January 16). Remarks by Amb. Henry A. Crumpton, U.S. coordinator for counterterrorism at RUSI Conference on Transnational Terrorism. London, UK. Retrieved August 12, 2008, from http://london.usembassy.gov/ukpapress17.html

Denney, J. (1998). *Emerging first responder threats: 911 target acquisition.* Emergency Response Research Institute.

Denney, J., & Lee, D. (1997). *The emergence and employment of tactical ultra-violence.* Emergency Response Research Institute. http://www.emergency.com/stratvio.htm

Department of Coroner. (1993). Emergency mortuary response plan: County of Los Angeles. Los Angeles, CA: Los Angeles County Department of Health Services.

Department of Homeland Security. (2009). *National infrastructure protection plan.* Washington, DC

Department of Justice. (2000). *Crime scene investigation: A guide for law enforcement.* Washington, DC: GPO.

Douglas, J. D. (1987). *America the vulnerable: The threat of chemical/biological warfare, the new shape of terrorism and conflict* (p. 29). Lexington, MA: Lexington Books.

Evan, W. M. (1972). An organization-set model of interorganizational relations. In M. Tuite, R. Chisholm, & M. Radnor (Eds.), *Interorganizational decisionmaking* (pp. 181–200), Chicago, IL: Aldine Publishing Company.

Evans, W., & Manion, M. (2002). *Minding the machines: Preventing technological disasters.* Upper Saddle River, NJ: Prentice Hall.

Federal Emergency Management Agency. (2004). Responding to incidents of national consequence: Recommendations for America's fire and emergency services based on the events of September 11, 2001, and other similar incidents (pp. 34, 46–48). Washington, DC: FEMA; Document ID FA-282. Retrieved November 30, 2009 from http://www.usfa.fema.gov/downloads/pdf/publications/fa-282.pdf

Fisher, B. J. (2000). *Techniques of crime scene investigation* (6th ed.). Boca Raton, FL: CRC Press.

Flanagin, A., & Lederberg, J. (1996). The threat of biological weapons—prophylaxis and mitigation. *JAMA, 276,* 410–411.

Fox, R. H., & Cunningham, C. L. (1973). *Crime scene search and physical evidence handbook.* Washington, DC: U.S. Department of Justice.

Fukiya, S., & Matsumura, K. (1992). Active and passive immunization for tetrodotoxin in mice. *Toxicon, 30,* 1631–1634.

Genig, V. A. (1965). Experience on mass immunization of human beings with the M-44 live vaccine against Q fever. Report 2. Skin and oral routes of immunization. *Voprosi Virusologii, 6,* 703–707.

Glasser, S. B. (2002, October 30). Russia confirms gas was opiate-based fentanyl. *The Washington Post.* Retrieved November 30, 2009 from http://www.washingtonpost.com/ac2/wp-dyn?pagename=article&contentId=A40202-2002Oct30&notFound=true

Hallett, M., Glocker, F. X., & Deuschl, G. (1994). Mechanism of action of *botulinum* toxin. *Annals of Neurology, 36,* 449.

Hanson, D. (1994). *Biological defense: Vaccine information summaries.* Frederick, MD: USAMRIID, Fort Detrick.

Harris, R., & Paxman J. (1982). *A higher form of killing* (pp. 75–81). New York: Wang and Hill.

Harris v. United States, 331 US 145 (1947).

Harrison, D. (2001, October 14). *Legacy of fear on blighted anthrax island.* Telegraph.co.uk. Retrieved October 1, 2009, from http://www.telegraph.co.uk/news/uknews/1359420/Legacy-of-fear-on-blighted-anthrax-island.html

Hatheway, C. L. (1995). Botulism: The present status of the disease. *Current Topics in Microbiology and Immunology, 195,* 55.

Hawthorne, M. R. (1999). *First unit responders: A guide to physical evidence collection for patrol officers.* Boca Raton, FL: CRC Press.

Horgan, J. (1994, January). Biowarfare wars: Critics ask whether the army can manage the program. *Scientific American, 22.*

Hornick, R. B., & Eigelsbach, H. T. (1966). Aerogenic immunization of man with live tularemia vaccine. *Bacteriological Reviews, 30,* 532–538.

Horrock, N. (1997). The new terror fear: Biological weapons. *U.S. News & World Report, 122*(18), 36. http://search.ebscohost.com.proxy1.ncu.edu

Hospital Emergency Incident Command System, Orange County Health Care Agency, Emergency medical services. (1991). San Mateo, CA: DHHS.

Hudson, R. A. (1999). The sociology and psychology of terrorism: Who becomes a terrorist and why? Washington, DC: Library of Congress, Federal Research Division.

Hughes, P. M. (1998). Global threats and challenges: The decade ahead. Senate Select Committee on Intelligence; High Reliability Theory. Retrieved November 30, 2009 from http://armed-services.senate.gov/statemnt/1999/990202ph.pdf

Hughes, R., & Whaler, B. C. (1962). Influence of nerve-ending activity and of drugs on the rate of paralysis of rat diaphragm preparations by *Cl. botulinum* type A toxin. *Journal of Physiology* (London), *160*, 221–233.

Improving NYPD emergency preparedness and response. (2002, August 19). New York, NY: McKinsey & Company. Retrieved November 30, 2009 from http://www.nyc.gov/html/nypd/pdf/nypdemergency.pdf

Interagency OPSEC support staff. The National OPSEC Program. (n.d.). Retrieved November 30, 2009 from www.IOSS.gov

Ivins, B., Fellows, P., Pitt, L., Estep, J., Farchaus, J. Friedlander, A., et al. (1995). Experimental anthrax vaccines: Efficacy of adjuvants combined with protective antigen against an aerosol *Bacillus anthracis* spore challenge in guinea pigs. *Vaccine*, *13*, 1779–1794.

Jaax, N., Jahrling, P., Geisbert, T., Geisbert, T., Steele, K., McKee, K., et al. (1995). Transmission of Ebola virus (Zaire strain) to uninfected control monkeys in a biocontainment laboratory. *Lancet*, *356*, 1669–1671.

Jankovic, J., & Brin, M. (1991). Therapeutic uses of *botulinum* toxin. *New England Journal of Medicine*, *324*, 1186–1194.

Japan-101. (n.d.). Sarin gas attack on the Tokyo subway. Retrieved from http://www.japan-101.com/culture/sarin_gas_attack_on_the_tokyo_su.htm

Joint Security Commission. (1994). *Redefining security: A report to the Secretary of Defense and the Director of Central Intelligence*. Washington, DC: Joint Security Commission.

The Joint Staff. (1991). *Doctrine for intelligence support to joint operations*. Washington, DC: Office of the Joint Chiefs of Staff.

Khan, M. (2001). *Terrorism and globalization*. Adrian College, MI. Retrieved November 30, 2009 from http://www.glocaleye.org/terglo.htm

Kaufman, B., Wright, D. C., Ballou, W. R., & Monheit, D. (1991). Protection against tetrodotoxin and saxitoxin intoxication by a cross-protective rabbit anti-tetrodotoxin antiserum. *Toxicon*, *29*, 581–587.

Kaufmann, A. F., Meltzer, M. I., & Schmid, G. P. (1997). The economic impact of a bioterrorist attack: Are prevention and post-attack intervention programs justifiable? *Emerging Infectious Diseases*, *3*, 83–94.

Kirk, P. L. (1974). *Crime investigation*. New York, NY: John Wiley & Sons Inc.

Kriner, S. (1999). Hurricane Floyd: Filled with sound and fury, signifying—traffic? Retrieved December 21, 2009 from http://www.disasterrelief.org/disasters/990928evacuations/

Lange, W. R. (1990). Puffer fish poisoning. *American Family Physician*, *42*, 1029–1033.

Laobhripatr, S., Limpakarnjanarat, K., Sanwanloy, O., Sudhasaneya, S., Anuchatvorakul, B., Leelasitorn, S., et al. (1990). Food poisoning due to consumption of the freshwater puffer *Tetradon fangi* in Thailand. *Toxicon*, *28*, 1372–1375.

Lebeda, F. J. (1997). Deterrence of biological and chemical warfare: A review of policy options. *Military Medicine*, *162*, 156–161.

Mackenzie, C. F., Smalley, A. J., Barnas, G. M., & Park, S. G. (1996). Tetrodotoxin infusion: Nonventilatory effects and role in toxicity models. *Academic Emergency Medicine*, *3*, 1106–1112.

Maggi, L. (2009, September 5). Federal probe digs deeper into NOPD's actions after Hurricane Katrina. *The Times-Picayune*. Retrieved September 5, 2009 from http://www.nola.com/crime/index.ssf/2009/09/federal_probe_digs_deeper_into.html

Malone, M. (1998). *Chemical biological incident response force*. Norfolk, Virginia: USMC-ASPD.

Maniscalco, P. M., & Christen, H. T. (2001). *Understanding terrorism and managing its consequences*. Upper Saddle River, NJ: Prentice Hall.

Marighella, C. (1969). *Mini-Manual of the Urban Guerilla*. Retrieved December 21, 2009 from http://www.latinamericanstudies.org/marighella.htm

Matsumura, K. (1995). A monoclonal antibody against tetrodotoxin that reacts to the active group for the toxicity. *European Journal of Pharmaceutics*, *293*, 41–45.

Mayer, T. N. (1995). The biological weapon: A poor nation's weapon of mass destruction. In: *The battlefield of the future*. Retrieved October 1, 2009, from www.airpower.maxwell.af.mil/airchronicles/battle/chp8.html

Medical Management of Biological Casualties Handbook, (2nd ed.) (1996, March). Frederick, MD: U.S. Army Medical Research Institute of Infectious Diseases, Ft. Detrick.

Meselson, M., Guillemin, J., Hugh-Jones, M., Langmuir, A., Popova, I., Shelokov, A., et al. (1994). The Sverdlovsk anthrax outbreak of 1979. *Science, 266*, 1202–1208.

Metzgar, C. (2001). Moderate sleep deprivation produces impairments in cognitive and motor performance equivalent to legally prescribed levels of alcohol intoxication. *Professional Safety 46*(1), 17.

Meyer, K. F. (1956). The status of botulism as a world health problem. *Bulletin of the World Health Organization, 15*, 281–298.

Meyer, K. F. (1970). Effectiveness of live or killed plague vaccines in man. *Bulletin of the World Health Organization, 42*, 653–666.

Mobley, J. A. (1995). Biological warfare in the twentieth century: Lessons from the past, challenges for the future. *Military Medicine, 160*, 547–553.

Molander, R. C., Riddile, A. S., & Wilson, P. (1996). *Strategic information warfare: A new face of war* (Doc. No.: MR-661-OSD). Santa Monica, CA: Rand Corporation.

National Emergency Management Association. (2009). Emergency Management Assistance Compact. Retrieved December 21, 2009 from http://www.emacweb.org/

National Guard. (n.d.). The National Guard's role in homeland security. Retrieved from http://www.ng.mil/features/HomelandDefense/cst/factsheet.html

National Research Council. (2002). *Making the nation safer: The role of science and technology in countering terrorism*. Washington, DC: National Academies Press.

National security decision directive 298; The National Operations Security Program. (1988, January 22). Washington, DC: The White House.

NATO handbook on the medical aspects of NBC operations. (1991). NATO.

Neal, R. (2003, September 11). Ground zero workers' health cloudy. *The Early Show*. Retrieved November 30, 2009 from http://www.cbsnews.com/stories/2003/09/10/earlyshow/contributors/emilysenay/main572586.shtml

NFPA. (2007). *Standard on protective ensembles for first responders to CBRN terrorism incidents*. Quincy, MA: National Fire Protection Association.

NFPA. (2005). *Standard on vapor-protective ensembles for hazardous materials emgergencies*. Quincy, MA: National Fire Protection Association.

Nozue, H., Hayashi, Y, Hashimoto, T., Ezaki, K., Hamasaki, K., Ohwada, K., et al. (1990). Isolation and characterization of *Shewanell alga* from human clinical specimens and emendation of the description of *S. alga* Simidu et al. *International Journal of Systematic Bacteriology, 42*, 628–634.

Office of the Inspector General, U.S. Department of State. (1997). *Major management challenges*. Washington, DC: U.S. Department of State.

The Oklahoma Department of Civil Emergency. (1996). After action report: Alfred P. Murrah Federal Building bombing. Retrieved November 30, 2009 from http://www.ok.gov/OEM/documents/Bombing%20After%20Action%20Report.pdf

Okumura, T., Suzuki, K., Fukuda, A., Kohama, A., Takasu, N., Ishimatsu, S., et al. (1998). The Tokyo subway sarin attack: Disaster management. Part II. Hospital response. *Academic Emergency Medicine, 5*, 618–624.

Operations security: Intelligence threat handbook. (1996). Greenbelt, MD: Interagency OPSEC Support Staff, The National OPSEC Program. Retrieved November 10, 2009 from http://www.fas.org/irp/nsa/ioss/threat96/part01.htm

Oyston, P. C., Williamson, E. D., Leary, S. E., Eley, S.M., Griffin, K.F., & Titball, R.W. (1995). Immunization with live recombinant *Salmonella typhimurium* aroA producing F1 antigen protects against plague. *Infection and Immunity, 63*, 563–568.

Pastika, Made Mangku (2003, January). Summary of the Bali blast case. *Feral News*. Retrieved November 10, 2009 from http://feralnews.com/issues/bali/bali_bombing_analysis.html

Rivera, V. R., Poli, M. A., & Bignami, G. S. (1995). Prophylaxis and treatment with a monoclonal antibody of tetrodotoxin poisoning in mice. *Toxicon, 33*, 1231–1237.

Robert T. Stafford Disaster Relief and Emergency Assistance Act, Pub. L. No. 93-288, as amended. (2009). Retrieved December 21, 2009 from http://www.fema.gov/about/stafact.shtm

Roberts, K. H. (1990, Summer). Managing high reliability organizations. *California Management Review, 32*(4), p 101–113.

Russel, P., Eley, S. M., Hibbs, S. E., Manchee, A.J., Stagg, A.J., & Titball, R.W. (1995). A comparison of plague vaccine, USP and EV76 vaccine induced protection against *Yersinia pestis* in a murine model. *Vaccine, 13,* 1551–1556.

Sandman, P. (2002). *Obvious or suspected, here or elsewhere, now or then: Paradigms of emergency events.* Retrieved November 30, 2009 from http://www.petersandman.com

Sato, S., Kodama, M., Ogata, T., Saitanub, K., Furuyaa, M., Hirayamac, K., et al. (1997). Saxitoxin as a toxic principle of a fresh-water puffer *Tetradon fangi,* in Thailand. *Toxicon, 35,* 137–140.

Schultz, D. O. (1977). *Crime scene investigation.* Upper Saddle River, NJ: Prentice Hall.

Sehnke, P. C., Pedrosa, L., Paul, A. L., Frankel, A. E., & Ferl, R. J. (1994). Expression of active processed ricin in transgenic tobacco. *Journal of Biological Chemistry, 269,* 22473–22476.

Shlyakhov, E. N., & Rubinstein, E. (1994). Human live anthrax vaccine in the former USSR. *Vaccine, 12,* 727–730.

Sims, J. K., & Ostman, D. C. (1986). Pufferfish poisoning: Emergency diagnosis and management of mild tetrodotoxication. *Annals of Emergency Medicine, 15,* 1094–1098.

Sudoplatov, P., & Sudoplatov, A. P. (1994). *Special tasks.* New York, NY: Little, Brown and Company.

Tambyah, P. A., Hui, K. P., Gopalakrishnakone, N. K., & Chin T. B. (1994). Central nervous system effects of tetrodotoxin poisoning. *Lancet, 343,* 538–539.

The White House. (2003, February). Homeland Security presidential directive-5, management of domestic incidents. Retrieved December 21, 2009 from http://www.fas.org/irp/offdocs/nspd/hspd-5.html

The White House. (2003, December). Homeland Security presidential directive-8, national preparedness. Retrieved December 21, 2009 from http://www.dhs.gov/xabout/laws/gc_1215444247124.shtm

The White House. (1997). *Critical foundations: Protecting America's infrastructures.* Washington, DC.

The White House. (1998). *Presidential decision directive 63.* Washington, DC.

The White House. (2003a). *National strategy for physical protection of critical infrastructures and key assets.* Washington, DC.

The White House. (2003b). *National strategy to secure cyberspace.* Washington, DC.

USA PATRIOT Act 2001, 42 USC 5195c(e).

U.S. Army. (1996). *Handbook on the medical aspects of NBC defensive operations* (FM 8–9), Part II—Biological (Annex B). Washington, DC: United States Government Printing Office.

United States Department of Defense, Office of Joint Chiefs of Staff. (1998). *Joint publication 3-07.2: Joint tactics, techniques, and procedures for antiterrorism.* Washington, DC: United States Department of Defense. Retrieved November 30, 2009 from http://www.dtic.mil/doctrine/jel/new_pubs/jp3_07_2.pdf

United States Department of Defense, Office of Joint Chiefs of Staff. (2003). *Joint publication 1-02: Department of Defense dictionary of military and associated terms.* Washington, DC: United States Department of Defense. Retrieved November 30, 2009 from http://www.dtic.mil/doctrine/jel/new_pubs/jp1_02.pdf

U.S. Department of Homeland Security, Federal Emergency Management Agency, National Response Framework. (2008, January). FAQs. Retrieved November 30, 2009 from http://www.fema.gov/pdf/emergency/nrf/NRF_FAQ.pdf

United States Department of Justice, Federal Bureau of Investigation. (n.d.). *Terrorism 2002–2005.* Retrieved December 21, 2009 from http://www.fbi.gov/publications/terror/terrorism2002_2005.pdf

United States Department of State. (2007). Legislative requirements and key terms. *In Country reports on terrorism.* Retrieved November 10, 2009 from http://www.state.gov/s/ct/rls/crt/2006/82726.htm

United States Department of State (2004). United States Code § 2656f(d) Title 22. Retrieved December 8, 2009 from http://www.state.gov/documents/organization/65464.pdf

U.S. Public Health Service. (1997). *Metropolitan medical strike teams: Field operations guide.* Rockville, MD: Office of Emergency Preparedness, U.S. Public Health Service.

Watson, F. M. (1976). *Political terrorism: The threat and the response.* Fairfield, CT: Robert B. Luce Co.

Wiener, S. L. (1996). Strategies for prevention of a successful biological warfare aerosol attack. *Military Medicine, 161,* 251–256.

Wittenberg, S., & Bennet, A. (1993). *The man who stayed behind.* New York, NY: Simon & Schuster.

WNBC.com. (2002, November 19). Small businesses cry foul after alleged lootings. Retrieved November 10, 2009 from http://www.wnbc.com/news/1424628/detail.html

Yasumoto, T. (1991). in *The Manual for the Methods of Food Sanitation Tests* (p. 296), Vol. for Chemistry, Bureau of Environmental Health, Ministry of Health and Welfare, Japan Food Hygenic Association, Tokyo, Japan.

Glossary

2 in 2 out A firefighting safety principle dictating that when two members enter a structure or high-hazard area, two additional members are standing by outside the hazard area for the purpose of immediate rescue and/or support.

Accountability The process of tracking and accounting for personnel and equipment resources on the incident scene.

Active shooter response The quick action by whatever group of law enforcement officers initially arrive on scene by aggressively entering a building or structure with the intent of engaging an active shooter or shooters. The primary objective is to save lives by neutralizing the shooter.

Air-purifying respirator (APR) A face mask with protective filtering canisters certified to meet the requirements for known agents and concentrations. Air from the outside atmosphere is drawn through the filtering canisters and into the face piece when the user inhales. APRs are not suitable in oxygen-deficient atmospheres.

Air-to-air nets Communications networks between aviation units using aviation radio frequencies.

All hazards A system that addresses a wide spectrum of threats including man-made hazards, natural disasters, and terrorist attacks.

Alpha particles Heavy and energetic radiation particles consisting of two protons; alpha particles interact readily with materials they encounter, including air, causing much ionization in a very short distance.

Ammonium nitrate A common civilian deflagrating explosive that detonates with great force when mixed with a catalyst.

Atom The smallest unit of an element that contains a nucleus of neutrons and protons with electrons orbiting the nucleus.

Beta particles Negatively charged radiation particles that weigh a small fraction of a neutron or proton; beta particles travel up to several meters in air, depending on the energy, and are stopped by thin layers of metal or plastic.

Biological terrorism The use of etiological agents (disease) to cause harm or kill a population, food, and/ or livestock.

Black powder A deflagrating explosive that detonates with extreme force when stored in a confined container.

Blast overpressure Air in the vicinity of an explosion is compressed and expands, creating a pressure higher than atmospheric pressure that causes barotrauma damage in the form of air embolisms and damage to tethered organs as well as structural damage to buildings.

Branch The ICS organizational level having functional, geographical, or jurisdictional branches that are responsible for major parts of incident operations. Branches are an effective tool for maintaining a narrow span of control.

Brisance A sharp and shattering effect produced by an explosive.

C4 A military explosive with high brisance.

Chain of command A clear line of authority within the structure of the ICS organization progressing from the command or unified command level to units or single resources.

Chemical/biological/radiological (CBR) An incident or threat involving chemical, biological, or radiological devices or weapons.

Class 1 ensemble Encapsulating suit with SCBA that provides vapor, liquid, and permeability protection. The protective suit covers the breathing apparatus and includes protective boots and gloves. Outer boots and gloves are required for additional protection. All seams and closures must provide protection from vapors and liquids.

Class 2 ensemble A protective ensemble with SCBA that is worn outside the protective garment and utilized when the agent is known and liquid or particulate hazards are at a concentration at or above the immediate danger to life and health.

Class 3 ensemble A garment with attached or separate gloves and footwear or booties with outer boots utilized in incidents with low levels of vapor, liquid, chemical, or particulate hazards with concentrations below the IDLH threshold. Respiratory protection can be PAPRs or APRs.

Class 4 ensemble Lightweight garment certified for protection against blood-borne pathogens and utilized when biological or radiological particulate hazards are below IDLH levels; APR or PAPR respiratory protection is permitted. Class 4 ensembles do not provide protection against chemical vapors or liquids and are designed for particulate protection only.

Command net A communications network between the incident commander, command staff, and general staff.

Communications unit A unit in the logistics section responsible for the effective use and maintenance of communications equipment during an incident.

Community emergency response team (CERT) An organized team of community citizens trained to respond to local disasters and perform actions that mitigate death, injury, property loss, and quality of life.

Community shielding An effective and unique preparedness strategy to engage individuals, communities, and government in a unified response to disasters and future acts of terrorism, in particular bioterrorism. Originating from the University of Virginia's Critical Incident Analysis Group, this strategy is being adopted widely as a means of community and organizational resilience.

Convergent responders Citizens or workers who witness a terrorism incident and converge on the scene, call 911, and take action before first responders arrive.

Crime scene Any area in which a crime may have been committed as well as anywhere the criminal was during the commission of the crime and the egress from the scene.

Critical infrastructure Systems and assets, whether physical or virtual, so vital that the incapacity or destruction of such may have a debilitating impact on the security, economy, public health or safety, environment, or any combination of these matters, across any federal, state, regional, territorial, or local jurisdiction.

Cyanide A toxic material, like the nerve agents, that can cause serious illness and death within minutes, but is also volatile and lighter than air.

Decontamination The process of removing or neutralizing a hazard from the environment, property, or life form.

Deflagration A very rapid combustion that is less than the speed of sound.

Deliberate decontamination Type of decontamination that is required when individuals are exposed to gross levels of contamination or for individuals who were not dressed in personal protective clothing at the time of contamination.

Demobilization unit A unit in the planning section responsible for the planning and execution of procedures for the release and return of incident resources.

Divisions An organizational level responsible for activities within a specified geographical area.

Documentation unit A unit in the planning section responsible for maintaining, administrating, and archiving all incident documents.

Dosimeters Instruments that measure radiation over time.

Dynamite A high explosive that generates a shock wave of 14,000 to 16,000 fps.

Electrons Negatively charged particles that orbit the nucleus of the atom.

Emergency decontamination Actions taken by first responders to establish and perform decontamination operations for victims in a field setting.

Emergency operations plan (EOP) A comprehensive interagency and interdisciplinary plan identifying the key elements of the terrorism response continuum using the NIMS and NRF as templates.

Emergency support function annexes Areas in the NRF that explain and outline emergency support functions.

Emergency support functions (ESFs) A defined set of actions and responsibilities for fifteen federal disaster support functions, including lead federal agencies and secondary support agencies for each function.

Enzyme-linked immunosorbent assay An immunological immunoassay technique for accurately measuring the amount of a substance, for example, in a blood sample.

Erythrocyte sedimentation rate Also called the sedimentation rate or Biernacki reaction, it is the rate at which red blood cells precipitate in a period of one hour; a common hematology test which is a nonspecific measure of inflammation. Anticoagulated blood is placed in an upright tube, known as a Westergren tube, and the rate at which the red blood cells fall is measured and reported in mm/h.

Evidence Something legally submitted to a competent tribunal as a means of ascertaining the truth in an alleged matter under investigation.

Explosive train A chain of events that initiate an explosion.

Facilities unit A unit in the logistics section responsible for the setup, maintenance, and demobilization of incident facilities.

Federal coordinating officer The focal point of coordination in the unified coordination group for Stafford Act incidents, ensuring integration of federal emergency management activities.

Forward-leaning posture A preparedness and response philosophy that advances from citizens/

households upward through governments to the federal level because incidents can rapidly expand and escalate.

Front-end plan Planning for anticipated incidents rather than waiting for an incident to occur before developing a plan.

Gamma rays High-energy radiation rays that travel significant distances; gamma rays can travel from one to hundreds of meters in air and readily travel through people and traditional shielding.

Globalization A measure of the ease with which labor, ideas, capital, technology, and profits can move across borders with minimal government interference.

Gross decontamination The process of removing clothing and flushing the affected area with water as quickly as possible to reduce contamination by a chemical or infectious agent.

Ground support unit A unit in the logistics section responsible for the maintenance, support, and fueling for vehicles and mobile equipment. This unit also provides transportation vehicles and support.

Ground-to-air net A communications network between ground functions and aviation units.

Groups An organizational tool in ICS used to divide the incident into functional areas of operation.

Hasty decontamination Type of decontamination that is primarily focused on the self-decontaminating individual using the M258A1 skin decontamination kit; this kit is designed for chemical decontamination and consists of wipes containing a solution that neutralizes most nerve and blister agents.

Homeland Security Advisory System A tool to improve coordination and communication among all levels of government, the private sector, and the American public that identifies the threat condition and protective measures that can be taken by partner agencies.

Homeland Security information bulletins Protection products that communicate information of interest to the nation's critical infrastructures that do not meet the timeliness, specificity, or significance thresholds of warning messages.

Homeland Security Operations Center (HSOC) Homeland Security center that serves as the nation's center for information sharing and domestic incident management by enhancing coordination among federal, state, territorial, tribal, local, and private-sector partners.

Homeland Security threat advisories Information analysis and actionable information about an incident involving or a threat targeting critical national networks, infrastructures, or key assets.

Hydroxocobalamin A vitamin B_{12} precursor that is now available in multiple countries as an antidote for cyanide poisoning.

Immediate danger to life or health (IDLH) The maximum hazardous substance concentration allowable for escape without a respirator within 30 minutes and without impairment or irreversible health effects.

Improvised explosive device (IED) An explosive device that is not a military weapon or commercially produced explosive device.

Improvised nuclear device (IND) An improvised explosive used to scatter a chemical, biological pathogen, toxin, or radiation source.

Incident action plan (IAP) A plan that contains objectives that reflect the incident strategy and specific control actions for the current or next operational period. An IAP is verbal in the early stages of an incident.

Incident annexes The description of the response aspects for broad incident categories (e.g., biological, nuclear/radiological, cyber, mass evacuation).

Incident command system (ICS) The combination of facilities, equipment, personnel, procedures, and communications under a standard organizational structure organized so as to manage assigned resources and effectively accomplish stated objectives for an incident.

Incident commander (IC or Command) Individual responsible for incident activities and functions including safety and the establishment of incident objectives and incident management.

Incident management teams The incident command organizations composed of the command and general staff members with appropriate functional units of an incident command system organized as regionally based interagency special response teams.

Intelligence The product resulting from the collection, collation, evaluation, analysis, integration, and interpretation of collected information.

Interagency Incident Management Group (IIMG) Senior representatives from DHS, other federal departments and agencies, and nongovernment organizations to provide strategic situational awareness, synthesize key intelligence and operational information, frame courses of action and policy recommendations, anticipate evolving requirements, and provide decision support to the secretary of Homeland Security.

Ionization A characteristic of the radiation produced when radioactive elements decay.

Joint field office (JFO) A temporary federal facility that provides a central location for the coordination of response and recovery activities of federal, state, tribal, and local governments. The JFO is structured and operated using NIMS and ICS as a management template. The JFO does not manage on-scene activities.

Joint task force commander Person designated by the Department of Defense to command federal military activities to support an incident.

Key asset Person, structure, facility, information, material, or process that has value.

Key resources Publicly or privately controlled resources essential to minimal operations of the economy and government.

Law enforcement incident command system (LEICS) Law enforcement incident management functions organized by the ICS template.

Lewisite An oily liquid with the odor of geraniums that contains arsenic and a heavy metal and is more volatile than sulfur mustard.

Liaison officer The position within the incident command system that establishes a point of contact with the outside agency representatives.

Logistics section The section within the incident command system responsible for providing facilities, services, and materials for the incident.

Lookout, awareness, communications, escape, and safety (LACES) Scene safety procedures based on having a lookout, situational awareness, functioning communications among units, and an escape route leading to a safe zone.

Marine nets A communications system for marine units using maritime radio frequencies.

Mass decontamination Type of decontamination for large numbers of victims exposed to unknown chemicals or infectious agents.

Multiagency coordination system (MACS) A system of coordinated entities and off-scene resource processes organized as a full-scale logistics system to support the resource requirements of single or multiple incidents in a local area or region. Entities in the MACS include government agencies, nongovernment agencies, volunteer organizations, and private-sector resources.

National Counterterrorism Center The primary federal organization for integrating and analyzing all intelligence pertaining to terrorism and counterterrorism and for conducting strategic operational planning by integrating all instruments of national power.

National incident management system (NIMS) A consistent, nationwide approach for federal, state, tribal, and local governments to effectively and efficiently prepare for, respond to, and recover from domestic incidents, regardless of the cause.

National Infrastructure Coordinating Center (NICC) Center that monitors the nation's critical infrastructure and key resources on an ongoing basis and provides a coordinating forum to share information across infrastructure and key resources sectors through appropriate information-sharing entities such as the information sharing and analysis centers and the sector coordinating councils.

National Military Command Center The nation's focal point for continuous monitoring and coordination of worldwide military operations.

National Operations Center (NOC) The primary national hub for situational awareness and operations coordination across the federal government for incident management.

National Response Coordination Center (NRCC) A 24/7 operations center that monitors potential or developing incidents and supports the efforts of regional and field components.

National response doctrine The five key principles that support national response operations that are engaged partnerships, tiered response, scalable/flexible/adaptable capabilities, unity of effort through unified command, and readiness to act.

National Response Framework A document outlining a coherent strategic framework for senior emergency response chiefs, emergency management practitioners, and senior executives in the private sector.

Nerve agents Toxic materials that produce injury and death within seconds to minutes.

Network of networks A system that directly supports the following operations within all sectors of the nation's economy: energy (electricity, oil, gas), transportation (rail, air), finance and banking, telecommunications, public health, emergency services, water, chemical, defense, food, agriculture, and postal.

Networking A process (formal and informal) of collaboration and relationship building leading to trust and mutual support among individuals, agencies, and organizations.

Neutrons Particles in the nucleus of an atom that are neutrally charged.

Operations section chief (operations chief) The general staff position responsible for managing all operations activities. It is usually assigned with complex incidents that involve more than 20 single resources or when command staff cannot be involved in all details of the tactical operation.

OPSEC A tool designed to promote operational effectiveness by denying adversaries publicly available indicators of sensitive activities, capabilities, or intentions.

Photons Bundles of radiation energy in the form of particles or waves.

Physical evidence Anything that has been used, left, removed, altered, or contaminated during the commission of a crime by either the victim or the suspect.

Pipe bomb A length of pipe filled with an explosive substance and rigged with some type of detonator.

Planning briefing cycle An 8-, 12-, or 24-hour cycle encompassing the development of the IAP and the conduct of an IAP briefing by the planning section chief in collaboration with the incident commander.

Planning section The section within the incident command system responsible for the collection, evaluation, and dissemination of tactical information related to the incident and for preparation and documentation of incident management plans.

Planning section chief (plans) The general staff position responsible for planning functions and for tracking and logging resources. It is assigned when command staff members need assistance in managing information.

Powered air-purifying respirator (PAPR) A face mask with protective filtering canisters certified to meet the requirements for known agents and concentrations that uses a battery-powered unit to pump air into the face mask, creating a positive pressure that offers leakage protection and makes breathing less labored than a nonpowered device. PAPRs are not suitable in oxygen-deficient atmospheres.

Preparedness cycle The cycle of planning, organizing, training, equipping, exercising, and evaluating for improvement that integrates with traditional emergency response training and exercising objectives.

Principal federal official The representative of the secretary of Homeland Security who is responsible for coordination of domestic incidents requiring a federal response.

Protons Positively charged particles in the nucleus of an atom.

Public information officer (PIO) The position within the incident command system responsible for providing information about the incident. The PIO functions as a point of contact for the media.

Pulmonary agents Chemicals that produce pulmonary edema (fluid in the lung), with little damage to the airways or other tissues.

Radiation A natural and spontaneous process by which the unstable atoms of an element emit or radiate excess energy in the form of particles or waves.

Radiation-absorbed dose (RAD) Measurement of absorbed radiation energy over a period of time.

Radioactivity A characteristic of materials that produce radiation because of the decay of particles in the nucleus.

Radiological dispersal device A device using conventional explosives to physically disperse radioactive materials over a wide area.

Readiness to act posture The NRF design intention enabling a rapid and timely response capacity to an attack or disaster.

Recovery The period of short and/or long-term assistance for individuals, households, critical infrastructures, and businesses for restoration and rehabilitation from the effects of a disaster.

Resilience The organizational elasticity to bounce back or recover from unexpected events.

Resource management The coordination and management of assets that provide incident managers with timely and appropriate mechanisms to accomplish operational objectives during an incident.

Resources unit A unit in the logistics section responsible for the check-in and tracking of personnel, equipment, and major items on the incident site.

Response The immediate actions to save lives, protect property and the environment, and meet basic human needs, including the execution of emergency plans and operations or actions that support short-term recovery.

Riot control agents Solids suspended in liquids as powdery particles; often used in spray devices and used commonly in the United States.

Risk communication Communicating disaster preparedness information and mitigation strategies to the public in order to minimize the potential effects of an event before said event occurs.

Roentgen equivalent man (REM) A radiation dose that takes into account the type of radiation producing the exposure and is approximately equivalent to the RAD for exposure to external radiation.

Roentgen A unit of radiation exposure.

Safety officer (SO) The position responsible for monitoring incident operations and advising the IC/UC on all matters relating to operational safety, including the health and safety of emergency responder personnel.

Secondary device Timed device or booby trap that is designed and placed to kill emergency responders.

Self-contained breathing apparatus (SCBA) A respiratory device with an internal air supply that provides breathing air in hostile or oxygen-deficient atmospheres. Certification standards require that devices have a positive-pressure face piece to ensure that during face piece leakage, air in the mask flows into the contaminated atmosphere instead of outside air flowing inward and harming the user.

Senior federal law enforcement official The official appointed by the attorney general to coordinate law enforcement operations related to the incident.

Service branch A branch in the logistics section responsible for communications, food, and basic medical services. This branch contains the communications, food, and medical units.

Shock wave A supersonic wave of highly compressed air that begins at the origin of detonation, travels outward in all directions, and dissipates with distance.

Situation unit A unit in the planning section that collects, organizes, and presents ongoing information and intelligence about the incident for use in the IAP.

Span of control The ratio of subordinates to a single manager or supervisor. The span of control should vary from three to seven subordinates per manager. A low span of control is recommended for dynamic/high-stakes incidents.

Staging A safe area near the incident scene where nonessential and support units, managed by a staging officer, stand by awaiting further orders or assignments.

Strategic information and operations center FBI focal point and operational control center for all federal intelligence, law enforcement, and investigative law enforcement activities related to domestic terrorist incidents or credible threats, including leading attribution investigations.

Strike teams A group of like units managed by a strike team leader.

Sulfur mustard (mustard) A light yellowish to brown oily liquid that smells like garlic, onions, or mustard and causes cellular damage and death with subsequent tissue damage.

Supply unit A unit in the planning section responsible for ordering, supplying, and processing all incident resources.

Support annexes Essential supporting aspects that are common to all incidents.

Support branch A branch in the logistics section responsible for transport, maintenance, facilities, and supplies for the incident. This branch consists of the supply, facilities, and ground support units.

Support net A communications network for logistics support units or entities.

Tactical net A communications network for tactical functions with the operations section.

Tactical violence The predetermined use of maximum violence to achieve one's criminal goals, regardless of victim cooperation, level of environmental threat to the perpetrator, or the need to evade law enforcement or capture.

Task forces A combination of unlike units directed by a task force leader.

Technical decontamination A process performed by hazardous materials teams to clean the members of the entry team once the members have entered a contaminated environment. The process involves a thorough cleaning of personnel and equipment that often involves the use of brushes and chemical-specific cleaning solutions.

Technical specialists A team of responders who serve as an information-gathering unit and referral point for both the incident commander and the assistant safety officer.

Terrorism Individual act(s) of reckless destruction to property or person(s) or decidedly complicated events perpetrated by organizations with extreme social, environmental, religious, economic, or political agendas.

Thermal wave A short-distance extreme heat wave near an explosive point of origin.

Unified coordination group and staff Group that provides coordination in accordance with the NIMS concept of unified command.

Unified planning A coordinated planning effort between multiple jurisdictions, agencies, and/or disciplines within the planning section.

Unity of command Situation in which every individual, unit, function, or entity in the ICS has only one supervisor at the incident scene.

Vehicle-borne improvised explosive device An explosive device that is not a military weapon or commercially produced explosive device and is placed inside a vehicle.

Vesicants Agents that cause vesicles or blisters.

Windshield survey Careful scan of the incident scene from a vehicle, especially the entire scene periphery, to determine hazards or threats.

Index

Figures and tables are indicated by *f* and *t* following the page number.

Blair, Dennis C., 4–5
Blast overpressure, 163–164, 169
Blood agents, decontamination requirements, 178
Botulinum toxins
   clinical effects of, 132, 138
   decontamination, 133*t*
   detection/diagnosis, 133*t*, 138
   signs/symptoms, 133*t*
   source of, 132
   treatment/prophylaxis, 133*t*, 138
Branches, 24–25, 32
Brisance, 163, 163*f*, 169
Brucellosis, 143–144
Bubonic plague, 125, 126, 145

C
C4, 163, 164, 169
Cable colocation, 52
California *FIRESCOPE Field Operations Guide,* 65
CAM (chemical agent monitor), 176
"Cardinal's cap," 142
Care under fire, 15
Casualty care, in combat environment, 14–15
CBRN terrorism agents
   improvised explosive devices, 165
   incidents, 11, 13, 184, 184*f*
      crowd control for, 100
      mass fatality management plans for, 15
      proper respiratory protection for, 185–186
      response to, 101
   respiratory protection, 185
   threat of, 5
   training for first responders, 14
Centers for Disease Control and Prevention (CDC), 128
Centers for Disease Control and Prevention Strategic National
   Stockpile, 62*f*
CERT (community emergency response team), 73, 83
Chain of command, 23, 32
Chain of custody, 199–200
Chain or line networks, 7, 7*f*
Chechen terrorists, 97
Chemical, nuclear and biological improvised explosive devices
   (IEDs), 165
Chemical agent monitor (CAM), 176
Chemical agents. *See also* CBRN terrorism agents
   accidental spills *vs.* deliberate releases, 106
   delivery/dissemination, 106–107
   early recognition of, 117–118
   historical background, 106
   incidents
      indicators of, 76–77
      wind change in, 80
   liquid, 106–107
   military, 106
   triage for, 116–118
   vapors, 106–107

Chemical/biological/radiological (CBR), 76, 83. *See also* CBRN
   terrorism agents
Chemical warfare agents. *See* Chemical agents
Chickenpox, 54
Choking agents, decontamination requirements, 178
Cholera, 133*t*, 144
Civil support teams (CSTs), 11
Civil unrest, after disasters, 96
Class 1 ensembles, 187, 188*t*, 191
Class 2 ensembles, 187–188, 188*t*, 191
Class 3 ensembles, 188, 188*t*, 191
Class 4 ensembles, 188, 188*t*, 191
Claymore mines, 163, 163*f*
Clostridium botulinum, 126, 132, 138
Clostridium perfringens, 138
Clostridium toxins, 138–139
Cobalt-60, 155
Cold War, end of, 4
Collection, in intelligence cycle, 88
Columbine High School, Littleton, Colorado, 75
Command net, 27, 32
Command post, with unified EMS/fire/law enforcement
   management, 61, 61*f*
Command responsibilities, 60–61
Communications
   capabilities, of civil support teams, 11
   in medical facilities, 81
Communications section, of national incident management
   system, 30
Communications unit, 27, 32
Community emergency response team (CERT), 73, 83
Community shielding, 131, 149
Computer systems, cable colocation, 52
Containment, of incident area, 101
Contract security, 82
Convergent responders
   agencies, 73
   awareness, 80
   definition of, 72–73, 83
   role of, 73
   training for, 73, 80
   vs. first responders, 73
Coordination of response activities, 60
Cost issues, logistic caches, 62
Countermeasures, appropriate, application of, 87–88
Counterterrorism conventions, 4
Covert intimidation, 10
Coxiella burnetii, 146
Crime scene
   analysis, 198
   definition of, 194, 201
   evidence at, 194–196, 194*f*, 195*f*
   law enforcement responsibilities, 198–199
   observations by initial responders, 196–197, 196*t*
   processing of, 199–200
Criminal activity, after disasters, 96

Photo Credits

Color Plate Inserts

3-1B Courtesy of Barry Bahler/DHS/FEMA; 8-1 Courtesy of the U.S. Chemical Safety and Hazard Board; 8-3 © Kyodo/Landov; 8-4 Mark 1 Nerve Agent Antidote Kit courtesy of Meridian Medical Technologies, Inc., a subsidiary of King Pharmaceuticals, Inc.; 8-5 DuoDote Kit courtesy of Meridian Medical Technologies, Inc., a subsidiary of King Pharmaceuticals, Inc.; 8-6 Cyanokit Antidote Kit courtesy of Meridian Medical Technologies, Inc., a subsidiary of King Pharmaceuticals, Inc.; 8-7, 8-8 Courtesy of Dr. Saeed Keshavarz/RCCI, Research Center of Chemical Injuries/IRAN; 9-1 Courtesy of Brian Prechtel/USDA; 9-2 Courtesy of Professor Robert Swanepoel/National Institute for Communicable Disease, South Africa; 9-3A, 9-3B Courtesy of CDC; 9-4 Courtesy of Dr. J. Noble, Jr./CDC; 10-1A, 10-1B, 10-1C Courtesy of the U.S. Department of Transportation; 11-1, 11-2 From *When Violence Erupts: A Survival Guide for Emergency Responders,* courtesy of Dennis R. Krebs; 11-3 © Jordanian TV/AP Photos; 13-4 Flame-resistant coverall made with DuPont TM Nomex® Brand fiber. Photo courtesy of Dupont.

Chapter 1

Opener Courtesy of Andrea Booher/FEMA

Chapter 2

Opener Courtesy of Captain David Jackson, Saginaw Township Fire Department; 2-1 © michael ledray/ShutterStock, Inc.

Chapter 3

Opener Courtesy of Jocelyn Augustino/FEMA; 3-2 Courtesy of Andrea Booher/FEMA; 3-3 Courtesy of Mark Wolfe/FEMA; 3-4 Courtesy of George Armstrong/FEMA

Chapter 4

Opener © AbleStock; 4-1 Courtesy of Win Henderson/FEMA; 4-3A © Larry Rana/USDA; 4-3B © AbleStock; 4-3C © Photodisc; 4-3D Courtesy of Gene Alexander/NRCS; 4-4 Courtesy of FEMA; 4-5 Courtesy of Photographer's Mate 2nd Class Bob Houlihan/U.S. Navy

Chapter 5

5-3 Courtesy of the Strategic National Stockpile/CDC

Chapter 6

Opener Courtesy of Andrea Booher/FEMA; 6-1 Courtesy of Journalist 1st Class Mark D. Faram/U.S. Navy; 6-3 © Jim Ruymen/Reuters/Landov; 6-4 © Photos.com

Chapter 7

Opener © Jim Ruymen/Reuters/Landov; 7-2 Courtesy of International Association of Emergency Medical Services Chiefs; 7-3 © Edward Keating, POOL/AP Photos; 7-4 © Mark C. Ide

Chapter 8

Opener Courtesy of Senior Airmen Julianne Showalter/U.S. Air Force; 8-1 Courtesy of Tim McCabe/USDA

Chapter 9

Opener Courtesy of CDC; 9-1A, 9-1B, 9-1C Courtesy of the FBI

Chapter 10

10-2 Courtesy of Berkeley Nucleonics Corporation; 10-3 Courtesy of S.E. International, Inc.; 10-4 © PhotoCreate/ShutterStock, Inc.

Chapter 11

Opener © Gershberg Yuri/ShutterStock, Inc.; 11-1 Courtesy of FEMA; 11-2 © Jason Boulanger/Dreamstime.com; 11-3 Courtesy of Tech Sgt. Brenda Nipper/U.S. Army

Chapter 12

Opener © U.S. Marine Corp; Staff Sgt. Bill Lisbon, HO/AP Photos; 12-2 Courtesy of Emergency Film Group; 12-6 © John Mokrzycki/Reuters/Landov; 12-7 © Marmaduke St. John/Alamy Images

Chapter 13

Opener Courtesy of Mass Communication Specialist 2nd Class Paul Honnick/U.S. Navy; 13-2 Courtesy of Fullyinvolvedfire.com; 13-3 Courtesy of Sperian Respiratory Protection; 13-4 Courtesy of The DuPont Company

Chapter 14

Opener © Loren Rodgers/ShutterStock, Inc.; 14-2 © Bill Fritsch/age fotostock; 14-3A © Kevin Chesson/Dreamstime.com; 14-3B © Kevin L. Chesson/ShutterStock, Inc.; 14-4 © Olivier Le Queinec/ShutterStock, Inc.; 14-5 © Jack Dagley Photography/ShutterStock, Inc.; 14-7 From *When Violence Erupts: A Survival Guide for Emergency Responders,* courtesy of Dennis R. Krebs

Unless otherwise indicated, all photographs and illustrations are under copyright of Jones and Bartlett Publishers, LLC, courtesy of Maryland Institute for Emergency Medical Services Systems, or have been provided by the authors.